The U205 Health and Disease Course Team

The following members of the Open University teaching staff and external consultants have collaborated with the authors in writing this book, or have commented extensively on it during its production. We accept collective responsibility for its overall academic and teaching content.

Basiro Davey (Course Team Chair, Lecturer in Health Studies, Biology)

Gerald Elliott (Professor of Bio-physics, Physics)

Alastair Gray (Senior Research Associate, Centre for Socio-legal Studies, Wolfson College, Oxford, and Senior Lecturer in Health Economics, London School of Hygiene and Tropical Medicine.)

Marion Hall (Course Manager)

Richard Holmes (Senior Lecturer, Biology)

Julia Johnson (Lecturer, School of Health and Social Welfare

Kevin McConway (Senior Lecturer in Statistics)

Perry Morley (Senior Editor, Science)

John Oates (Lecturer in Developmental Psychology, School of Education)

Stephen Pattison (Senior Lecturer, School of Health and Social Welfare)

Clive Seale (Lecturer in Medical Sociology, Department of Sociology, Goldsmiths' College, University of London)

The following people have contributed to the development of particular parts or aspects of this book.

Sylvia Abbey (course secretary)

Jane Ashley (indexer)

Mel Bartley (Research Fellow, Social Statistics Research Unit, City University, London) (critical reader)

Gail Block (BBC producer)

Martin Brazier (cover design)

Eric Brunner (Research Fellow, Department of Epidemiology and Public Health, University College London Medical School) (critical reader)

Mike Bury (Professor of Sociology, Department of Social Policy and Social Sciences) (critical reader)

Bill Bytheway (Researcher, Centre for Advanced Studies in the Social Sciences, University of Wales, Cardiff) (critical reader)

Gary Elliott (picture researcher)

John Greenwood (librarian)

Pam Higgins (designer)

Jeanne Sampson Katz (Lecturer, School of Health and Social Welfare) (critical reader)

Patti Langton (BBC producer)

Mike Levers (photographer)

James McCarthy (photographer and picture researcher)

Jonathan Montgomery, (Senior Lecturer in Law, Faculty of Law, University of Southampton) (critical reader)

Rissa de la Paz (BBC producer)

Sheila Peace, (Senior Lecturer, School of Health and Social Welfare) (critical reader)

Naomi Pfeffer (Senior Lecturer in Health Studies, University of North London, School of Health Studies) (author and critical reader)

Mary Renfrew, (Professor of Midwifery Studies, Institute of Epidemiology and Health Services Research, University of Leeds) (critical reader)

Helen Roberts, (Co-ordinator, Research and Development, Barnardos) (critical reader)

Mercia Seminara (BBC production assistant)

Moyra Sidell (Research Fellow, School of Health and Social Welfare) (critical reader)

Liz Sugden (BBC production assistant)

John Taylor (graphic artist)

Doreen Tucker (text processing compositor)

Peter Wilson, (Director, 'Young Minds', the National Association for Child and Family Mental Health) (critical reader)

Gavin Young (General Practitioner, Cumbria) (author and critical reader)

Authors

The following people have acted as principal authors for the chapters listed below.

Chapters 1 and 14

Basiro Davey, Lecturer in Health Studies, Department of Biology, The Open University.

Chapter 2

Alastair Gray, Senior Research Associate, Centre for Socio-legal Studies, Wolfson College, Oxford and Senior Lecturer in Health Economics, London School of Hygiene and Tropical Medicine.

Chapter 3

Gavin Young, General Practitioner, Cumbria, and Kevin McConway, Senior Lecturer in Statistics, Department of Mathematics and Computing, The Open University.

Chapter 4

Jim Stevenson, Reader in Psychology, Institute of Child Health and Great Ormond Street Hospital for Children NHS Trust, London, and John Oates, Lecturer in Developmental Psychology, School of Education, The Open University.

Chapter 5

Judith Green, Senior Lecturer in Sociology, Department of Legal, Political and Social Sciences, South Bank University, London.

021293

Chapter 6

Viviane Green, Child Psychotherapist, Anna Freud Centre, and the Marlborough Family Service, London, and Basiro Davey, Lecturer in Health Studies, Department of Biology, The Open University.

Chapter 7

Naomi Pfeffer, Senior Lecturer in Health Studies, School of Health Studies, University of North London.

Chapter 8

Howard Kahn, Lecturer in Organisational Psychology, Department of Business Organisation, Heriot-Watt Business School, Heriot-Watt University, Edinburgh; Cary Cooper, Professor of Organizational Psychology, Manchester School of Management, University of Manchester Institute of Science and Technology; and Basiro Davey, Lecturer in Health Studies, Department of Biology, The Open University.

Chapter 9

Mike Hepworth, Reader in Sociology, Department of Sociology, University of Aberdeen.

Chapter 10

Robert Slater, Lecturer, School of Psychology, University of Wales, Cardiff.

Chapter 11

Julia Johnson, Lecturer, School of Health and Social Welfare, The Open University.

Chapters 12 and 13

Clive Seale, Lecturer in Medical Sociology, Department of Sociology, Goldsmiths' College, University of London.

External assessors

Course assessor

Professor James McEwen, Henry Mechan Chair of Public Health and Head of Department of Public Health, University of Glasgow.

Book 5 assessor

Professor Mildred Blaxter, Professor of Medical Sociology, School of Social and Economic Studies, University of East Anglia.

Acknowledgements

The Course Team and the authors wish to thank the following people who, as contributors to the first edition of this book, made a lasting impact on the structure and philosophy of the present volume.

Lynda Birke, Nick Black, David Boswell, Rosemary Lennard, Anne Murcott, Jennie Popay, Steven Rose, Phil Strong.

We would also like to acknowledge the help of the following: Marian Hall, Graham McCune, Geoffrey Baruch and the Brandon Centre.

We wish to remember, with warm affection, our colleague and friend, Richard Holmes, who died while working on this book.

The Open University Press, Celtic Court, 22 Ballmore, Buckingham, MK18 1XW.

First published 1985. This completely revised edition first published 1995. Reprinted with corrections 1995.

A catalogue record of the book is available from the British Library.

Library of Congress Cataloging-in-Publication Data

Birth to old age: health in transition/edited by Basiro Davey.

p. cm. — (Health and disease series: Book 5)

Completely rev. ed. first published in 1985.

Includes bibliographical references and index.

ISBN 0-335-19207-6 (pbk.) 1. Health. 2. Developmental biology. 3. Aging. 4. Child development. I. Davey, Basiro. II. Series.

RA776.B595 1995

613 — dc20   94–27569

CIP

Edited, designed and typeset by the Open University.

Printed in the United Kingdom by The Alden Press, Oxford

ISBN 0 335 19207 6

This text forms part of an Open University Second Level Course. If you would like a copy of *Studying with the Open University*, please write to the Central Enquiry Service, PO Box 200, The Open University, Walton Hall, Milton Keynes, MK7 2YZ.

2.2

12055C/u205b5prelimsi2.2

BIRTH TO OLD AGE: HEALTH IN TRANSITION

Edited by Basiro Davey

7-

5|

PUBLISHED BY THE OPEN UNIVERSITY PRESS
IN ASSOCIATION WITH THE OPEN UNIVERSITY

 OPEN UNIVERSITY PRESS

 The Open University   Health and Disease Series, Book 5

Contents

About this book

A note for the general reader

Birth to Old Age: Health in Transition is a unique account of some of the major issues affecting the health of the present population of the United Kingdom, seen through the eyes of an unusually varied collection of authors. The book traverses the human lifespan, from the moment of conception to the moment of death, focusing on the overlapping generations of individuals—from the new-born to the very oldest—who inhabit the British Isles as the twentieth century draws to a close.

This book contains fourteen chapters; the first two and the last one consider the whole of the lifespan, but each of the intervening chapters focuses on a particular age-group. The interests and expertise of the author of a given chapter have strongly influenced their choice and interpretation of the major health issues affecting the age-group on which they have focused: some are practitioners from within the caring professions, others are academic researchers with certain disciplinary allegiances, and some combine both these perspectives. The professional and academic affiliations of the authors are given in the Study Comment box at the start of each chapter.

Chapter 1 gives a general introduction and sets out three coherent themes for the book: shifting definitions of what constitutes health, illness or disability; shifting social expectations about health and behaviour in each age-group; and shifting levels of dependence, interdependence and autonomy experienced as each person progresses through the lifespan. Chapter 2 describes the ways in which social and economic circumstances vary during a lifetime and assesses these trends for the economy and society as a whole.

Chapters 3 to 5 deal with the period from conception to just before puberty. Chapter 3 examines antenatal care, the medical management of childbirth and the newborn baby and considers the extent to which common practices have been evaluated. Chapter 4 looks at child development and the contribution of biological, social and psychological influences on health in childhood. Accidents—the largest single cause of mortality and disablity in children—are the subject of Chapter 5.

Chapters 6 to 9 focus on the period from adolescence to mid-life. In Chapter 6, we consider the psychological tasks that adolescents must negotiate in making the transition, through puberty, to an adult social and sexual identity, and examine the possible causes of risk-taking behaviour among teenagers. Sex and fertility are the subjects of Chapter 7, which discusses the social pressures on adult men and women to conform to certain expectations about their sexual and reproductive behaviour. Chapter 8 considers another common source of strain in adult life—stress at work, from unemployment and from conflicting domestic and occupational roles. The ambiguous status of mid-life, both as a time of fulfilment and as a period of crisis, are investigated in Chapter 9.

Growing older is the central concern of Chapters 10 and 11, the first of which describes the experiences of older people in the context of negative social expectations about health and behaviour in later life. In Chapter 11, the emphasis shifts to the experience of disability among older people. Chapters 12 and 13 discuss death, dying and bereavement in the changing social environment in which most deaths occur in the United Kingdom in the 1990s. In Chapter 14, the book is brought to a conclusion with a brief look at the ways in which events at one stage of the lifespan can have long-term reverberations, even affecting health in later generations.

Birth to Old Age: Health in Transition is the fifth in a series of eight books on the subject of health and disease. The book is designed so that it can be read on its own, like any other textbook, or studied as part of U205 *Health and Disease*, a second level course for Open University students. General readers do not need to make use of the study comments, learning objectives and other material inserted for OU students, although they may find these helpful. The text also contains references to a *Reader*[1] of previously published material and specially commissioned articles prepared in association with the OU course: it is quite possible to follow the text without reading the articles referred to, although doing so will enhance your understanding of the contents of this book. The book is fully indexed and referenced and contains an appendix of abbreviations and an annotated guide to further reading.

[1] *Health and Disease: A Reader* (Open University Press, second edition 1995).

A guide for OU students

Birth to Old Age: Health in Transition is the fifth book in the 'Health and Disease' series and the first to deal exclusively with the United Kingdom. It takes a lifespan perspective and is focused principally on the present decade. It assumes familiarity with the major influences on the epidemiological, biological and sociological profile of health, illness and disability in the United Kingdom, derived from the course books that you have already studied earlier in the academic year; *World Health and Disease,* Chapters 9 and 10 are particularly relevant and you could usefully re-read them before commencing this book.

Study comments, where appropriate, are given in a box at the start of chapters. These primarily direct you to important links to other components of the course, such as the other books in the course series, the *Reader*, and audiovisual components. Major learning objectives are listed at the end of each chapter, along with self-assessment questions (SAQs) that will enable you to check that you have achieved those objectives. The text and the index display key terms by printing them in **bold** type; the index indicates (also in bold) the page on which a definition or explanation of that term can be found, enabling you to look it up easily as an aid to revision as the course proceeds. Abbreviations are listed at the end of the book. There is also a list of further reading for those who wish to pursue aspects of study beyond the scope of this book.

The time allowed for studying *Birth to Old Age: Health in Transition* is four weeks, or about 40–48 hours. The following table gives a more detailed breakdown to help you to pace your study. You need not follow it slavishly, but try not to let yourself fall behind. Depending on your background and experience, you may well find some parts of this book much more familiar and straightforward than others. If you find a section of the work difficult, do what you can at this stage, and then return to the material when you reach the end of the book.

There is a tutor-marked assignment (TMA) associated with this book; about three hours have been allowed for completing it, *in addition to* the time spent studying the material that it assesses.

Study Guide for Book 5 (total 40–48 hours, including time for the TMA, spread over 4 weeks). The chapters vary in length, for example, Chapters 1 and 14 are very short, but Chapters 2 and 3 are the longest in the book, about twice the length of most of the other chapters. There are two television programmes and two audiotape bands (each of which lasts about 25 minutes) and several 'set' Reader articles, as well as some optional ones. You should pace your study accordingly.

1st week

A television programme 'First steps to autonomy' is relevant to your study of Chapters 3–5

Chapter 1	**The life-course perspective**, including *Reader* article by Blaxter (1990)
Chapter 2	**The changing fortunes of the life course**, including *Reader* article by Laslett (1989)
Chapter 3	**Care in pregnancy and childbirth**, including optional *Reader* articles by Oakley (1980), Cornwell (1984) and extracts from the House of Commons Health Committee Report (the 'Winterton' report) (1992)

2nd week

Chapter 4	**Child health and development**
Chapter 5	**Children and accidents**, including *Reader* article by Roberts, Smith and Bryce (1993)
Chapter 6	**Adolescent development and risk taking**, including audiotape 'Exploring adolescent development' and revision of *Reader* article by Bogin (1993)
Chapter 7	**Sex, fertility and adulthood**, including *Reader* article by Pfeffer (1987)

3rd week

A television programme 'Accumulating years and wisdom' is relevant to your study of Chapters 10 and 11

Chapter 8	**Work and stress in adult life**, including audiotape 'Working lives: choices and conflicts' and optional *Reader* article by Paterson (1981)
Chapter 9	**Change and crisis in mid-life**
Chapter 10	**Experiencing later life**
Chapter 11	**Living with disability in later life**, including *Reader* article by Parker (1983)

4th week

Chapter 12	**Dying**, including *Reader* article by Field (1984)
Chapter 13	**Society and death**, including *Reader* article by Vincent (1994)
Chapter 14	**Health in transition**, including optional *Reader* article by Morris (1990)

TMA completion

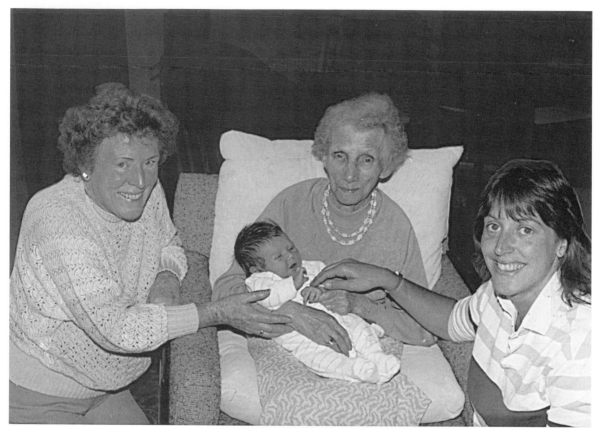

Birth to old age. Four generations of women from the same family: great-grandmother, grandmother, mother and newborn daughter. (Photo: courtesy of Tony Boucher)

1 The life-course perspective

During your study of this chapter you will be asked to read an article entitled 'What is health?' by Mildred Blaxter, which appears in the Reader.[1]

The author of this chapter, Basiro Davey, chairs the Open University Course Team associated with this book and others in the **Health and Disease** *series.*

A multi-disciplinary approach to the life course

This book is about the health experience of people living in the United Kingdom in the 1990s. It is an unusually varied collection of insights, observations and predictions contributed by academic researchers and professional practitioners from a wide range of disciplines. The aim of the book is to shed light on the major factors affecting health and well-being at all stages of the human lifespan, from birth to old age, at the end of the twentieth century. We asked each author to write about a certain period of the lifespan from the perspective of their particular discipline, and to reflect on some of the most important and interesting issues arising from contemporary academic research or professional practice. Inevitably, this has produced a collection of 'personal accounts', which vary greatly in the subjects covered, the concepts and terminology used, and in the style of writing. The aim of this unusual multi-disciplinary approach is to reveal the richness of the material available when human lives are viewed through the eyes of such a varied group of commentators. But despite this variation in the authors' 'gaze', the book has been written with three guiding principles in mind.

First, we share the belief that human lives can be understood *both* as the subject of rigorous social and scientific research on representative samples and occasionally censuses of the whole population, *and* as the often intangible experiences of the 'hearts and minds' of individuals, as expressed in personal accounts, literature, letters and a host of other idiosyncratic and unrepresentative sources.

Second, we recognise that the health status of an individual is continually in *transition*, changing from day to day throughout the 70–80 years that, on average, the present inhabitants of the United Kingdom can expect to live. The individual grows and develops, degenerates and self-repairs and experiences long periods of good health interspersed with episodes of illness, injury or disability, which may be minor and self-limiting, acute and life-threatening, or may develop slowly and perhaps become chronic. These fluctuations in health and well-being are multi-dimensional in the sense that people may consider themselves healthy in certain areas of their lives and simultaneously unwell in others. We cannot 'sum up' an individual's state of health; we can only shed a limited light on it.

Third, we believe that the health status of an individual at any point in the lifespan is determined by the *interaction* of many influences, principally arising from their biology, their social and economic circumstances, their personal psychology and behaviour, and the occurrence of 'random' events. Some of these influences were active only briefly in that person's earlier development but have left their mark, some have been persistent influences over many years, and others are quite recent in their effects. Note that our 'snapshot' of the population in the last quarter of the twentieth century includes several generations of individuals, the oldest of whom were born before World War I and the youngest only yesterday. It is self-evident that the range of influences on health will vary from one generation to the next; each has its own unique characteristics (as Chapter 2 will illustrate).

Taken together, these guiding principles help to explain why this chapter—which sets the scene for the whole book—is called 'The life-course perspective'. **Life course** is a term devised by sociologists to convey the fluctuating but rhythmic course of a human life, marked out by key events, as distinct from *lifespan* which merely

[1] *Health and Disease: A Reader* (Open University Press, revised edition, 1995).

5

refers to the number of years it contains. A life-course perspective acknowledges that the trajectory from birth to death is at once highly personal and unique to each individual, and yet contains experiences and events that tend to be common to most members of a social group. The most significant of these shared experiences are often referred to as **life-course transitions**; they can be thought of as bringing about significant and long-lasting changes in a person's status as seen by the outside world and in their own 'self concept' or identity. Many of these key transitions are located at certain points in the lifespan and shared by almost everyone at around the same age: for example, puberty occurs at roughly 11–15 years in most people in the current population; the changes associated with puberty are profound and long-lasting, both in their biological impact and in their social and personal significance (a more detailed account appears in Chapter 6).

☐ Can you think of other events that might qualify as life-course transitions?

■ Being born, reaching school-age, leaving school, getting a first job, leaving home, getting married, becoming a parent, experiencing the menopause, retiring from work or drawing a pension. There is room for debate about the relative significance of these events and some of them (like getting married) occur at quite a wide spread of ages, but for most of the population there is a 'peak age' for passing through these transitions and coming out a changed person.

Within the framework of this life-course perspective, the authors of this book highlight the interaction of a wide range of influences on health from birth to old age. The following exercise should help you to organise your thoughts about the varied influences at work in the United Kingdom in the 1990s.

☐ On a blank sheet of paper, jot down as many of the influences on health status that occur to you in the space of a few minutes. Then try to organise the items on your list into related groups. Finally, write a few sentences describing each group.

■ We identified four major groups of influences, which have been mentioned many times in earlier books in the *Health and Disease* series. They are highly interacting, so you may quite reasonably have grouped the items in your list somewhat differently from ours.

(a) *Biological factors:* these include a person's genetic inheritance and the past and current biological functioning of their body. Genetic factors may directly cause certain relatively rare inherited diseases, but may also influence the chances of an individual developing a certain disease if he or she is exposed to particular 'threats' in their environment at a critical stage in the lifespan. Events in the past as well as in the present may cause a long-lasting change in the biological functioning of a person's body, which increases their vulnerability to certain health disorders in the future.[2]

(b) *Socio–economic circumstances:* these can be roughly distinguished into those material factors relating to the immediate personal environment of individuals, for example, their income, nutrition, housing quality, clothing, access to a car, etc. and those relating to the wider social environment, for example, the availability of and access to health care, social services, education and training, shops, civic amenities, play-spaces, entertainment and public transport, the provision of workplace and road-safety measures, sewage and rubbish disposal, air and water quality controls, etc.[3]

(c) *Psycho–social circumstances:* these include cultural, ethical and religious values; personal beliefs and attitudes; educational history and attainment; the availability of supportive social networks; relationships with significant others; individual personality 'traits' and coping styles; perceived levels of stress; numbers of dependents; traumatic or rewarding events in one's personal history, etc.[4]

(d) *'Lifestyle' or personal behaviour:* these include tobacco smoking, levels of exercise, consumption of alcohol and other drugs, observance of speed-limits when driving, participation in risky sports, etc. The likelihood that an individual will display any of these behaviours is very strongly influenced by all three groups (a)–(c): for example, social class as measured

[2]Biological influences on health are primarily discussed in another book in this series, *Human Biology and Health: An Evolutionary Approach* (Open University Press, 1994).

[3]Socio–economic influences on health are primarily discussed in another book in this series, *World Health and Disease* (Open University Press, 1993).

[4]The major discussion of psycho–social influences on health occurs in this book, but see also *Experiencing and Explaining Disease* (Open University Press, 1985, and revised edition 1996).

by occupation and high levels of stress are strongly associated with the likelihood of smoking tobacco, whereas a history of heart disease may lead a person to quit smoking.[5]

If we had attempted to give a comprehensive multi-disciplinary account of all these influences and their interactions at all parts of the life course, the reader of this book might have collapsed under its weight. An alternative strategy would have been to examine the life course from the perspective of a single discipline, for example sociology. This approach has the merit of coherence and consistency, but there is a serious drawback: it would tend to elevate the *apparent* importance of the influences on health that lie 'close to the heart' of sociologists, for example, the effects of social class or income, and down-play other important influences such as individual psychology or biology, which fall outside the expertise and interests of social researchers. Precisely the same partiality would have occurred if we had asked only biologists or psychologists to write about the life course: they would have focused on the traditional concerns of their discipline, usually without much reference to the social and economic context in which individuals live out their lives.

So, in assembling material for this book, we have given a limited space to *all* the major disciplines currently investigating contemporary human health in the United Kingdom. We invited a wide range of authors each to contribute a chapter on the age-group that is the main focus of their research or professional practice. As you might expect from the title of this book, it includes chapters on life before birth and the newborn, the pre-school child, children from school-age to puberty, adolescents, adulthood, middle-age and old age, followed by a discussion of death and dying. What is unique is the variety of interests and disciplinary allegiances of its contributors. This strategy has the merit of keeping alive the inter-disciplinary emphasis which is the hallmark of the *Health and Disease* series, while avoiding the bulk of a truly comprehensive account in which all parts of the lifespan are subjected to the gaze of every contributing discipline.

Two drawbacks arise from this compromise, which you should bear in mind as you study the book. First, as

noted above, in drawing on the work of many different authors, each writing about a certain period of the lifespan, we risk fragmenting the course of human lives into distinct 'age-groups' (like Shakespeare's 'Seven Ages of Man'), which appear to have some objective reality. This should not be allowed to obscure the cultural and historical relativity of some of these divisions: the lifespan has not always been divided into the stages we commonly recognise today. For example, in the words of the British social anthropologist, Frank Musgrove, 'The adolescent was invented at the same time as the steam-engine' (Musgrove, 1964, p. 33). The age between childhood and adulthood has undergone continuous 're-invention' ever since. Very different standards of dress and behaviour were considered appropriate for teenagers in, for example, the 1950s; even in the present day, adolescent 'lifestyles' accepted in the white majority population of the United Kingdom differ from those sanctioned by some other ethnic groups, and there are variations between regions and between social classes. Variations must be kept in view across the whole life course.

Second, the choice of author for a certain chapter may create a misleading impression that each of these age-groups is best investigated by the practitioners of a certain academic discipline or occupation. For example, the principal author of the chapter on adolescence (Chapter 6) is a psychotherapist who, inevitably, has focused primarily on the inner psychology of individual adolescents and only secondarily on the wider social context in which the transition through puberty and the teenage years is negotiated; by contrast, the chapter on adult sexuality and fertility (Chapter 7) has been written by a social historian, who has given much less attention to the inner world of personal emotions in examining the wider social and legal pressures that influence sexual identity and sexual behaviour. It would be quite wrong to conclude from this that social context is relatively unimportant in determining health status during adolescence but suddenly becomes crucial in adult life, or that the psychological development of adults can be ignored but is of paramount importance when considering the health of teenagers.

In studying this book, the reader should remain aware that the insights it offers into health during the life course are the unique product of this particular group of authors: a different 'cast list' would have produced a quite different book. Nonetheless, it offers an unusual range of perspectives not normally found within the same volume. Yet, despite the very different backgrounds of the authors, you might be surprised to find three consistent themes emerging from these chapters.

[5]See several chapters in *World Health and Disease* and also *Dilemmas in Health Care* (Open University Press, 1993), particularly Chapter 10 on coronary heart disease.

A thematic approach to the life course

Shifting definitions

The first theme concerns the shifting definitions of states such as 'healthy', 'ill', 'normal', 'abnormal', 'disabled' or 'injured'. At least one of these terms arises in every chapter of this book and each, in their different ways, illuminates the contested nature of these states. There are fundamental disagreements about what healthy or sick *means*, which become apparent when the definitions used by different governments and international organisations, academic disciplines and health care occupations, individual researchers and practitioners, and lay people of different ages, sexes, ethnic groups and social classes are compared. To illuminate this point you should now read the article 'What is health?', which appears in the *Reader*; it is taken from the sociologist Mildred Blaxter's book *Health and Lifestyles*, published in 1990.

☐ Identify some major differences in the ways that people in Blaxter's study conceptualised 'health'.

■ Some could not conceptualise it at all, either because they never thought about their health or because to have a chronic illness was a normal state for them. Others defined health as 'not being ill', while some responded that they were healthy 'despite disease'. Concepts that contain some positive affirmation of health as a state in its own right were evident in those who saw it as a 'reserve' to draw on, or in terms of physical fitness, energy and vitality, or a sense of well-being. Some people saw health in terms of behaviour and 'living a healthy life' or of being able to function 'normally' and do the usual things; others saw it as a statement about being able to cope psychologically with their relationships and responsibilities. Few people have just *one* definition of health; most of them recognise that health has many dimensions.

Complexity of meanings such as these have to be taken into account when designing research studies or interpreting their results. Health research usually involves carefully chosen operational criteria to act as indicators or proxies for states of health, illness, injury or disability. For example, injuries might be measured in terms of attendance at a hospital accident and emergency clinic; an illness might be defined by the presence of certain measurable signs and symptoms; a disability might be assessed in terms of reliance on others for help in performing certain tasks. But operationalising complex states of health with measures such as these has serious practical limitations, which have been discussed elsewhere in this series,[6] *and it does not resolve the fundamental disagreements in meaning.*

As an example, consider the following definitions of 'disability'.

Disability: in the context of health experience, a disability is any restriction or lack (resulting from impairment) of ability to perform an activity in the manner or within the range considered normal for a human being. (World Health Organisation, 1980, pp. 27–9)

Disability: is the disadvantage or restriction of activity caused by a contemporary social organization which takes little or no account of people who have physical impairments and thus excludes them from participation in the mainstream of social activities. (Union of the Physically Impaired Against Segregation, 1976, p. 14)

☐ How would you summarise the major differences between these two definitions?

■ The WHO definition relies on an assumption that the physical and mental abilities displayed by the majority of the population represent what is considered 'normal for a human being', and hence that disability is a consequence of restriction or lack of those abilities in an *individual*. It makes no mention of the organisation of the society in which the disabled person lives. By contrast, this is central to the UPIAS definition, which is based on the premise that it is normal for a society to contain individuals with physical or mental impairments. Disability is a consequence of restriction or lack in *society's* provision of the means to include all such people in mainstream activities.

These conflicting definitions point to the simultaneous existence of disability as a physical or mental reality and as a social construction[7]. The debate about

[6]See *Studying Health and Disease* (Open University Press, 1994), Chapter 5.

[7]The social construction of disease, and of the body as the site of disease, is discussed in another book in this series, *Medical Knowledge: Doubt and Certainty* (Open University Press, 1994), Chapter 7.

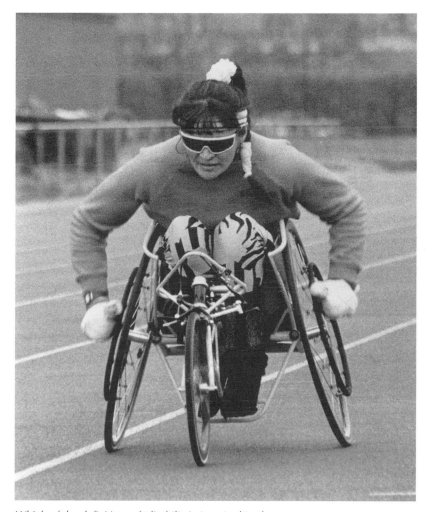

Which of the definitions of 'disability' given in this chapter seems most appropriate when you consider the Olympic Gold Medal winner, Rose Hill? (Photo: Mike Attwood)

'how much' of the disablement arises from each of these sources appears many times in this book, and can also been seen in conflicting definitions of states of health, of injury and of disease. Several authors draw attention to the fact that what is regarded as normal or healthy in one place, at a certain time, may not be so regarded elsewhere.

The shifting boundaries of 'normal health' create new disease categories and destroy others: for example, the list of children's health problems has been extended to include their behaviour, and diseases such as attention deficit disorder and hyperactivity have become accepted diagnoses in developmental psychology; in adolescents, anorexia nervosa has become commonplace, whereas medical and (to a lesser extent) lay opinion no longer considers homosexuality to be a disease; in adult women, infertility and the menopause are frequently represented in terms that closely resemble states of disease rather than states of female biology; and will the hitherto unremarkable forgetfulness of later life come to be re-named early dementia?

Shifting expectations

This leads us to another theme that penetrates every chapter of this book: the shifting expectations of health experience and health-related behaviour during different parts of the lifespan. Even within the overlapping generations of the same population, there may be sharp differences of view: for example, the health expectations we have for toddlers in the 1990s have changed significantly since today's middle-aged people were in their infancy, and these in turn are different from the expectations shared by people who grew up in the 1920s.

    ☐ What do you think might have contributed most to changing expectations about the health of young children?

    ■ The dramatic decline in infant mortality, particularly from infectious diseases, has created an expectation that serious illness or death in childhood is a 'thing of the past' (a subject we return to in Chapters 5 and 12). The increasing availability of health and social care reinforces the expectation that children's illnesses, even minor ones, should get professional attention.

Shifting expectations are also evident in notions of 'age-appropriate' behaviour, which tend to dominate the way a society views people of a certain age. **Stereotyping** can be defined as displaying attitudes that reinforce a standardised image of a certain social group. Stereotypes apply powerful and different pressures on the sexes: in Chapters 5 and 6 we ask to what extent do cultural expectations underlie the prevalence of eating disorders among adolescent girls while protecting them from the accidents that claim so many of their brothers' lives. Chapter 7 investigates the 'social norms' that people are pressured to live up to in their sexual and reproductive behaviour. Chapter 8 is partly concerned with the stereotypes of the 'working man' and the 'working woman'. Expectations about each age-group are apparent throughout the lifespan, but are nowhere more damaging than in the negative assumptions about older people (reviewed in Chapters 9 and 10), which make it harder to adapt positively to physical and mental difficulties in later life and may even foster dependency and loneliness as a 'normal' part of getting old (Chapter 11). And at the end of life, we consider how social expectations shape the ways in which dying people and their companions experience this unavoidable event (Chapters 12 and 13).

Shifting dependencies

Finally, and perhaps the most important of the emergent themes, is the emphasis on the shifting level of dependency as each individual follows his or her personal trajectory from birth to old age. As the life course unfolds, we emerge from high dependency on others to a state of interdependence in which areas of individual autonomy expand; as we age, so autonomy tends to decline and dependency often increases again. How much of this fluctuation is due to physical or mental changes and how much to cultural expectations and degree of social support?

It may seem that a newborn baby is totally dependent on its parents, but even as an embryo it performs certain biological tasks for itself (as Chapter 3 describes). Its dependency on others is extremely high nonetheless, but as the infant grows and develops it gradually acquires areas of competence and there begins a time of complex negotiations with parents to attain new freedoms (Chapter 4). The outcome of these negotiations can have a profound impact on later psychological and physical health; a balance has to be struck between protecting the child and restricting its development. And if something goes wrong in the gradual transition from dependency to increasing autonomy, who is 'to blame'? For example, accidents to children are often represented as the consequence of inadequate parental supervision, but in Chapter 5 we ask if urban environments are now too dangerous for children to explore? Risk-taking among teenagers can be interpreted as self-damaging rebellion against parental control, but some experimentation with risky behaviours may be an essential step in the transition from adolescence to adulthood (Chapter 6).

The tension between personal freedom and conformity is also apparent in adult life, particularly in issues of sexual identity and fertility (Chapter 7), and in the conflicting demands of paid work and domestic life (Chapter 8). Women during pregnancy, childbirth and infertility treatment often experience their autonomy as independent adults being eroded by medical interventions, some of which have dubious efficacy, and by the attitudes of the doctors and nurses on whom they are encouraged to depend (Chapters 3 and 7). Another prominent feature of adulthood is the restriction of autonomy that comes with responsibility for an increasing circle of others; women have a particularly difficult path to tread, given the prevalence of households in which they have paid work outside the home and carry the main share of domestic responsibility within its walls (Chapter 8).

In later life, physical and economic restrictions on mobility in an unsupportive environment may create a spiral of increasing dependency that, under more supportive circumstances, might have been slowed down (Chapters 10 and 11). At the end of the book, we explore the social and personal organisation of death, dying and bereavement—experiences that may be faced at any point in the life course (Chapters 12 and 13). Dying usually involves high levels of dependency on others for support and palliative care but, in the case of suicide and voluntary euthanasia, it may be seen on the one hand as the ultimate act of personal autonomy and on the other as a desperate response to lack of social and psychological support.

Conclusion

We offer this book as an illumination of the life course at 'this time'—the 1990s—and in 'this place'—the United Kingdom. It will not always match your own experiences of living here and now, nor reflect your own views, but we predict that in studying it you will acquire a greater appreciation of contemporary lives, from birth to old age.

2 The changing fortunes of the life course

During your study of this chapter, you will be asked to read an article entitled 'A new division of the life course' by Peter Laslett, which appears in the Reader.[1] The author of this chapter, Alastair Gray, is a Senior Research Associate at the Centre for Socio-Legal Studies, Wolfson College, Oxford University, and a Senior Lecturer in Health Economics at the London School of Hygiene and Tropical Medicine. He has been a major contributor to several books in this series, both in their first and second editions.

A theme running through this book is that an individual's health is closely linked to a series of significant *transitions* occurring over the life course. These transitions have different dimensions: for example, some concern biological changes such as puberty, menopause or the onset of age-related diseases such as senile dementia. Others concern economic or social circumstances, such as employment and retirement, marriage or divorce. Often these factors are intertwined: for example, the social context powerfully influences the impact of biological changes and the ways in which we view and respond to them.

This chapter focuses primarily on the social and economic circumstances of individuals, and how these vary during a lifetime. It begins by examining the life course within the family, and how this has changed over time. The chapter then considers life-course transitions relating to work. Finally, it considers some broader questions about the implications of these life-course events and trends for the economy and society as a whole.

---

[1] *Health and Disease: A Reader* (second edition, 1995).

The life course and the family

The *family* is possibly one of the oldest and certainly one of the most ubiquitous of all social institutions. It can exert a powerful influence on an individual's experience of health and disease, which may in turn strongly affect an individual's experience of family life. For example, the family plays a fundamental role in the nurture and socialisation of children (as Chapter 4 describes), and is consequently the focus of a great deal of surveillance by the health and social services. The family is also an important source of nursing care and of information about health and disease. Finally, adult members of the family may play an important role in deciding when to seek professional help in caring for the health of children and older people.

Though definitions of a **family** may vary over time and between places, all societies have some such concept, and membership of one or more family units is something most people experience over their lifetime. Social scientists usually reserve the word 'family' to refer precisely to groups of people related by blood or marriage, whether or not they live together—that is, **kinship groups**. A **nuclear family**, for example, consists of mother, father and children, whereas the **extended family** includes other kin, such as uncles, aunts, cousins and grandparents. The term **household** is used to refer to people living under one roof, whether kin or not. In popular usage, 'family' refers to both kinship groups and living arrangements. In this chapter we are primarily concerned with the family situation *in which people live* and we will be using the word 'family' in this sense most of the time.

Family types and family life courses in modern Britain

The family and its history have been flourishing research areas in recent decades, and one very clear fact emerges from this literature:

...there is not, nor has there ever been, a single family system. The West has always been characterised by diversity of family forms, by diversity of family functions and by diversity in attitudes to family relationships not only over time but at any one point in time. There is, except at the most trivial level, no Western family type. (Anderson, 1980, p. 14)

A summary of the types of household arrangements prevailing in Britain in 1992 is given in Table 2.1, which also shows how the pattern has changed in recent decades.

Table 2.1 Households by type, Great Britain, 1961 and 1992

Household type	Percentage of population in		Percentage of house-holds in
	1961	1992	1992
living alone	4	11	27
married or cohabiting couple with:			
no children	18	23	28
dependent children	52	40	24
non-dependent children	12	11	8
lone parent with children	2	10	9
other households	12	5	4

Source: derived from Central Statistical Office (1994b) *Social Trends 24*, HMSO, London, Tables 2.5 and 2.6, p. 36.

☐ What does the table show to be the type of family in which most people live, and how has this changed since 1961?

■ The first two columns of the table show that the married couple with dependent children—probably still the most common view of a 'typical' family—is indeed the most common type, but that only 40 per cent of the population now live in this kind of family arrangement, a proportion which has been falling in recent decades. In contrast, the proportion of the population living alone or in families consisting of a lone parent and dependent children, has been rising quite rapidly.

The final column calculates the percentage of *households* of different types rather than the percentage of the population who live in these households, and so it shows a slightly different pattern. In particular, the 'married couple with dependent children' arrangement is shown to account for less than a quarter of all households, and to be less common as a household type than one-person households or households containing couples with no children.

Although family types are presented as separate categories in the table, over time a family will change and may pass through several of the categories shown, as individuals are born, age and die, come together and separate. These sequences are sometimes termed the **family life cycle**, a title that suggests the process has a continuous cyclic nature, in contrast to the finite *lifespan* of individual family members. However, such sequences are not purely cyclical: as living patterns alter, the 'typical' sequence, or the length of time spent at any point in the sequence, may change. Hence the expression favoured here is the **family life course**.

☐ What are likely to be the key transition points in a 'typical' family life course, starting from the decision of a young adult to leave the parental home and begin a new family?

■ A simplified sequence of key transitions might be: (i) finding a partner, leading to marriage or cohabitation; (ii) childbearing and rearing; (iii) children leaving home; (iv) retirement from work; (v) death of spouse; (vi) own death.

☐ Can you suggest some variations on this sequence?

■ There are many possible variations—childlessness (chosen or involuntary), divorce, remarriage, children who do not leave home, children from different marriages, premature death of a spouse, and so on. Gay relationships passing through these transitions should also be borne in mind.

But every family passes through at least some of these transitions, and the sequence forms a useful framework for considering current patterns of family life and how they are changing.

Marriage and cohabitation

Marriage has traditionally been seen as the event that marks the beginning of a new family. Over recent decades, patterns of marriage have changed quite dramatically in Britain. First, the average age at which people first get married has been rising steadily. If we look at the cohort of women born in 1946, half had married by the age of 21.5 years (that is, 21.5 years was the median age of marriage). But for the cohort of women born in 1964, the median age of marriage had risen to just under 25 years of age (Kiernan, 1989, p. 28). As a result of this change, teenage brides have almost vanished: in 1980 they made up almost a quarter of all marriages, but by 1990 barely one in ten.

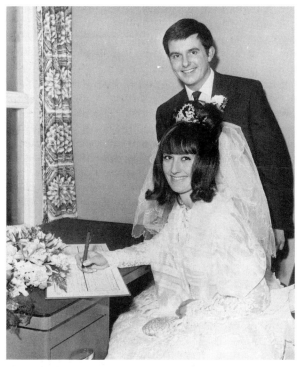

Teenage brides have declined steadily as a proportion since their high point in the 1960s, when this 18-year-old married, and are a rarity in the 1990s. (Photo: Edward Ede)

Second, there has been a steady rise in the proportion of people who do not get married at all, and the total number of marriages each year has been falling steadily. In 1971 only 7 per cent of men and 4 per cent of women who reached the age of 50 had never been married. But during the 1990s, if present marriage rates continue, around one in five people will reach the age of 50 without ever having married. However, people who remain unmarried do not necessarily live alone, and it has become increasingly common for people to cohabit for some time before marriage or to cohabit and never get

married. Only 7 per cent of women marrying for the first time at the beginning of the 1970s had cohabited before their marriage, but by 1994 this had risen to almost two-thirds.

The third major change in recent decades has been the number of marriages that end in divorce. Before World War II the annual number of divorces in Britain seldom rose above 5 000, and in 1951 it was less than 30 000. But by 1991 divorces had risen to over 170 000. It is still the case that the majority of marriages are ended by the death of a partner, but if the divorce rates prevailing in the 1980s continue, around 37 per cent of marriages—more than one in three—will end in divorce.

However, divorce is not always a permanent state for individuals. In fact almost three-quarters of men and more than half of all women remarry within five years of a divorce. One result is that more than a third of all marriages in 1992 involved at least one partner getting married again.

Although patterns of marriage in Britain have changed dramatically over recent decades, they may not be so striking within a longer historical perspective. For example, Figure 2.1 casts some interesting historical light on the proportion of marriages now broken by divorce.

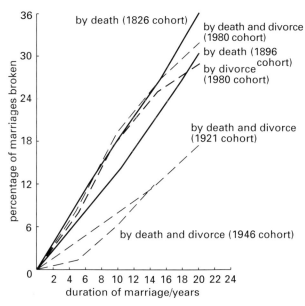

Figure 2.1 *Percentages of marriages broken by death or divorce for cohorts of people marrying in 1826, 1896, 1921, 1946 and 1980. (Source: British Society for Population Studies, 1983,* The Family, *Occasional Paper 31, OPCS, London, p. 5)*

☐ What does Figure 2.1 reveal about the proportion of marriages broken by death or divorce since the early nineteenth century?

■ Throughout the nineteenth century as many marriages were broken by death as were broken in the 1980s by divorce.

Because family size was greater in the nineteenth century, an even higher proportion of children might have been affected by the loss of a parent than they are today. It is also worth considering that, as a result of rising life expectancy, a twentieth-century marriage unbroken by divorce may commonly continue for 40 or 50 years, which would have been much more unusual in the nineteenth century. Queen Victoria, for example, was widowed after just 21 years of marriage (during which she had nine children) and lived on as a widow for a further 40 years.

Similar historical points have been made about age at first marriage, which was generally even higher than in the 1990s (probably somewhere between 25 and 27 for men and women) in England for a long period from the sixteenth century onwards (Anderson, 1980, p. 18), implying that the period around the 1950s was unusual in its very low average age of marriage partners.

Despite changes in recent years, the United Kingdom still has one of the youngest age patterns of marriage in Western Europe, and cohabitation is still much less common than in most European Union countries. For example, the proportion of young women cohabiting is twice as high in France, Germany and the Netherlands as it is in the United Kingdom, and in Denmark and Sweden it is even higher (Kiernan, 1989, pp. 32–3). These patterns elsewhere suggest that the changes seen in British marriage patterns have far from run their course.

Raising children

Changing patterns of marriage, divorce and cohabitation have major implications for the next stage of the family life course: childbearing and childrearing. The first major change in the twentieth century has been a major fall in the **average completed family size**. In the late nineteenth century each marriage resulted, on average, in six children, although many did not survive infancy or childhood. But this fell dramatically around the beginning of the twentieth century, so that marriages contracted in the period 1925–9 had on average fewer than two and a half children. The average completed family size has not changed a great deal since then, although it did rise during the 1960s 'baby boom' before falling again.

These changes over the course of this century are likely to have made a major contribution to the increased life expectancy experienced by women: the hazards of childbirth and the frequency of confinement were greatly reduced, and fewer women being worn out by almost constant childbearing meant that fewer women succumbed to diseases such as tuberculosis and pneumonia. The decline in completed family size has also been associated with—and may in part be a consequence of—a rising proportion of women joining the labour force, as you will see shortly.

There are, however, differences in family size among the different ethnic groups in the United Kingdom. Women born in the Indian subcontinent for example are more likely to have larger families than those born in either the United Kingdom or the West Indies, though there has been a decline in the frequency of births of three or more children in all the minority ethnic groups in recent years. These differences, plus variations in the proportion of people living alone, help to explain why average household size varies by ethnic group: the average Bangladeshi or Pakistani household in the United Kingdom contains more than five people, and the average Indian household more than four, while the average white household contains between two and three people.

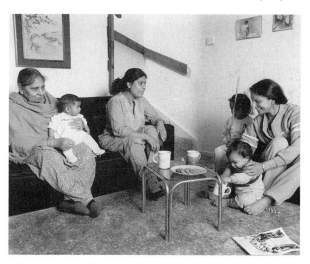

The proportion of Asian people living alone in the United Kingdom is lower than for other ethnic groups, partly because older people tend to live within their extended family. (Photo: Mike Levers)

Alongside the fall in completed family size, other changes in childbearing have become more pronounced in recent decades. First, couples have been delaying starting their families, so that the average age of the mother at first birth has gone up from 24 years in 1970 to almost 27 years by 1990. In parallel with this, the average parental age at the *final* birth has gone down, a fact of some biological significance as older parents carry and pass on more mutations.[2]

Second, an increasing number of women have started childbearing before (or, in a smaller proportion of cases, without) subsequent marriage. As a consequence, the number of births taking place outside marriage has increased markedly. Table 2.2 shows the proportion of all live births taking place outside marriage in the United Kingdom and other European Union (EU) countries, and how this has changed in recent decades.

Table 2.2 Live births outside marriage as a percentage of all births in 1960 and 1991: European Union

Country	Percentage in	
	1960	1991
Denmark	7.8	46.5
France	6.1	31.8
United Kingdom	5.2	29.8
Irish Republic	1.6	16.6
Portugal	9.5	15.6
Germany	7.6	15.1
Luxembourg	3.2	12.2
Netherlands	1.4	12.0
Belgium	2.1	10.7
Spain	2.3	9.6
Italy	2.4	6.6
Greece	1.2	2.4

Source: Central Statistical Office (1994b) *Social Trends 24*, HMSO, London, Table 2.22, p. 40.

☐ What changes does Table 2.2 reveal about births outside marriage across the European Union?

■ In every EU country there has been a substantial increase in the proportion of births occurring outside marriage. In the United Kingdom, the proportion was almost one in three births in 1991, which was higher than in most other EU countries.

[2]See *Human Biology and Health: an Evolutionary Approach*, Chapter 11, for a discussion of this point.

Despite this increase, there is some evidence that the nature of illegitimacy itself is changing. Three-quarters of all the births which took place outside marriage in 1992 were registered on the joint information of *both* parents, compared to under one-half in 1971. And almost two-thirds of these joint registrations were made by parents living at the same address. This suggests that many of these births are occurring within stable relationships where the child will have contact with both parents, and it reflects at least in part the increasing popularity of cohabitation before or instead of marriage. Accompanying these changes, there is some evidence that cohabitation and having children outside marriage are becoming more socially acceptable than in the past. For example, in 1987 the Family Law Reform Act removed all remaining differences in the legal rights of children born within and outwith a marriage, and made it impermissible to use the term 'illegitimate' to refer to such children in any legal document.

Lone parents

Although many children are now born outside marriage but to a cohabiting couple, around one in ten households consists of a lone parent with at least one dependent child, as you saw in Table 2.1. There has been a sharp increase in the number of children living for some of their childhood in these **lone-parent families**, compared to the experience of children born in the later 1940s and 1950s. In the United Kingdom in 1971, around 1 million children lived in families headed by a lone parent, but by 1992 lone-parent families contained more than 2.2 million children or about one in six of all children (Haskey, 1993, p. 29). Partly because of their rising numbers, lone-parent families became a major focus of debate, research and media attention during the early 1990s.

Over 92 per cent of these lone-parent families are headed by mothers, with fewer than 8 per cent headed by fathers. In the majority of cases, lone-parent families have arisen because of marital breakdown, leading to separation or divorce. But there has also been a sharp increase in the proportion of lone parents who are single (that is, unmarried) mothers: up from 16 per cent of all lone parents in 1971 to 34 per cent in 1993. One clear change is that, whereas in the past a substantial proportion of lone-parent families arose because of widowhood, this only accounted for about 6 per cent of such families in 1993.

Beyond these stark facts, the circumstances of parents and children in lone-parent families are hard to establish, and as with all family types there is a tremendous amount of variation. It is clear that lone-parent families are less likely than other families to be owner-occupiers, and lone mothers are less likely to be working than are married or cohabiting mothers. Lone parents are also much more likely than are married couples to be on low household incomes: in 1991 only ten per cent of married couples with dependent children received a weekly household income of less than £150, compared with 70 per cent of lone-parent families.

A growing concern in recent years has been whether children who grow up in lone-parent families, or in families which have broken up, have poorer health and wellbeing.

☐ Why might lone-parent families face greater hazards to their health and wellbeing than other types of family?

■ The lower incomes of many lone-parent families may result in poorer material circumstances, nutrition and other factors which may adversely affect health.[3] Second, if there has been a divorce or separation or a partner has died, there may be damaging stresses and strains associated with the disruption of the family. Finally, the physical and emotional pressures of caring for children alone may also take their toll of the health of parents or of children.

The evidence on these topics is complex. A recent review of research findings by the social policy analyst Louie Burghes stressed that

… there is neither a single outcome, nor explanation for the outcomes for children who experience family disruption and who live in one parent families (Burghes, 1994, p. 39)

However, despite these qualifications Burghes did conclude that

It is an uncomfortable fact that, almost without exception, children are upset when families break up. It would, presumably, be surprising if they were not. Frequently this is accompanied by psychological stress and changes in their

[3]The effect of material deprivation on health is discussed in several chapters of *World Health and Disease* (1993), particularly Chapters 9 and 10.

socio–economic circumstances. These were thought, generally, to have short term, but now, possibly, longer-term consequences. (Burghes, 1994, p. 39)

In her review of outcomes relating to lone parenthood, Burghes found a number of studies in which the *perinatal mortality rate* was higher amongst children born to separated, widowed, divorced and single women compared with married women. A higher proportion of babies born to non-married women were also of low birth weight. Both these outcomes may be related to a later and lower use of antenatal services amongst non-married women and/or to differences in their material circumstances. However, the subsequent physical development of children born to non-married women does not seem to show any such differences: they tend to reach the same developmental points at similar times, and their sight and hearing is as good.

Burghes also found a number of studies which showed that children whose parents had separated or divorced were significantly more likely to have lower educational attainment than children with married parents, but that no such underachievement existed among children whose mothers had been widowed. And women whose parents' marriage had broken down by the time they were 16 years old have been found to be more likely to leave home early, have a child by the age of 20, or to have a baby themselves outside marriage, suggesting one way in which such patterns may sustain themselves.

Almost all studies in this area stress that it is not possible to generalise across *all* lone-parent families, which vary tremendously in their circumstances. Also, life in a lone-parent family is not inevitably a greater threat to health than life in any other sort of family. Some lone parents and their children may feel that their situation is considerably improved, especially if they had previously lived within insecure or unhappy marriages.

These complexities are reflected in social attitudes to lone parents. Most surveys have found a consistent majority expressing the view that '…a child needs a home with both a father and a mother to grow up happily': indeed, the proportion of a British sample who agreed with this view rose between 1981 and 1990 from 67 per cent to 73 per cent. Similarly, the 1989 British Social Attitudes Survey found that only 30 per cent of respondents agreed that 'a single mother can bring up her child as well as a married couple'. But the same survey also found that 60 per cent of respondents thought it was better or much better for the children of an unhappy marriage if it were ended (quoted in Burghes, 1994, p. 14).

Old age and the death of a spouse

The number of people in Great Britain aged over 65 has risen from fewer than 2 million in 1901 to almost 9 million in 1991. And within this older population, the number of very old people has also been rising steeply: in 1901 there were fewer than 60 000 people over the age of 85, but in 1991 this age-group had risen to well over half a million.

Table 2.3 shows the household characteristics of all older people living in private households (that is, not in institutions such as nursing homes) in Great Britain in the late 1980s.

Table 2.3 Household circumstances of older people in private households in 1986, Great Britain

Living:	All males and females aged 65+ (%)	Females aged 80+ (%)
with spouse only	45	11
alone	36	61
with spouse and others	7	1
with children/ children-in-law	7	21
with siblings	3	3
with other relatives	1	2
with non-relatives	1	1

Source: derived from Central Statistical Office (1987) *Social Trends 17*, HMSO, London, Table 2.8, p. 44.

□ What are the main features of the data in Table 2.3?

■ First, the very high proportion (81%) of men and women aged 65 or over who live alone or solely with their spouse; and second, the high proportion (61%) of women aged 80 or over who are living entirely alone.

Although widowhood has declined as a cause of lone parenthood, marriage partners often lose their spouse later in life and are faced with long periods of living alone. This is particularly so for women, who not only have a significantly longer life expectancy than men to begin with, but also tend to marry men older than themselves.

As a result, while only 17 per cent of men aged 65 or over are widowers, 50 per cent of women in the same age group are widows.

This transition between living in a family and living alone has significant consequences for health: for example, widowed or divorced people on average suffer more ill-health than their married counterparts, and these differences appear to be greater for men.[4]

The ageing of the population also has many important implications for the family's role as a source of nursing care, and on the nature of *kinship ties,* such as the number of relatives a person has. Look at the quotation below, for example, taken from a study of patterns of family and kinship ties in a South Wales town by two anthropologists in the 1960s.

Trevor Jones was 69 and was thus born in 1891. He was the last but one of thirteen children (two of whom died in infancy), covering an age span of twenty-two years. His wife, Maud, whom he married in 1917, was one of eleven children covering a span of nineteen years. Two very large families. Trevor was the son of a blacksmith, and his wife the daughter of a collier. Trevor and Maud had just two daughters (now in their thirties) and have three grandchildren. Not one of the twenty uncles and aunts of these two daughters (that is, the brothers and sisters of Trevor and Maud) had more than three children. Five of them remained unmarried into old age, and four more had just one child each. The familial experience of these three generations— that of Trevor Jones's own generation, and of his grandchildren—within a single Swansea family is markedly different. His own generation was thickly peopled with relatives; his grandchildren in comparison have remarkably few. (Rosser and Harris, 1965, p. 117–8)

These changes in *kinship networks* are sometimes used to support the view that families now don't look after their elderly members as well as they did in the past. But before reaching that conclusion we need to know more about the stability of communities and the geographical proximity of kin in the past. According to an analysis of the 1851 census undertaken by the sociologist Michael Anderson, well under half of the population at that time were living where they had been born:

[4]Potential explanations for such differences are discussed in *World Health and Disease*, Chapter 9.

… with these rates of population turnover, the likelihood that people would have had many relatives living in the same village as themselves was quite low right into the twentieth century. (British Society for Population Studies, 1983, p. 3)

Larger kinship networks in the past, therefore, do not necessarily imply that families in the past were much more likely to care for their elderly relatives. We also know that the proportion of old people who are in institutional care is no higher now than it was a century ago: in 1906 almost 6 per cent of the population over 65 were living in Poor Law institutions—today the proportion in institutional care is around 5 per cent.

In fact the evidence suggests that, with the ageing of the population, *increasing* numbers of families are pro-

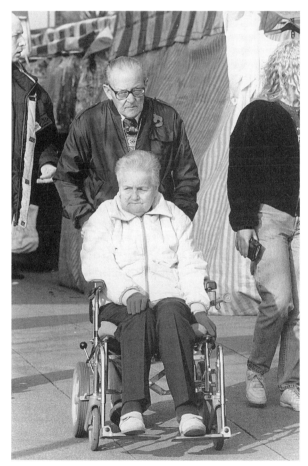

Increasing numbers of adults are caring for sick, elderly or handicapped relatives in 'the community' in the 1990s. (Photo: Mike Levers)

viding care and support for elderly and infirm relatives. Recent surveys suggest that such *informal care-giving* is a major activity, with up to 14 per cent of all adults in Great Britain looking after or regularly helping people who are sick, elderly or handicapped (Green, 1988). And although the majority of these carers are women, around 40 per cent are men. Researchers have also found that such activity can have a far-reaching financial impact on the care-givers, leading them into prolonged expenditure on items such as food, laundry, and equipment, and often causing them significant loss of earnings as a result of shorter working hours, missed promotion prospects, or having to retire or temporarily stop paid employment altogether (Glendenning, 1992).

The ageing population has also led many researchers to consider the meanings attached to old age. The historian Peter Laslett, for example, has explored the historical meanings of old age in the context of our current demographic circumstances. An extract from his 1989 book, *A Fresh Map of Life*, entitled 'A new division of the life course', is included in the Reader, and you should read this now.

□ What does Laslett suggest is the main historical association of old age in Western culture?

■ He argues that it is associated with dependence and decrepitude, in a way that permeates our language, culture and social policies.

□ Why might this association be damaging?

■ Demographic changes in Western industrialised nations such as the United Kingdom have resulted in large numbers of healthy and active people beyond the current retirement age. According to Laslett (a viewpoint explored further in Chapter 10 of this book), their talents and experience are being seriously damaged and undervalued.

□ What proposal does Laslett make to begin remedying this situation?

■ He proposes a new ordering of the life course into four stages: first, dependence and socialisation; second, responsibility, earning and saving; third, personal fulfilment; and fourth, dependence and death. By reordering the way we divide the life course, he hopes to break the inaccurate perception of most of the older population as dependent.

Laslett has clearly identified a problem in the way we tend to think of older people. But his advocacy of the 'third age' as a proposed solution has in turn been criticised. In particular, it has been argued that his approach may further marginalise those in the fourth age—the dependent, decrepit and dying, as he describes them. Sociologist Michael Young and the gerontologist Tom Schuller, for instance, while in agreement that chronological age is not a useful basis on which to divide the life course into stages, have argued that in Laslett's schema

> … elevating the third [age] by the comparison is only done by treading down the fourth. The labelling problem is wished on to even older and more defenceless people. (Young and Schuller, 1991, p. 181)

If Laslett's proposed division of the life course is indeed interpreted in this way, then its positive intentions may be accompanied by some negative consequences.

The life course and work

Let us now turn to another aspect of the life course that is closely linked to the family but can be considered separately for convenience: the life course and work. Paid employment is a central feature of our society, though not everyone who works gets paid for doing so. We often ask people what they 'do', and 'doing' has become so synonymous with paid employment that many people not paid for their work tend to answer that they 'don't work', or that they are 'just' a housewife (a subject we return to in Chapter 8). Of course, the reason why the question is so frequently asked is that a great deal about a person can be discovered or guessed from the answer: their background, education, status, power, earnings, and so on. A person's health can also depend on their work: people in different occupations are exposed to very different levels of risk or health hazard, and their income and *occupational class* has an important influence on such things as life expectancy or infant mortality.[5]

Commencing work

The ages at which employment begins and ends have varied considerably over time and across different societies. At present in the United Kingdom the beginning of **working age**—the age at which full-time paid employment is legally allowed—is 16, but the trend in industrialised countries has been for this starting age to be pushed up (and, as you will see, for the retirement age to be drawn down).

These very clearly defined ages of transition both into and out of working life are a recent phenomenon. In non-industrial societies the labour of children is often used in or around the home or in agricultural activity, is supervised by parents, and is likely to change almost imperceptibly into adult work without a set age of transition.

However, the Industrial Revolution involved a move away from rural agricultural life towards urban life, away from domestic production to factory production regulated by the clock, and wage labour.[6] As this system developed in England, children were increasingly drawn into factory employment by the need for money to supplement family income, or were pushed into it by officials anxious to avoid the need to support them with public funds. As is well known, the result was a rapid growth of child employment, often in dangerous or unhealthy occupations such as mining, machine-minding or chimney-sweeping. Brutality, ill-treatment, exploitation and fear became commonplace. The dread of punishment for lateness felt by a young mill-worker in eighteenth-century Derby is graphically conveyed in the following recollection:

> I did not awake … till daylight seemed to appear. I rose in tears for fear of punishment, and went to my father's bedside to ask what was o'clock? 'He believed six'; I darted out in agonies, and from the bottom of Full Street to the top of Silkmill Lane, not 200 yards, I fell nine times! Observing no lights in the mill, I knew it was an early hour and the reflection of the snow had deceived me. Returning, it struck two. (William Hutton, quoted in Challis and Elliman, 1979, p. 23)

Throughout the nineteenth century, controls over the kinds of work children were permitted to do and over their conditions of employment were gradually tightened. By the end of the century, full-time factory work had been replaced by full-time compulsory education, and the idea of what a normal, healthy child could do had radically changed. But our assumptions and images concerning child labour are still influenced by this episode of British history. Full-time factory work is illegal, as in most other industrial countries, but other forms of part-time work are still common: around three-quarters of all children aged between 13 and 15 in the United Kingdom have some form of part-time employment, a third of them in paid work such as delivery rounds or work in shops, the remainder in domestic or voluntary work.

[5]See *World Health and Disease*, Chapter 9.

[6]See *World Health and Disease*, Chapter 5.

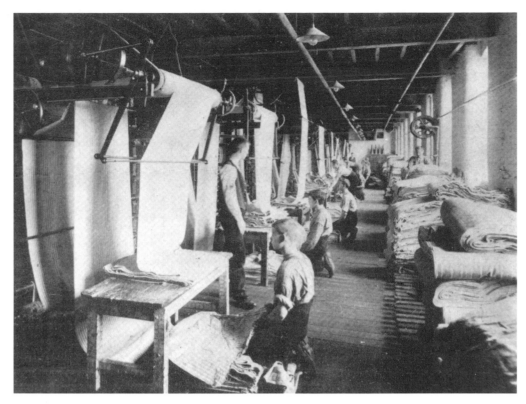

(a)

Controls over the kind of work that children are allowed to do have increased during the twentieth century, but in the 1990s three-quarters of children aged 13–15 years have some form of part-time work. (a) Boys employed to raise the nap on cloth woven at Samuel Heap's Spotland Bridge Mills in Rochdale in about 1910. (Photo: Rochdale Local Studies Library) (b) A boy employed to deliver newspapers in Milton Keynes in 1995. (Photo: Mike Levers)

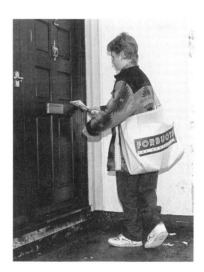

(b)

□ Why should the working conditions of children be of particular concern?

■ First, developing children may be particularly susceptible to chemical, radiological or other hazards, and may be in need of longer hours of sleep, etc. Second, in the past they were given jobs which were particularly dangerous, but which only they could do because of their size: climbing into machines, along pipes or up chimneys, for example. Third, because they are relatively powerless they need the protection of the law.

At the same time, however, it is important to ask if the bad conditions sometimes experienced by labouring children are a problem of *age*. In many instances, the occupations that children were eventually prevented from doing in

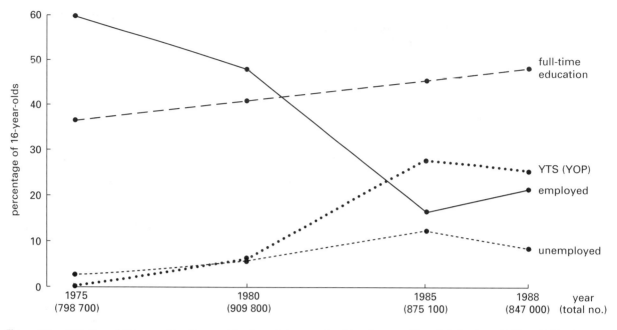

Figure 2.2 *Activities of 16-year-olds after reaching the minimum school leaving age, Great Britain, from 1975 to 1988. (Source: Kiernan, K. and Wicks. M., 1990,* Family Change and Future Policy, *Family Policy Studies Centre, London, Figure 13, p. 24)*

Victorian Britain were taken over by adults, who then experienced the same hazards. The problem was the working conditions, rather than the age of the person doing the job.

It is also worth noting that not all child labour is injurious to health, and that obtaining even a small income may be an important source of independence and freedom. The gradual abolition of many forms of child labour in industrialised countries such as the United Kingdom, and the rise of compulsory and supervised education, brought freedom from some forms of exploitation, but also created new forms of regulation and control.

In recent years, although there has been no change in the official school-leaving age, there have been dramatic changes in the early life experience of school-leavers, as Figure 2.2 shows.

The main change that has occurred is a very sharp decline in the numbers of school-leavers going into employment: in 1975 over 60 per cent did so, but by 1988 this had fallen to around 20 per cent. Instead, they are now much more likely to become unemployed, to go into a youth training scheme (YTS), or to stay on in full-time education.

The proportion of the population that does enter formal employment (that is, people who are in or are actively seeking employment) is normally called the **participation rate** (or *economic activity rate*). Figure 2.3 shows the participation rate for men and women in Great Britain in 1992.

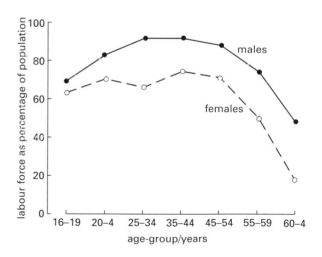

Figure 2.3 *Labour force participation rates for males and females, by age, Great Britain 1992. (Source: derived from Central Statistical Office (1994b) Social Trends 24, HMSO, London, Table 4.5, p. 57)*

□ What strikes you about the different patterns for women and men shown in Figure 2.3?

■ The participation rate for women is lower at all ages than that of men.

The average participation rate of all women aged between 16 and 59 years in the United Kingdom was 71 per cent in 1992. This compares with 40 per cent in Spain, for example, but over 79 per cent in Denmark. The average across the European Union is around 54 per cent. Despite these variations, the participation rate of women has been rising quite steeply since World War II in most industrialised countries (in the same age group, it was around 36 per cent in the United Kingdom in 1950). Almost all of this increase, certainly in the United Kingdom, has been due to an increase in part-time employment.

□ What reasons can you think of for the slight decline in the female participation rate between the ages of 20–4 and 25–34 as shown in Figure 2.3?

■ There are two main reasons. First, many women leave the labour market in order to have children, and some of them subsequently return to employment once children are going to school. Second, some women stop work when they get married and thereafter depend on their husbands for financial support.

However, the decline in the participation rate of this age group is now much less pronounced than it was in the past, as a result of factors such as delayed age of first birth and more women recommencing work after childbirth.

Lifetime earnings

Let us now look more closely at those who are in paid employment during their working years. Not only do the earnings of people in employment vary widely depending on occupation, sex and ethnicity, but they also vary considerably according to age. These patterns of earnings at different ages are normally called **lifetime earnings profiles**. Figure 2.4, which is based on work by the economic demographer Heather Joshi, illustrates such earnings profiles for three hypothetical individuals, each of whom is assumed to have left school at the age of 17: a man in full-time employment, a woman who has no children, and a woman who has two children.

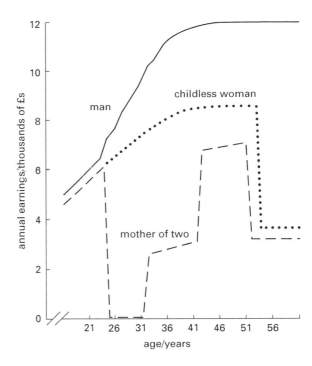

Figure 2.4 *Illustrative lifetime earnings profiles for a man, a childless woman, and a mother of two, Britain, 1980s. (Source: Joshi, H. (ed.), 1989, The Changing Population of Britain, Blackwell, Oxford, Figure 10.6, p. 170)*

The absolute value of earnings (on the vertical axis of Figure 2.4) is based on earnings in the late 1980s, and is less important than the shape and relative position of the profiles. The top profile in the Figure is for a male worker in a full-time lower-paid manual job. His pay gradually increases with age and experience until around the age of 40, when it levels off. The woman without children starts in a full-time non-manual job, from which she earns substantially less than the man. She then switches to part-time work in her mid-50s before retiring at age 59. Finally, the woman who has had two children has taken eight years out of paid employment to provide pre-school care, and then works part-time for most of the years when they are at school. Eventually she returns to full-time employment but because of her employment history her pay is lower than that of the woman who has not interrupted her employment to have children. The woman with children finally returns to part-time work in her early 50s.

The result of these different earnings profiles is that, between the ages of 17 and 59, the man earns almost half as much again as the woman without children, who in turn earns almost twice as much as the woman with

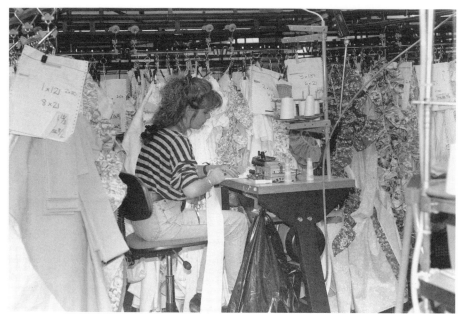

Women's employment in the 1990s tends to be predominantly in relatively low-paid part-time manual work, which can be combined with heavy domestic responsibilities. (Photo: Mike Levers)

children. Put another way, the difference between the top and middle lines shows that women typically are less well rewarded for entering the labour market than are men of similar qualifications. The difference between the middle and bottom lines is one measure of the cost to a woman of becoming a mother.

☐ If lost earnings are a 'cost' of becoming a mother, what differences in childbearing might you expect to find between well qualified and poorly qualified women?

■ As a well-qualified woman is likely to have higher earnings, the 'cost' to her of stopping work to have children is greater, and she is more likely to postpone having children or to have fewer children.

This is indeed the pattern of recent changes: the trend towards older age at first birth, for example, is particularly evident among women with more years of formal education.

One of the main points that can be drawn out of the lifetime-earnings profiles in Figure 2.4 is that there is a close link between family responsibility and pay. Women do far more unpaid domestic work than men, including childcare, care of older relatives and housework. For example, parenthood has a dramatic effect on women's, but almost no effect on men's, earnings and participation rates. Getting married tends to give men a pay advantage over unmarried men, perhaps because they can rely on their spouse to maintain their domestic foundations and thus can devote more of their time to their career[7]. Moreover, the community care policy of the 1990s is heavily dependent on the unpaid caring work of women[8]. Consequently, as Heather Joshi has argued, if progress towards equality of opportunity is to continue, it is not sufficient to focus on equal pay in the labour market:

… measures to improve women's access to education, training and remunerative jobs need to be complemented by measures to give families more choice about the management of their unpaid responsibilities. (Joshi, 1989, p. 173)

Such measures include a wider provision of day nurseries, and supportive domiciliary services for older relatives.

[7]An audiotape for Open University students, associated with Chapter 8 of this book, illustrates this point by comparing the domestic arrangements of two senior civil servants, one male and one female, both married with children.

[8]Community car is discussed in *Dilemmas in Health Care* (1993), Chapter 8.

Finally, it should be noted that in addition to differences between males and females, there are many other variations in lifetime-earnings profiles. In most manual jobs—including the male example in Figure 2.4—there is little scope for promotion after the first few years, and earnings tend to reach a plateau by the early 40s, if not sooner. Earnings may indeed decline towards the end of the working life if a manual job is physically demanding and so becomes progressively more difficult for older workers. Salaried white-collar and management jobs, in contrast, tend to be accompanied by a package of inducements, promotions and increments that ensure a fairly steady increase in earnings throughout most of the working life.

Unemployment over the life course

Like earnings, unemployment is strongly influenced by age, and the likelihood of experiencing unemployment varies significantly at different points in the life course. Figure 2.5 shows the rate of unemployment by sex in each age-group in the United Kingdom in 1993.

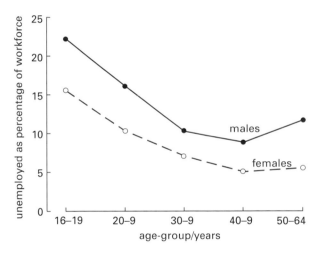

Figure 2.5 *Unemployment rates by sex and age, United Kingdom, 1993. (Source: derived from* Central Statistical Office, 1994b, Social Trends 24, *HMSO, London, Table 4.20, p. 62)*

☐ What does Figure 2.5 reveal about unemployment over the life course?

■ The unemployment rate forms a 'U-shape' with increase in age: that is, it is high among young people, then falls to a low point for the age group 40–9, then starts to rise again, especially among males, as people approach the end of their working life. The 'U' is shallower for women than for men.

Unemployment has become a particular problem among young people in recent years (a subject we return to in Chapter 6). Even in earlier periods of prolonged high unemployment, for example the inter-war years, the U-shape shown in Figure 2.5 was much less pronounced. And in the decades after World War II, 15–18 year olds accounted for only around 4 per cent of the total numbers unemployed; by comparison, in 1993 over 11 per cent of the total numbers unemployed were aged 16–19. In contrast, unemployment rates have been falling over time amongst the older age-groups in the labour force.

Retirement

The transition that occurs at the end of a working life is usually referred to as **retirement**, commonly defined as being in permanent and voluntary withdrawal from the labour force and in simultaneous receipt of a pension income. In the United Kingdom our view of retirement is heavily influenced by the National Insurance scheme, which currently provides a state retirement pension to insured men and women at the age of 65 and 60 respectively. This will gradually be equalised at 65 for all in the early part of the twenty-first century. But retirement is often much less clear-cut than these set ages and definitions would suggest, as the following six cases taken from Johnson and Falkingham (1992) illustrate:

1 John M, aged 67, self-employed electrician, draws state retirement pension but still works 'now and again, for friends, like'.
2 Arthur B, aged 59, former miner, suffering from acute lung failure, in receipt of a disability pension.
3 William S, aged 58, accountant, took early retirement (and large 'golden handshake') from a multinational corporation when it was rationalizing its staff. He now works in a small accountancy partnership in a provincial town 'just to keep my mind alert; I don't need the money, but it's more interesting than golf'.

ISLE COLLEGE
RESOURCES CENTRE

4   Frank G, aged 64, former steelworker, made redundant when his company went bankrupt earlier in the year, not able to find alternative employment, drawing unemployment benefit, and considered by the Department of Employment to be 'early retired'.

5   Daphne R, aged 62, housewife, mother and grandmother 'and proud of it', has not worked since the birth of her first child thirty-seven years ago and has 'no intention of starting now!'. Her civil servant husband has another 18 months to go before he retires.

6   Mary L, aged 61, used to do a lot of local cleaning jobs, 'all cash-in-hand stuff, of course', but has stopped now her husband has taken early retirement (at 64) from the local engineering factory.

(From Johnson and Falkingham, 1992, pp. 84–5)

☐ How many of these people would you consider to be retired?

■ Opinions will vary, but most people would probably consider all these individuals to be retired or at least 'semi-retired'.

☐ How many of the six fit the general definition of retirement given earlier?

■ None of them. Neither Arthur nor Frank withdrew from work voluntarily or receives a state pension. Daphne and Mary have not paid National Insurance contributions and so will not receive a pension until their husbands retire at the age of 65. And John and William are drawing pensions but are still working from time to time.

These complexities are not allowed for in most official statistics, which usually classify people simply as being in the labour force or in retirement. But despite their limitations, official statistics do show whether major changes have been taking place, and some patterns are very clear. Among men, retirement at the age of 65 was very unusual at the beginning of the twentieth century: in 1921, around 60 per cent of all men in the United Kingdom aged over 65 were still economically active. But this has steadily fallen until in 1990 only 8 per cent of all men aged 65 or over are economically active. More recently, a similar change has been occurring amongst men in the 60–5 age group. As recently as 1970 almost 90 per cent of this group were classified as economically active, but this slumped to barely one-half by 1990. Among women, economic activity in these age groups has also been falling, but it has never been particularly high: even in 1911 only 11 per cent of women over 65 years of age were economically active in the United Kingdom, compared with 3 per cent by 1990.

The reasons for these changes—which are not confined to the United Kingdom, but have also occurred in countries such as France, Germany and the USA—are not simple. The trend towards earlier retirement has been encouraged by the growth of occupational pension schemes which have enabled members to retire while maintaining a reasonable standard of living, and by early retirement schemes or forced redundancy schemes devised by some employers to reduce their workforces in the face of declining demand or improved productivity. Older workers have often seemed an attractive target of such schemes because they tend to have higher earnings and therefore the potential savings are higher. However, in recent years such policies have been increasingly questioned: older workers have come to be seen as more reliable and experienced, the cost to pension funds of early retirement has become a cause for concern, and in some countries, such as the USA, anti-age discrimination legislation has made it illegal to make someone redundant on the grounds of age.

As with the official beginning of working age, then, there is a good deal of evidence that the end of working age is relative to time and place. It is also strongly influenced by a particular set of social, psychological and economic circumstances (as the six cases mentioned above illustrate), and has little direct association with the biological capacity to sustain work effort.

The life course and the economy

In this final section we look in more detail at some of the broader links between the life course and the economy, focusing in particular on the life experience of birth cohorts and the role of welfare spending in redistributing resources across the life course. Focusing on these topics helps to illuminate the fact that the life course of each generation has a unique character, over and above the variations between individuals.

The life experience of cohorts

Many aspects of the life course examined so far in this chapter have had to rely on data which may be misleading as a description of the lifetime experience of an *individual*.

For example, lifetime-earnings profiles are often based on *cross-sectional* rather than *longitudinal data*.[9] That is, they compare the earnings of, for example, one group of people aged 30 with *another* group aged 40, rather than making a comparison with the same group 10 years later. Because the cohort currently aged 40 has a particular rate of earnings, it does not necessarily follow that the cohort currently aged 30 will have the same rate of earnings 10 years later: an age-cohort can have its own characteristics that make it different from older or younger cohorts.

Cross-sectional data are frequently the only source of lifespan information, as longitudinal data on cohorts are difficult and expensive to obtain, involving the monitoring of large groups of people for long periods. The crucial point to remember is that a generalised life course constructed from cross-sectional data might not accurately describe the lifetime experience of any one individual.[10]

One longitudinal study that does provide a wealth of information on a particular cohort has followed for over 40 years the development of around five and a half thousand children born in England, Wales and Scotland in 1946. This study has allowed researchers to demonstrate the ways in which

> ... the imprint of each stage of the individual's development affects later life, and is, in turn, affected both by previous stages and by previous generations in the same family, and by the world in which development is taking place (Wadsworth, 1991, p. vi)

The world into which this particular cohort was born—the immediate post-war period—was

> ... a period of great innovation in education and in health care ... the National Health Service began two years after the study began. Two years before the study began the 1944 Education Act sought to eliminate barriers to educational opportunity. (Wadsworth, 1991, p. v)

Consequently, the members of this cohort share an experience of the world in which they were children that is unique to them, and this is one important influence on their lifetime experience.

Of all the reasons that might make cohorts differ in their lifetime experiences, one of the more interesting suggestions is that the *size* of the cohort exerts a strong influence. Figure 2.6 shows clearly the changes in the average number of annual births in the United Kingdom this century.

□ From Figure 2.6, how much variation has there been over time in birth cohort size: that is, the numbers born in any one period?

■ The variation has been substantial, forming a wave-like pattern of peaks and troughs: in the early years of the century over a million babies on average were born each year. This fell to less than three-

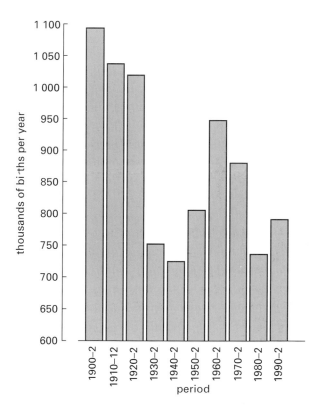

Figure 2.6 *Average number of annual births, United Kingdom, 1900–2 to 1990–2 (Source: derived from* Central Statistical Office, 1994a, *Annual Abstract of Statistics,* HMSO, London, Table 2.16 p. 26)

[9]*See Studying Health and Disease* (revised edition 1994), Chapter 6.

[10]Problems associated with analysing cross-sectional data are discussed in *Studying Health and Disease* (revised edition 1994), Chapter 6. An example of a cohort effect in the incidence of lung cancer is described in *World Health and Disease*, Chapter 9.

quarters of a million in the periods prior to and during the war, then rose again to almost a million in the early 1960s (the 'baby boom'), before falling back again in the early 1980s. This suggests that, for example, the early-1960s cohort is substantially bigger in relation to the rest of the population than the early 1950s cohort or the early 1980s cohort.

How might cohort size influence an individual's life course? One suggestion is that members of a large cohort—that is, a cohort born at a peak in the birth-rate—will face higher unemployment, lower wages, and poorer promotion prospects, because of their relatively abundant numbers. In contrast, members of a small cohort—that is, a cohort born at a trough in the birth-rate—will encounter much better labour market conditions because of their relatively scarce numbers. This argument has been applied especially in the context of post-war America, where a small war-time cohort was followed by the 'baby-boom' generation born in the 1950s and early 1960s. It has even been argued by some observers that the 'baby boomers' will face such unfavourable prospects that they will become the first American generation to be less well off than their parents.

In 1980 the American economist Richard Easterlin took these arguments even further, suggesting that a large cohort—for example the post-war baby boomers—will experience a high degree of stress from 'crowding' at different stages of life, leading to higher rates of suicide, murder, drinking, and other drug use, longer-term higher mortality rates, and even higher levels of 'political alienation' and general dissatisfaction. Easterlin noted that among the largest post-World War II American cohort there has been a rise in violent deaths (suicides, homicides, and accidents) producing a

> ... change in overall mortality for this group that contrasts noticeably with that for other age groups in the population. ... We have dramatic testimony to the growth in mental stress among young adults. (Easterlin, 1980, p. 107)

☐ Is this the only conclusion you could draw from the rise in violent deaths among young adults? Think about the main causes of death in these age-groups.

■ One of the largest single causes of death among young adults in the USA, as in the United Kingdom, is from motor vehicle accidents.[11] The increased mortality might simply be because the greater prosperity of the post-war period gave more young adults access to vehicles.

There are many similar criticisms that can be levelled at these **'cohort size' theories**. For example, the number of school places available and the degree of classroom crowding is clearly influenced by such things as public expenditure and social policy decisions, irrespective of changes in cohort size. Similarly, the number of jobs available to a cohort reaching employment age is strongly influenced by the state of the national and international economy, the economic policies being pursued, and many other factors.

More recently, Easterlin has returned to this subject and reached slightly different conclusions. The evidence so far, he argues, is that the income of baby boomers is higher than was the income of their parents at the same stage of the life course. Partly this is because of economic growth and rising living standards, which in general have made each generation more materially wealthy than their predecessors. But it is also, Easterlin argues, because the decisions the baby boomers have made about their family circumstances are very different from those made by their parents. More of them have remained single, more of them have remained childless, they have had fewer children and many more of them have combined child-rearing with mother's employment. These decisions have helped them to maintain their economic welfare, but may result in less leisure and fewer family members to whom they can turn for care when they reach retirement age. In short:

> ... on balance, while the boomers in retirement will typically do better than their parents in terms of material well-being, their advantage from a total welfare viewpoint may be less. (Easterlin et al., 1993, p. 520)

The life course and welfare expenditure

We have already noted the 'ageing population' and some of its implications for families and employment patterns. Its implications for welfare services have also attracted considerable attention.

---

[11]This is discussed in World Health and Disease, Chapter 9, and is given further attention in Chapters 5 and 6 of this book.

As individuals make their transit over the life course, their demands on the core services of the welfare state in the United Kingdom—health, education and social security—are constantly changing. Figure 2.7 summarises this pattern by showing spending per person on each of these services at different ages.

▢ Describe and interpret the patterns of spending shown in Figure 2.7.

■ Birth is associated with a block of health spending, which then falls to very low levels before increasing steadily from the age of around 60 onwards. Among those aged 85 and over, health expenditure outweighs all other welfare spending. The pattern of education spending is quite different: this is by far the largest item of welfare spending between the ages of 5 and 20, but from the age of 30 onwards is virtually non-existent. Finally, social security spending begins in the late teens, and thereafter is the largest component on welfare spending until very old age when it is overtaken by health expenditure. Social security spending rises particularly sharply around retirement age as people begin to receive their old age pensions.

Because welfare spending overall is focused mainly on older people, it follows that a rise in the proportion of the population who are old will tend to increase welfare expenditure. This has indeed been happening in the United Kingdom, and is projected to continue well into the twenty-first century. But the process is fairly gradual, and as the United Kingdom already has an older population than do many other Western countries, the impact is likely to be much less pronounced than has sometimes been claimed. On one set of calculations, if Britain continued to spend the same amount on welfare services on each person of a given age, but the population's age-structure continued to alter, then by the year 2041 total welfare spending would be 17 per cent higher than it was in 1991. Spread over 50 years, this would amount to no more than an increase in welfare spending of one-third of one per cent each year (Hills, 1993).

There is another very important aspect of welfare spending in relation to the life course. It is often assumed that old people are in some sense a burden on the welfare state, benefiting from it at the expense of others who are paying in. Welfare spending does involve an element of redistribution from rich to poor, but in some ways a more important feature of it is a redistribution *across the life course*. We have already looked at the way in which

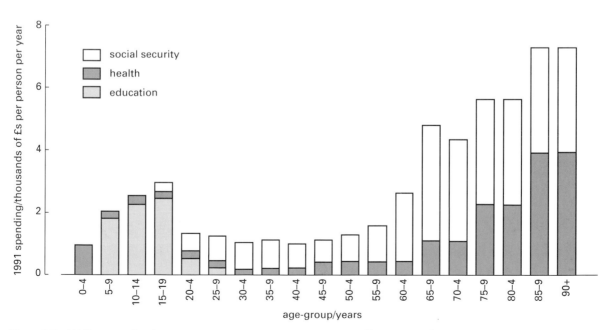

Figure 2.7 *Welfare spending by age group, Great Britain, 1991. (Source: Hills, J., 1993,* The Future of the Welfare State: A Guide to the Debate, *Joseph Rowntree Foundation, York, Figure 5, p. 11)*

earnings change over the life course: one way to view the welfare system is as a 'savings bank', which people pay into during periods when their income is relatively high, and draw from during periods of their life course when their income is relatively low.

Figure 2.8 illustrates this. The solid line shows an average profile of *original* income—that is, income before payment of any taxes or receipt of any benefits are taken into account. This rises to a peak around the age of 50–5, then falls sharply in the later stages of life as people retire from paid employment. The dashed line shows the profile of *net* income—that is, after taxes and cash benefits are taken into account. These reduce income before retirement (taxes), but boost it after retirement (pensions), and so flatten out the profile. Finally, the dotted line shows *final* income—that is, also taking into account benefits in kind such as education and health. This smooths out the profile even further.

So by means of this 'savings bank' effect, the welfare system reduces variations in standards of living over the life course. How important is this effect? Detailed research based on a computer model that simulates the life histories of around 4 000 individuals, suggests the following conclusions:

... *most* benefits are self-financed over people's lifetimes, rather than being paid for by others. Of the £133 000 average gross lifetime benefits from the system, an average of £98 000 is self-financed. Nearly three-quarters of what the welfare state does looked at in this way is like a 'savings bank'; only a quarter is 'Robin Hood' redistribution between different people. (Hills, 1993, p. 19)

Summary

In this chapter you have seen that the various events and transitions that occur during a lifetime—such as the beginning of working age, age of marriage, having children, and retirement—have changed significantly in the United Kingdom in the twentieth century.

In particular, you should note the following points:

1   The 'typical' family, consisting of a married couple with dependent children, is the most common family type, but only 40 per cent of the United Kingdom's population lives in this kind of family arrangement.

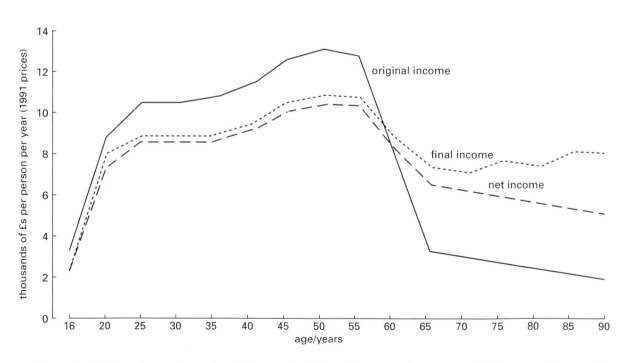

Figure 2.8 *An illustration of the way in which tax and social security even out incomes over the life course. (Source: Hills, J, The Future of the Welfare State: A Guide to the Debate, Joseph Rowntree Foundation, York, 1993, Figure 11, p. 18)*

2 The average age of marriage has been rising, and so has the proportion of marriages that end in divorce. An increasing number of people do not get married, and cohabitation and lone-parent families have become much more common.

3 The average completed family size has fallen, while the average age at first birth has gone up and the average age at final birth has gone down.

4 The participation rate of women has risen, mainly in part-time jobs. Levels of income and likelihood of being unemployed are strongly associated with different ages. Unemployment is a particular problem among the young.

5 The lifetime experience of individuals is likely to be influenced by the size of the cohort to which they belong, with some evidence that prospects are *relatively* poorer for those born into comparatively large cohorts.

6 An important function of the welfare state is to redistribute resources across different stages of the life course. Most welfare benefits are self-financed over people's lifetimes.

These changing patterns and their implications will be encountered again at many points in this book, as we explore in greater detail the lifetime experience of health and disease.

OBJECTIVES FOR CHAPTER 2

When you have studied this chapter, you should be able to:

2.1 Describe changes in family structure in the United Kingdom in recent decades, paying attention to age-effects and patterns of reproduction, marriage and divorce.

2.2 Outline the main lifetime characteristics of employment and earnings in modern Britain, noting individual variations particularly between men and women.

2.3 Briefly describe the relationship between the life course and the welfare state in the United Kingdom in the 1990s.

QUESTIONS FOR CHAPTER 2

Question 1 (*Objective 2.1*)

Fewer than one in four households now conforms to the traditional image of a married or cohabiting couple with children … evidence of the continuing erosion of conventional family patterns. (Brindle, 1994)

Assess this comment in the light of information in the first section of this chapter.

Question 2 (*Objective 2.2*)

What are the main differences in the participation rates of women and men in formal employment in the United Kingdom in the early 1990s?

Question 3 (*Objective 2.2*)

Why might data showing lifetime profiles of participation rates or earnings be a misleading guide to the lifetime experience of an individual?

Question 4 (*Objective 2.3*)

How does Figure 2.7 support the view that the welfare state may have an important role to play as a 'savings bank'?

ISLE COLLEGE
RESOURCES CENTRE

3

Care in pregnancy and childbirth

This chapter makes reference to the material on the safety of childbirth, on folic acid supplementation and on the programming hypothesis in Chapters 6, 8 and 10 of Studying Health and Disease, *and to the discussion of genetic disorders and prenatal diagnosis in Chapters 4 and 9 of* Human Biology and Health: An Evolutionary Approach. *Some aspects of this chapter relate to the discussion of medicalisation and de-medicalisation of childbirth in Chapter 8 of* Medical Knowledge: Doubt and Certainty.[1] *The television programme 'First steps to autonomy' is relevant to this chapter.*

The principal author of this chapter, Gavin Young, is a general medical practitioner based in Cumbria, who has a long-standing interest in the provision of health care in pregnancy and childbirth. He was a member of the 'Expert Maternity Group' set up by the Department of Health and chaired by Baroness Cumberlege, which reported in 1993. He helped to found and chairs the Association for Community-Based Maternity Care. (However, the opinions in this chapter are not necessarily those of either of these bodies.) Kevin McConway, from the Open University Course Team, made substantial contributions to this chapter by developing the distance-teaching aspects. Two other members of the Course Team, Richard Holmes and Basiro Davey, contributed to the biological sections of the chapter.

[1]*Studying Health and Disease* (revised edition 1994), *Human Biology and Health: An Evolutionary Approach* (1994) and *Medical Knowledge: Doubt and Certainty* (revised edition 1994).

Pregnancy and childbirth: what health care?

We have all experienced being born, though it is uncertain whether any of us can remember this event. In a matter of just a few minutes we move from a controlled environment where we were fed, oxygenated and kept warm in a liquid bath inside the mother's womb (uterus) into a much more hostile environment where we must breathe for ourselves, then feed and, to some extent, control our own temperature. It is therefore perhaps not surprising that such a crucial event should be accompanied by some secrecy and that the attendants should be considered to have special expertise, even magical powers. We wish to examine the ways in which professional expertise and control have affected pregnancy and childbirth in the United Kingdom in the 1990s.

Western-style health care claims considerable success. Only 4.1 women per 1 000 000 aged 15–44 years died in the United Kingdom (1988–90) from causes related to pregnancy and childbirth (Department of Health, 1994, p. 1). This can be expressed in another way: fewer than 8 women died from these causes per 100 000 maternities (pregnancies) in 1990. (In absolute numbers, 49 women died.) Things were very different in other times and places. In 1930–2 in the United Kingdom, 454 women died from causes related to pregnancy and childbirth per 100 000 maternities (Central Statistical Office, 1994). The average figure for African countries at present is about 600 deaths per 100 000 maternities (Tonks, 1994). In the United Kingdom, during a woman's pregnancy and childbirth, her male partner is more likely to die than she is (taking into account deaths from all causes). For babies too, birth is safer than it was (see Figure 3.1)—in 1990 the perinatal mortality rate in England and Wales was 8 per 1 000 births, compared to 62 per 1 000 births in 1931 (Office of Population Censuses and Surveys (OPCS), 1992a and 1993c). (Perinatal mortality rate is defined as the number of babies born dead after 24 weeks' gestation (stillbirths) and deaths in

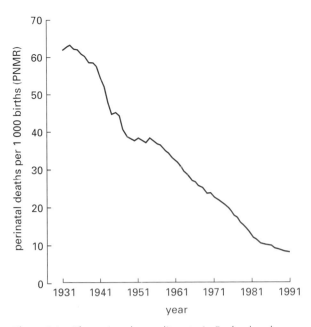

Figure 3.1 *The perinatal mortality rate in England and Wales, 1931 to 1990. (Data from annual OPCS reports)*

the first week of life, per thousand total (live and still) births.[2])

The apparent success of Western-style health care has, ironically, now led many to doubt whether medicalisation of pregnancy and birth[3] is necessary when birth is seen as safe. Opposing this view are others—particularly some health professionals—who argue that no birth is safe until it is over. We wish to examine how such opposing views arose and on what evidence these views are based.

The chapter begins with a brief outline of the biology of development in the womb and childbirth. We then turn for most of the chapter to look at the health care that is provided in the first nine months of life, and to investigate the rationale for its provision. Broadly speaking, the chapter moves through pregnancy and childbirth in the appropriate biological order. First we describe antenatal care, and then what happens during birth itself. Finally,

[2]Before October 1992, the length of gestation in the official definition of a stillbirth was 28 weeks. Definitions and further discussion of maternity statistics appear in Chapters 6 and 7 of *Studying Health and Disease* (revised edition 1994).

[3]The question of the medicalisation of childbirth is also discussed in *Medical Knowledge: Doubt and Certainty* (revised edition 1994), Chapter 8.

we look briefly at the care available to newborn babies and mothers in the period shortly after birth.

Biological development in the first nine months

Fertilisation and implantation

The point at which an individual human life is judged to have begun continues to be hotly debated: different 'dates' are recognised by different religions, laws and personal consciences. From a biological viewpoint, the unique genetic constitution of each new individual is complete within a single cell, at the moment when the chromosomes in a human egg (ovum) combine with the chromosomes from the sperm at **fertilisation**.[4] But there is a long and hazardous developmental road to travel if a baby is to be born nine months later. Figure 3.2 (*overleaf*) shows the first ten days.

The process can begin only if an egg and a sperm meet in ideal conditions for fertilisation to take place. In the United Kingdom, about 10 per cent of couples who want to have children experience long-term difficulty in doing so, and for many of them the underlying reason is a problem in achieving fertilisation. Mature eggs may not be shed from the woman's ovaries, or may not find their way into, or be able to pass along, one of the Fallopian tubes leading to the womb (or uterus, as labelled in Figure 3.2); mature sperm may not be produced in sufficient quantity by the man, or they may be killed by excess acid or antibodies in the woman's vaginal fluids.

☐ Can you think of a possible advantage to the human species of the vaginal fluids containing acids and antibodies?

■ The 'hostile' fluids give some protection against infectious organisms, such as bacteria and fungi, from getting into the womb during sexual intercourse and threatening the health of the woman and any baby she conceives.

Sperm are usually protected by the seminal fluid ejaculated at orgasm, which also supplies nutrients for the first part of the long swim that follows. Fertilisation is a chancy business: it can take several hours for sperm to

[4]The structure of chromosomes, genes and DNA, and their behaviour during fertilisation and cell division are described in *Human Biology and Health: An Evolutionary Approach*, Chapters 3 and 4.

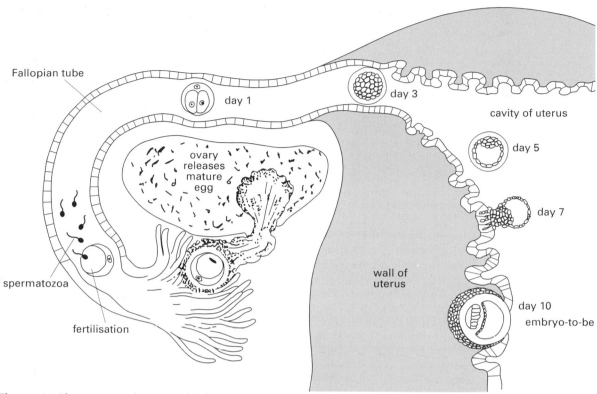

Figure 3.2 *The sequence of events in the development of a human embryo, from fertilisation in the Fallopian tube to implantation in the uterus about 10 days later.*

reach the top of the Fallopian tube and the egg remains viable for only about 24 hours after it has been shed from the ovary.

Various 'assisted conception techniques' have been devised to overcome infertility problems, including *in-vitro* **fertilisation** or **IVF** (*in vitro* means 'in glass'; the social and political aspects of infertility treatment are discussed in Chapter 7). In IVF, hormones are given to induce the ovary to shed several mature eggs at once, and these are collected by inserting a fine suction tube into the woman's abdomen; the eggs are kept alive in nutrient fluid in a culture vessel ('in glass') and freshly-collected sperm from the woman's partner or a donor are added. A single sperm penetrates the egg, just as it does in the Fallopian tube in unassisted conception, and the surface membrane of the egg immediately undergoes a profound structural change which makes it impenetrable to other sperm.

☐ What is the biological significance of this change in the egg?

■ It would make it unlikely that any further sperm could fertilise the egg; were they to do so, the potential embryo would have too many sets of chromosomes from the father and would fail to develop.

The fertilised egg has to *replicate,* that is make identical copies of all the chromosomes inherited from both parents (via the egg and sperm) and then divide into two identical cells, each with a complete set of chromosomes. These 'daughter' cells divide in their turn to give four identical cells, and so on. After about three days a ball of small, unspecialised cells looking rather like a blackberry has formed (see Figures 3.2 and 3.3), but cell divisions thereafter produce increasingly complex patterns as the cell mass begins to develop discernible structures.

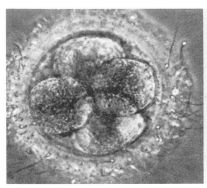
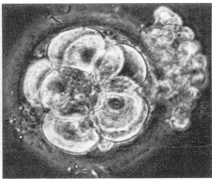
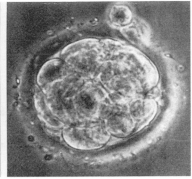

Figure 3.3   Three stages in the earliest development of a human embryo, from the four-cell stage (left) to the cell mass about three days after fertilisation (right). (Photos: Professor R. G. Edwards)

By five days, a space has opened in the centre of the mass, with a thickened disc of cells on one side; in a few days some of the cells in this disc will form the embryo, others will become the embryo's contribution to the placenta, and the outer sphere of cells will form the membranes that surround the embryo within a bag of fluid. Before that can happen, the replicating cell mass has to *implant*. Around day seven it drifts against the wall of the womb and begins to burrow into the lining, which is richly supplied with blood vessels. This is the stage known as **implantation**; without it, the potential embryo will continue down the

reproductive tract to be lost in the next menstrual period, without anyone knowing it had ever existed. The period during which an embryo is most likely to suffer a spontaneous abortion is during the first 15 days, prior to and just after implantation. Probably as many as 50 per cent of pregnancies fail at this stage; the causes include genetic abnormality in the embryo and failure to implant because of incorrect hormone balances in the mother. If implantation occurs, cells from the lining of the womb start to surround the embryo, and food and oxygen begin to diffuse into it from the mother's tissues.

An important legal as well as biological transition occurs between two and three weeks after fertilisation, soon after the embryo implants. A groove is formed in the embryonic disc, which then deepens and rolls up to form the neural tube. Over the next two weeks, this develops into the embryo's spinal cord and brain (Figure 3.4). In the United Kingdom, the Human Fertilisation and Embryology Authority (HFEA) prohibits research on, or manipulation of, human embryos *in vitro* beyond 14 days after fertilisation: a watershed chosen because it precedes the earliest signs of neural development and hence putative 'consciousness'.

The first trimester

Among health care professionals, pregnancy is thought of as consisting of three 'trimesters', or 3-month periods. The first trimester is the most critical: most of the organ systems the baby will require are established within the first eight *weeks*, as Figure 3.5 (*overleaf*) reveals. The ball of implanted cells continues to replicate, but some of the new cells become specialised to fulfil certain tasks in the growing embryo; in the process, they lose the ability to contribute to other functions. They also move around in the embryo until they reach their 'correct' location in the

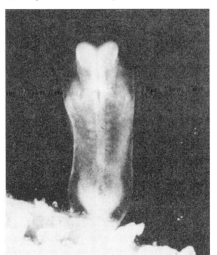

Figure 3.4   A human embryo at about 3 weeks after fertilisation. The embryo has its 'back' towards the viewer, showing the 'ribbed' surface of the neural tube, which will form the spinal cord, and the bulge at the top which is soon to form the brain. (Photo: Carnegie Institution of Washington and the Human Developmental Anatomy Center of the National Museum of Health and Medicine of the Armed Forces Institute of Pathology)

emerging organs and tissues. For example, some cells become contractile and organised into muscles in the arms and legs, others become secretory cells and migrate to the developing gut, or become sensory cells in the eyes. These linked processes are called **differentiation** (when cells 'become different' from their unspecialised predecessors) and **morphogenesis** (the development of functional organs and characteristic physical forms, such as limbs, ears and toes). Very little is known about the signals that 'orchestrate' this seemingly miraculous emergence of form and function from an unspecialised ball of cells. One counter-intuitive aspect is the programmed *death* of huge numbers of cells to create some of the essential 'spaces' in the body, for example between the fingers and toes.

While these early developmental processes are occurring, the embryo is at its most vulnerable to damage from toxic chemicals, radiation, inadequate nutrition or infection. The peak 'risk periods' can be very precisely defined for different organs: for example, the drug thalidomide, taken to combat morning sickness, had its greatest effect on limb bud development, which occurs between days 20 and 38, a peak period of sickness for some mothers. Neural-tube defects (the most common of which is spina bifida), are caused by failure of the neural tube to close up completely; any preventative steps, such as the mother taking extra folic acid, have to be started early, preferably prior to conception, as the tube normally develops and closes between 20 and 30 days.

☐ Look at Figure 3.5 and explain why active rubella infection (German measles) in a non-immunised mother in the first trimester can lead to blindness or deafness in her baby, but generally has little effect if she becomes infected in the last trimester.

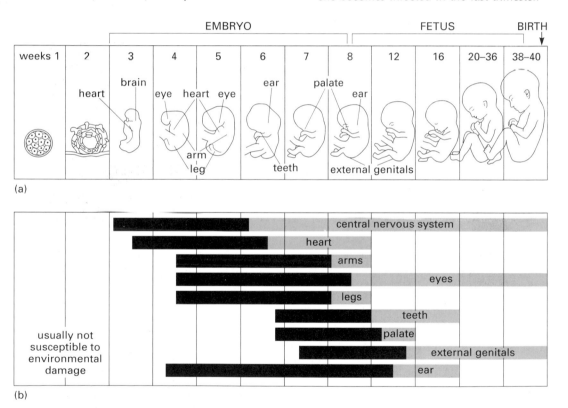

Figure 3.5 *(a) Development and organ formation in a human baby during a normal pregnancy. (b) Periods of particular vulnerability to damage from environmental factors occur as the organ is being formed (dark bars), but some susceptibility may persist thereafter (light bars). Note the variation in vulnerability between organs.*

■ The eyes form between 4 and 8 weeks of pregnancy, and the ears between 4 and 12 weeks, and are much less susceptible to damage after these periods. (Infection between days 28 and 49, when the lens of the eye develops, may lead to cataract (opaque lens), whereas later infection leaves the lens clear, but may result in deafness, as parts of the inner ear differentiate between days 42 and 56.)

As the weeks pass, the embryo becomes increasingly humanoid in appearance (Figure 3.6). It is genetically destined to be male or female from the moment of fertilisation, but external genitals do not develop until about seven weeks after fertilisation, when the embryonic testes in the male begin to secrete the hormone testosterone, promoting the development of male genitals. If testosterone levels stay low, female genitals develop. At eight weeks, soon after the mother discovers she is pregnant, her baby already has a face and clearly defined fingers and toes. From this point until birth it is referred to as a **fetus** in medical science.

The second and third trimesters

The main distinguishing features of the last six months of pregnancy are the maturation of organs and systems already formed in the first trimester, and their rapid growth. At implantation the embryo weighs about 1 µg (one thousandth of a gram); at birth, an average baby weighs about 3 400 gm (see Figure 3.7 *overleaf*). Biologically, the important distinction is between the initial *development*, or formation, of the organ systems and their later *growth*, or increase in size. However, development continues throughout life in the womb, albeit at a slower pace, as the organ systems become more complex and approach those of the mature adult. Some organ systems do not complete their development until several years after birth; for example, those involved in reproduction do not mature until puberty, as Chapter 6 describes.

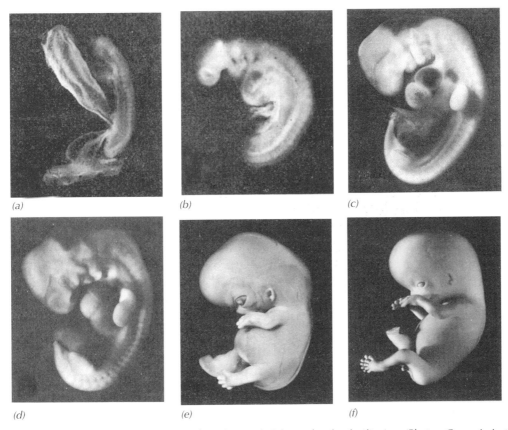

(a)   (b)   (c)

(d)   (e)   (f)

Figure 3.6 *Stages in fetal development, between about four and eight weeks after fertilisation. (Photos: Carnegie Institution of Washington and the Human Developmental Anatomy Center of the National Museum of Health and Medicine of the Armed Forces Institute of Pathology)*

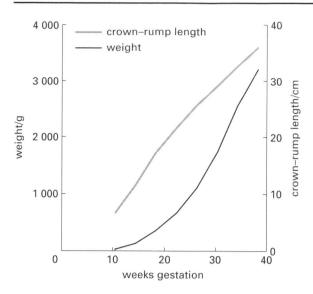

Figure 3.7 *Estimated change in average length and weight of the fetus, from 10 weeks after fertilisation until birth.*

The growing baby is connected by the *umbilical cord* to a mass of intertwined blood vessels and connective tissue, the *placenta*. A large vein in the cord carries blood rich in oxygen and nutrients from the placenta to the baby, and two arteries bring blood from the baby's body back to the placenta, where they discharge wastes, including carbon dioxide, the waste product of respiration. The placenta is the 'interface' between mother and unborn child: their blood vessels do not actually join up, but lie so closely entwined that small molecules can diffuse (flow passively) through the vessel walls and pass from one circulation to the other.

☐ What biological 'tasks' do you think the mother is performing for the baby in the womb, which it must do for itself as soon as it is born?

■ She is maintaining the baby at a constant body temperature, supplying oxygen and nutrients from her bloodstream, as it lies close to the baby's in the placenta, and removing wastes from its bloodstream. The unborn baby does not have to eat or breathe.

The circulation of blood in the fetus is different in several key respects from that of the newborn baby in the route taken by 'bright' blood, which is high in dissolved oxygen and nutrients, and 'dark' blood which is high in dissolved carbon dioxide and other wastes. (We are avoiding the terms 'arterial' and 'venous' blood because, in the fetus,

some arteries carry blood high in carbon dioxide and some veins carry blood rich in oxygen, e.g. in the umbilical cord.) The fetus gets its oxygen and nutrients in blood arriving from the placenta; this is very different from the situation after birth, when oxygen will be picked up by blood as it passes through the lungs, and nutrients will be absorbed into the bloodstream from the gut and liver.

The circulation relating to the lungs is strikingly different before and after birth.[5] The fetus is under water and cannot breathe; its lungs are collapsed and offer very high resistance to the small amount of blood that reaches them, bringing just enough nutrients and oxygen to keep the lung tissue alive. Most of the fetal bloodstream bypasses the lungs altogether, by means of two mechanisms (see Figure 3.8a). The first is a 'valve' (the *foramen ovale* or 'oval hole') which allows about half of the blood entering the fetal heart from the placenta to pass directly from one side of the heart to the other, missing out the 'loop' in the circuit that will take blood through the lungs after birth. The rest of the blood starts along the route towards the lungs, but before it arrives it meets the second mechanism, a bypass-duct (the *ductus arteriosus*), which shunts about 90 per cent of it away from the lungs and directs it into the *aorta*, the large artery supplying blood to the rest of the body. As soon as the newborn baby takes its first breath, the 'hole-in-the-heart' closes and the bypass duct begins to collapse and seal itself; the lungs inflate, reducing their resistance to blood-flow, and all of the baby's bloodstream is routed through the lungs (Figure 3.8b).

Other shunting mechanisms allow most of the blood to bypass the fetal liver and gut, which only require enough oxygen and nutrients to maintain their own growth while the baby is in the womb. After birth, when it begins to feed for itself, these shunts will close and the organs involved in digestion will receive a full blood supply, which fuels their increased activity and picks up the products of digestion for transport around the body.

This glimpse into the biological development of the fetus in the womb may give you some insight into the rationale behind antenatal care, as it has evolved in the United Kingdom in the twentieth century. Doctors, midwives and medical scientists have striven to scrutinise fetal development to detect the earliest possible signs of anything amiss. They have also given increasingly close attention to the health of the pregnant woman, partly for

[5]An animation sequence showing changes in the baby's circulation before and after birth is part of a television programme for Open University students, entitled 'First steps to autonomy', which is associated with this book.

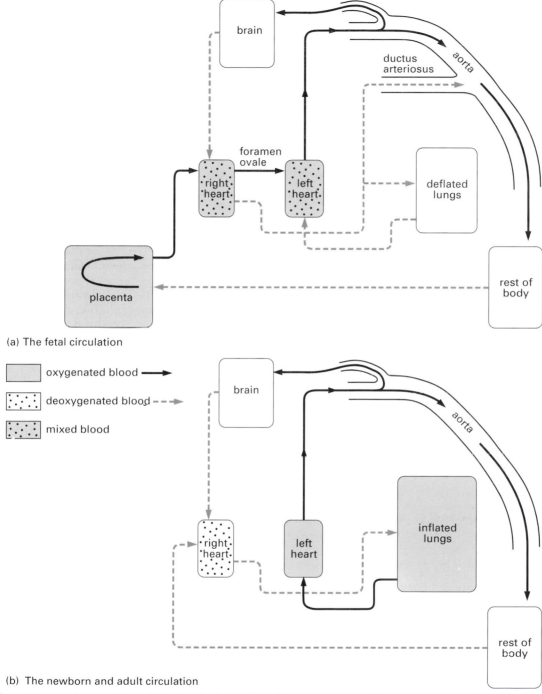

(a) The fetal circulation

oxygenated blood ⟶

deoxygenated blood - - ➤

mixed blood

(b) The newborn and adult circulation

Figure 3.8 *(a) The circulation of blood in the human fetus; by convention, circulation diagrams are always drawn with the subject's chest facing the viewer, so the left side of the fetal heart is on the right of the diagram, and vice versa. Note the foramen ovale connecting the right and left sides of the fetal heart and the ductus arteriosus diverting blood away from the lungs and into the aorta. (b) The circulation after birth.*

her own sake and partly to preserve the baby within. Even in the 1990s, the 'tools' available to assess the progress of mother and unborn child are still rather crude; practices have been maintained by tradition rather than by proof of effectiveness, as you will see in the next section of this chapter.

The antenatal period

Although the term **antenatal care** is usually restricted to care *after* conception, formal health care is beginning to include limited interventions before the baby is even conceived, with the intention of improving its health during and after a planned pregnancy. Such *pre-conception care*, with the exception of a few clear examples such as immunisation against rubella before pregnancy and the use of folic acid supplements to prevent recurrence of neural-tube defects such as spina bifida,[6] generally has no proven medical value and in any case has not yet become a regular or popular feature of United Kingdom health care.[7]

After the conception the story is different. Over 99 per cent of pregnant women in the United Kingdom have some antenatal care.

What is antenatal care?

The great reduction in maternal mortality and perinatal mortality in the Western world in the past 60 years has coincided with a rise in the amount of surveillance of pregnant women by health workers. Systematic antenatal care in the United Kingdom began around the time of World War I. In many respects the pattern and basic content of antenatal care has altered little since the 1920s. Women were (and still are, generally) seen at regular intervals, from about 12 weeks gestation— monthly to 28 weeks, fortnightly to 36 weeks and then weekly until delivery. Most women are seen about 12–14 times. They are weighed, have their urine checked for sugar and protein, have their blood pressure checked and the womb is felt through the woman's abdominal wall to assess fetal growth. The main purpose of urine checks and

[6]Further information on folic acid supplementation and on the malformations called neural-tube defects can be found in *Studying Health and Disease*, Chapter 8, and in a collection of papers on 'Ethical dilemmas in evaluation' in *Health and Disease: A Reader* (second edition, 1995).

[7]There are likely to be changes in the future, particularly in connection with the increased use of genetic techniques to predict hereditary disease. See *Human Biology and Health: An Evolutionary Approach*, Chapter 9.

blood-pressure measurement was and is to detect the early onset of a condition called *pre-eclamptic toxaemia* which can cause a marked reduction in placental circulation, leading to poor growth and ultimate death of the baby, as well as severe hypertension (raised blood pressure) and death of the mother. Hypertensive disease of this kind in pregnancy is still the biggest single cause of the very few maternal deaths in the United Kingdom.

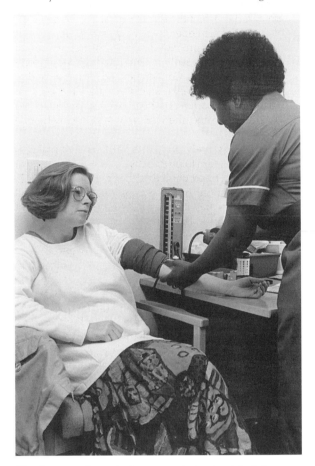

Blood pressure is routinely measured at antenatal clinics, largely to detect pre-eclamptic toxaemia. (Photo: Mike Levers)

Even though the general pattern of care has not changed much, antenatal care in the 1990s attempts far more than it did in the 1920s and 1930s. Newer technologies such as ultrasound scanning and genetic tests are available to investigate much more closely or make predictions about the condition of the fetus, and as a result pregnant women can be offered advice about the likelihood of inherited disorders such as thalassaemia, sickle-cell disease, muscular dystrophy, and of certain malformations and Down's syndrome.

Tests for genetic disorders and malformations[8]

Blood taken from the mother at about 15 weeks gestation can indicate, by the presence of certain proteins, whether she is at high risk of carrying a baby with a neural-tube defect or Down's syndrome. The categorisation of 'high' risk in these tests is arbitrarily set at about 1 in 200. If the woman has a higher risk than this, on the basis of the blood test, she is generally offered *amniocentesis* at about 18 weeks. In this procedure, fluid from around the baby is withdrawn by a needle inserted through the abdominal wall into the womb. Cells in the fluid are grown and show the chromosomal make-up of the fetus. If the fetus has an extra chromosome number 21, the characteristic of Down's syndrome, the woman will generally be offered an abortion.

Such tests rely on health workers giving unbiased, clear information to prospective parents—allowing them to make informed choices about their pregnancy. Such tests also impose more responsibility on the expectant parents. This has its negative side. Pregnancy, though now safer than in the past, is seen by some women as a series of very difficult choices followed by anxiety-ridden weeks awaiting the results of tests. The tests are not without hazard. A major randomised clinical trial of amniocentesis in Denmark (Tabor *et al.*, 1986) involved 4 600 women whose pregnancies were considered, on the basis of the woman's age and other factors, to be at low risk of chromosomal abnormalities like Down's syndrome. On the basis of this trial and other studies it is estimated that the additional risk of miscarriage associated with amniocentesis is about 1 in 100.[9] If 'high risk' of Down's syndrome (on the basis of the blood test) is taken as more than 1 in 200, roughly two healthy pregnancies will end spontaneously after amniocentesis for each Down's baby discovered and aborted.

[8]For more on prenatal screening for genetic and chromosomal disorders, using techniques such as amniocentesis and chorionic villi sampling (CVS), see *Human Biology and Health: An Evolutionary Approach*, Chapter 9.

[9]In the Danish study, the relative risk of miscarriage in women randomised to receive amniocentesis, compared to those who did not receive it, was 2.3. The concept of relative risk is discussed in *Studying Health and Disease*, Chapter 8. It must be borne in mind, however, that the results cannot necessarily be generalised to apply to women whose pregnancies are at high risk of Down's syndrome because of age or other factors.

Is antenatal care effective?

Early observational studies in the 1920s indicated that women who attended doctors or midwives for antenatal care had healthier babies and fewer miscarriages or still-births than those who did not attend. Many assumed the connection was causal.

□ What other interpretation of this evidence is possible?

■ There may have been other reasons for the observed differences. Perhaps women who attended differed from those who did not attend in terms of other factors such as social class or education, which in turn influenced the outcome of their pregnancies. It can be difficult to rule out such *confounding factors* in observational studies.[10]

One problem in assessing the efficacy of antenatal care is that the main outcome measures that have been used by medical researchers are maternal and perinatal mortality. There are always difficulties in using mortality as an outcome measure[11]—it takes no direct account of illness that does not result in death, nor of more general matters such as parents' or children's subjective feelings of wellbeing.

Most of the early antenatal clinics were set up by Labour municipal authorities in the 1920s and women attending them tended to be working-class—middle-class women tended to go to a GP or a private facility for antenatal care. However, even among working-class women it is plausible that those attending the new clinics were better educated and better off than those who did not receive any antenatal care. The finding of improved outcome may be an example of Julian Tudor Hart's 'Inverse Care Law' (Tudor Hart, 1971): those who receive care need it least, whereas those who do not receive it need the care most.

From 1920 to 1935 maternal mortality actually rose. This was a matter of considerable social and political concern. One reaction was that some people, understandably, doubted the value of antenatal care. From then on, there was a sharp decline in maternal mortality.

[10]There is further discussion of confounding factors and the difficulties they may cause in observational studies in *Studying Health and Disease*, Chapters 5 and 8.

[11]There is further discussion of the problems of using mortality measures in evaluating health in *Studying Health and Disease*, Chapters 6 and 7, as well as in Chapters 2 and 3 of *World Health and Disease*.

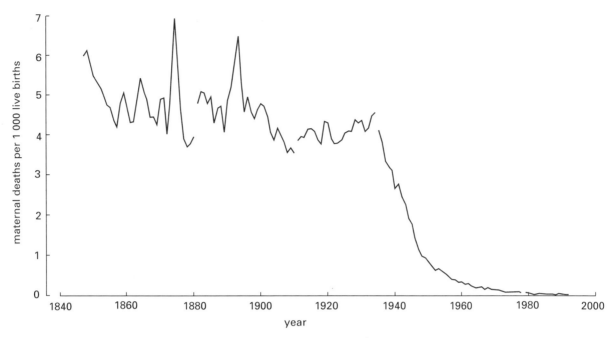

Figure 3.9 *Maternal mortality (deaths from causes related to pregnancy and childbirth) in England and Wales, 1847–1992. Note that definitions of maternal mortality have changed somewhat over the years as different definitions and different versions of the ICD (International Classification of Diseases) have come into use. Gaps in the line denote when these changes took place. (Source: revised from Figure 10 of Campbell, R. and Macfarlane, A., 1994, Where to be Born? The Debate and the Evidence, 2nd edn, National Perinatal Epidemiology Unit, Oxford. The graph is based on OPCS mortality statistics.)*

☐ Does the graph (Figure 3.9) and information above show a causal connection between medical care and a reduction in maternal deaths?

■ Not necessarily—these are observational data only, and tell us nothing directly about the cause of the decline. However, there was no sudden improvement in the overall standard of living from 1935. Advances in medicine such as blood transfusion, safer anaesthesia and antibiotics may well be part of the explanation, but we cannot conclude that they *caused* the decline.

There are other reasons for being cautious about mortality data. In the United Kingdom at present, maternal and perinatal deaths are rare events and to concentrate on them is to ignore the vast majority of pregnancies. Finally, both maternal and perinatal mortality may be influenced by care during birth ('intrapartum care') as well as by antenatal care, and it is difficult to separate the effects of one part of care from another.

Non-technological antenatal care

Later in the chapter we will examine the effectiveness of one of the more technological ways of assessing the fetus—ultrasound scanning. But we begin by examining more straightforward care as carried out by midwives, general practitioners and obstetricians in the 1990s. Such care encompasses the giving of advice, education and reassurance, as well as assessment of maternal and fetal wellbeing. Are the health of the mother and baby improved by advice and education?

Advice about diet, smoking, alcohol, work, exercise, sexual activity, use of medicines and drugs is regularly proffered. There is evidence that the acceptance of anti-smoking advice may increase the birthweight of some babies. Against that must be set a long list of general advice now known to be without good foundation, including the prohibition of alcohol, restricting weight gain, care of nipples, restriction of sexual activity and bed-rest for threatened miscarriage (Chalmers *et al.*,

1989, Enkin *et al.* 1995).[12] Advice is not always beneficial. It can lead to worry and guilt.

However, women want information from their carers and a consistent complaint of pregnant women is that they do not feel free to ask questions during their antenatal care. This criticism is especially so of hospital clinics, compared with care given by midwives and GPs. For instance, in an extensive study of antenatal care in Aberdeen, an obstetrician, Marion Hall, and two sociologists, Sally Macintyre and Maureen Porter (Hall *et al.*, 1985, p. 57) found that women asked no questions at all in about two-thirds of the 547 hospital antenatal consultations studied. If one aim of antenatal care is to educate the woman, deal with her needs for advice and reassurance, and help her feel good about herself in pregnancy, it is not doing very well—not in the hospital setting anyhow. Hall and her colleagues suggest that centralisation and specialisation in antenatal care, which has been carried out in order to improve its efficiency at predicting and diagnosing problems and disorders, 'may have militated against the achievement of antenatal care's other set of goals' (i.e. the provision of advice and reassurance; Hall *et al.*, 1985, p. 111).

Standard antenatal care can thus fail on psychological and educational aims. Does antenatal care do better at assessing the physical wellbeing of the mother and her baby?

Routine antenatal checks

Much time is spent by pregnant women, midwives and doctors in the antenatal clinic, checking the urine, weighing the mother, measuring her blood pressure and the size of her womb. Philip Steer, Professor of Obstetrics at Charing Cross Hospital, London (Steer, 1993) wrote in an editorial in the *British Medical Journal* in 1993, 'Almost all of these routine antenatal procedures are of dubious value'. As described earlier, one of the purposes of antenatal checks is the early detection of hypertensive disease in pregnancy. In 1988–90 there were 11.5 hypertensive deaths per million maternities compared with 17.7 in 1973–5 (Department of Health, 1994, p. 23). Though this is in accord with care becoming more effective, it is not clear how much of this reduction is due to improved early detection and how much is due to skilled care of seriously ill women on intensive care units. It is probably in part due to early detection, as the perinatal mortality associated with hypertensive disease has fallen even more sharply. Some argue that blood pressure and urine should be checked *more* often than at present, but

against this must be set the extra work to carers and the extra disruption to all pregnant women, most of whom will never develop hypertensive disease in pregnancy. A less disruptive way of improving the early detection would be for women to do their own urine tests and blood-pressure measurements at home.

☐ How could this innovation be evaluated, and why would evaluation be difficult in practice?

■ A randomised controlled trial of women undertaking 'self-testing' versus women receiving conventional clinic testing could be set up. However, given the rarity of the condition, the trial would have to involve a very large number of women.

Another important aim of antenatal care is to detect poor fetal growth, because it is believed that by delivering such a baby early, it may be saved from dying in the womb before the onset of labour. Can poor fetal growth be detected by routine antenatal checks? Women were (sometimes still are) routinely weighed at every visit, partly in an attempt to assess fetal growth. It is not clear that this is a reasonable activity. One is trying to detect a weight change in the fetus of, say, 200 grams in two weeks by weighing the container—a mother of maybe 80 kilograms.

There are other ways of assessing fetal size—by measuring the size of the womb. This is usually done by placing a hand on the mother's abdomen, or using a tape measure stretched over the abdomen. Such a measure is of size (a 'one-off' measure) not growth (a change over time). Measuring growth requires serial assessments. Can such measures detect small babies? In the Aberdeen study by Marion Hall and others (Hall *et al.*, 1985, p. 30), the records of all babies weighing the lowest 10 per cent of birthweights at each stage of gestation were reviewed to see if anyone had detected a small baby before birth. Only 44 per cent of these small babies had been correctly detected. For each *true* small baby, 2.5 babies were said to be small but actually weighed above the 10th percentile. In other words this method of detecting small babies had poor predictive value, and must therefore have resulted in much needless anxiety for mothers of babies wrongly assessed as small.

Another example of routine antenatal checks is the detection of *breech* babies before labour. Being born bottom (breech) first is less safe for a baby than the normal head-first position, and if carers have prior knowledge of a breech presentation, they can plan care accordingly. It is considered a failure of antenatal care to 'miss' a breech,

---

[12]For more information on these important sources, see the Further Reading list at the end of this book.

yet in Marion Hall's study 12 per cent of breeches were not detected until labour began (Hall *et al.*, 1985, p. 30). Though most were detected, this is far from perfection.

There is some hope that antenatal care will become more appropriate as the results and implications of trials become more widely available, for example, through the publication of easily-accessible literature reviews.[13] However, scientific evidence does not necessarily alter the behaviour of doctors and midwives. Here is an example where evidence has had little effect.

Kick charts

Fetal deaths before labour begins (antepartum stillbirths) now account for about half of perinatal deaths. The rate of this very distressing event has hardly diminished in the past few decades and medical science continues to look for some means of detecting babies who are ill in the womb before they become terminally ill. There is a clear association between decreased fetal movement and death in the womb. This, reasonably, led many to hope that mothers could monitor their own babies in the womb, by recording movements over a given time on *kick charts*. This was a very appealing idea—inexpensive, not requiring highly-trained staff and non-invasive. Unfortunately, a huge trial showed *no* decrease in antepartum deaths in mothers using kick charts (Grant, Elbourne *et al.*, 1989). For years after this trial, many doctors and midwives were still directing mothers to complete kick charts.

Ultrasound scanning: a cautionary tale

We turn now to look at an important example of modern, technological, pregnancy care to see what benefit—if any—has resulted from its use.

Using high-frequency sound (*ultrasonic*) waves it is possible to get an 'echo picture' of the baby inside the womb (Figure 3.10). In most Western countries this is carried out on all women as a routine measure at about 18 weeks, when it is possible to detect many malformations, e.g. heart and kidney abnormalities and defects in the formation of the brain and spine. The detection of lethal malformations, as with tests for genetic anomalies, allows the woman to choose if she wishes the pregnancy to be ended rather than bear a baby that will die in the womb, often around the time of birth, or in early infancy. **Ultra-sound scanning** also allows more accurate *dating* of the pregnancy (some women are unsure about their last menstrual period or have an irregular cycle, making it difficult to estimate date of delivery). It is also used to localise the placenta. Sometimes the placenta overlies the opening of the womb and is therefore a 'before-birth' (*placenta praevia*), which can cause severe bleeding and means the baby must be delivered by caesarian section.

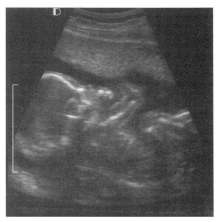

Figure 3.10 *An ultrasound picture of an 18-week-old fetus. (Picture: Milton Keynes General Hospital)*

How good is ultrasound at detecting malformations?

How can the efficacy of routine ultrasound be measured? It is clear that such an assessment may be complicated, because ultrasound scanning has more than one aim. In relation to the use of ultrasound to detect malformations, one measure is to look at changes over time in the rate of perinatal deaths caused by congenital malformation.

☐ How might this number change if routine ultrasound is effective in detecting malformations?

■ If ultrasound is effective, one would expect the rate of *perinatal* deaths caused by malformations to drop. This is because many malformed fetuses who would otherwise have died around the time of birth would be aborted earlier in pregnancy.

In England and Wales, from 1981 to 1991 (the period during which routine ultrasound scanning became widespread), the rate of perinatal deaths caused by congenital malformations halved from 249 per 100 000 births to 127 per 100 000 births (OPCS, 1984, 1993a and 1993b).

[13]In the antenatal context, such reviews of trials are now constantly updated and widely distributed as computer software, 'The Cochrane Database: Childbirth and Pregnancy Module'.

☐ Does this mean that ultrasound is effective in detecting malformations?

■ The data are in accord with that hypothesis, but they do not *prove* it—there may be some other reason for the decline, such as improvements in diet.

In fact, there is other evidence that ultrasound has some success in detecting abnormality. However, it does not increase the number of live births. Does one judge it a success to abort an abnormal fetus? Many women who have had such a termination of pregnancy are distressed by the experience but relieved not to have to bear the pregnancy to term. However, like any diagnostic test, ultrasound is not perfect. Sometimes it will fail to detect a malformation—a *false-negative* test[14]—and parents might well be more upset to have a malformed baby whom they were expecting to be normal. Also, ultrasound will sometimes 'detect' a malformation that is not actually present—a *false-positive* test—and parents would be distressed to learn that their baby showed signs of abnormality, even if they were reassured by later, more precise, tests. In a trial of over 9 000 women in Helsinki, (Saari-Kemppainen *et al.*, 1990) 2.4 women per 1 000 had such anxiety caused by false-positive scans, while 2.7 women per 1 000 were spared delivering a malformed baby.

Does accurate dating help?

It is clear that babies not yet born by 42 weeks (*postmature* babies) have a slightly higher chance of dying than babies born at 40 weeks (the usual length of pregnancy). Labour can be started artificially—*induced*—to try to overcome this problem.

☐ What effect would you expect routine ultrasound to have on rates of induction for postmaturity?

■ You might expect the induction rates to be lower (and in fact it was hoped that this would be the case when routine ultrasound was being introduced.) Without accurate dating, one might expect some women whose babies were not in fact postmature to be induced anyway to 'be on the safe side'.

In only one of four trials jointly reviewed by the doctors Heiner Bucher and Johannes Schmidt (Bucher and

Schmidt, 1993) was there a reduction in the number of inductions as a result of routine ultrasound scanning.

Does placental localisation help?

The placenta is found to be low enough partly to cover the opening (*os*) of the womb in 5–6 per cent of early pregnancy scans. Yet several studies have found that most of these women (at least 83 per cent of them, and more in some studies) will not have a placenta praevia at the end of pregnancy, as the lowest part of the womb grows most, thus 'pushing' the placenta up, away from the os. Conversely, less than half of placenta praevias present at the end of pregnancy are found on early scans. The power of routine early scans for predicting placenta praevia at the end of the pregnancy is so poor that an editorial in the *Lancet* in 1991 (*Lancet*, 1991) concluded that placental localisation at the initial routine scan cannot be recommended, and when a low placenta is noted during a routine scan, it is not necessary routinely to order a late pregnancy scan. (None of this rules out using ultrasound for placental localisation on a non-routine basis, for women who are specifically suspected of having placenta praevia.)

To sum up, the only medical benefit of routine ultrasound scans, and it is doubtful how important the benefit is, is to contribute to the detection of malformed fetuses. There remains, for some, anxiety about possible adverse effects of the sound waves themselves on the developing fetus. However, there is no firm evidence of harm, though some suggestion of an increase in left-handedness (Salvesen *et al.*, 1993), implies a possible effect on the brain control of 'handedness'. Overall, the evidence from a major review (Bucher and Schmidt, 1993) and a very large randomised trial published after the review (Ewigman *et al.*, 1993) is that routine ultrasound scans do *not* improve the live birth rate (the proportion of pregnancies that leads to a live birth), or reduce perinatal morbidity (improve the health of newborn babies). Ultrasound scanning is an example of a technology widely introduced before randomised controlled trials had defined its value. Many women, however, enjoy their early scan and like to keep the 'echo picture' of their baby. More importantly, many are greatly reassured when their scan detects no abnormality, or confirms that they are not carrying twins. It would therefore be unpopular to withdraw the universal service in the United Kingdom.

There are many unanswered questions. What do women believe is the purpose of ultrasound scanning? Do they understand that scanning does not increase the number of healthy babies born? Should women be entitled to further scans if they request them 'to see how the baby's doing', or 'to see what sex my baby is'?

---

[14]For a discussion of the terminology of tests used for screening for disease, see *Human Biology and Health: An Evolutionary Approach*, Chapter 9. Further discussion of screening is given in *Dilemmas in Health Care*, Chapter 9.

(Ultrasound scans do not provide an error-free method of determining the sex of a fetus.) There are resource implications of providing routine ultrasound scanning which could deplete the service in other, more important, areas.

The future of antenatal care

There was much criticism of antenatal care in the United Kingdom in the 1980s and early 1990s—much of it from women themselves, who gave up time to attend distant clinics and perhaps saw different personnel each time, underwent tests without proper explanation or informed consent, or felt rushed and overawed so that they could not ask questions. They sometimes had anxiety needlessly raised as a result of antenatal care. Following widespread concern, the House of Commons Health Committee chaired by Nicholas Winterton decided to look at maternity services.[15] Following its critical report in 1992, the government set up an 'Expert Maternity Group' chaired by Baroness Julia Cumberlege. This Group not only examined 'hard' measures such as perinatal death, but also concerned itself with a much broader look at maternity care. For example, the Group's report *Changing Childbirth*, published in August 1993, suggested that:

> The woman must be the focus of maternity care. She should be able to feel that she is in control of what is happening to her and able to make decisions about her care, based on her needs, having discussed matters fully with the professionals involved. (Department of Health, 1993, p. 9)

and recommended that:

> Antenatal care should take place as far as is practicable in the local community, with ready access to specialised advice, should it be necessary. The woman should feel confident that the antenatal consultations have a specific purpose, and that any tests and investigations have a clearly defined and valid objective, relevant to her particular circumstances. (Department of Health, 1993, p. 6)

This report marks a shift in emphasis from professionals to the mother herself. This is symbolised by the recommendations that the mother should carry her own pregnancy notes.

[15]Extracts from the Health Committee report are presented in *Health and Disease: A Reader*. You may like to read them at this point, though they are not essential reading for this chapter. (You will be asked to read them during study of *Dilemmas in Health Care*, Chapter 6.)

You might well wonder why has it taken professionals such a long time to recognise that the mother herself is the main carer for her unborn baby[16].

We have spent some time evaluating the goals of certain routine aspects of antenatal care and whether these are being achieved. Now we turn to birth itself: first to its biology and then to health care during this critical transition from womb to world.

The biology of birth

Labour and delivery

Towards the end of pregnancy, a number of factors interact to increase the likelihood of labour commencing and being maintained until the baby is born (the biological term for this sequence is *parturition*). It is the best example of a relatively rare phenomenon in biology: a positive feedback circuit. The small changes that take place at the onset of labour trigger others which increase the pace and magnitude of events, and these in turn promote even stronger responses. The biological signals governing labour are still incompletely understood and the subject of controversy, although no one disputes that certain of the mother's hormones are critically involved.

As pregnancy proceeds, the levels of the hormones progesterone and oestrogen rise in the woman's bloodstream. The 'balance' between progesterone and oestrogen is critical in maintaining a pregnancy to full term, and in preventing the mother from ovulating (releasing a mature egg from her ovaries), and hence from conceiving a second baby part way through a pregnancy.[17] Towards the end of the nine months, the balance between these hormones changes (disagreements centre on the exact details), and the muscles of the womb become increasingly 'twitchy'. The degree to which the muscles are stretched by a large baby and placenta may also contribute to their sensitivity to hormonal signals. Another group of hormones, the prostaglandins, seem to be essential promoters of muscular contractions in the womb. As contractions increase, the baby's head is

[16]A detailed examination of this question from the perspective of a feminist sociologist is given in a book by Ann Oakley, 1980, *Women Confined*. An extract from this book appears in *Health and Disease: A Reader* under the title 'Doctor knows best'. You may like to read it at this point, though it is not essential to do so.

[17]This property is exploited in the contraceptive 'pill', which contains oestrogen and progesterone in amounts that mimic their action in pregnancy.

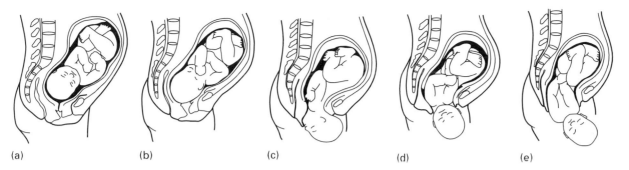

Figure 3.11 *Diagram of a normal labour and delivery (the mother is shown in an upright position). Note the shortening and thickening of the womb as labour progresses. (a) shows the beginning of labour; (b) part-way through Stage 1; (c)–(e) Stage 2 progresses towards birth.*

pushed harder against the cervix (neck of the womb), which dilates and triggers the release of yet another hormone, oxytocin, which strongly stimulates contraction of the womb. If labour is started artificially (medically induced), or fails to progress, the mother may be given an intravenous 'drip' containing oxytocin, a practice that is discussed later.

Although the precise details of these maternal factors are uncertain, they seem adequate to account for the *progress* of labour and birth, but not its accurate *timing*. There has been much research on the possibility that hormones produced by the fetus are involved in the onset of labour, and although fetal hormones *are* involved in the birth of some other large mammals, such as calves, in humans the evidence remains weak. There is still much to be explained about the biology of childbirth.

Labour is commonly described in three stages (Figure 3.11). Stage 1 begins with the onset of regular, powerful contractions of the middle and upper parts of the womb. After each contraction the muscles fail to relax back to their original length, so the space inside gradually decreases and the baby's head is forced against the cervix. The cervix dilates and allows the head to protrude into the birth canal. Stage 1 usually takes several hours, often more with a first baby; it is said to have ended when the cervix is fully dilated and the rim has 'rolled back', exposing the full circumference of the baby's head. Stage 2 is from this point until the baby is pushed out along the birth canal into the outside world, often as little as 20 minutes later and usually within two hours. Stage 3 is the gap between the birth of the baby and the expulsion of the placenta. The duration of labour is very variable: the average time for a first birth is about 14 hours, and about 7 hours for subsequent births.

Biological changes in the baby at birth

The process of birth involves very important changes for the baby as it moves from the liquid environment inside the womb to the air outside. Until the last few weeks of pregnancy, the thin wet walls of the air sacs in the lungs (*alveoli*) will be stuck together by surface tension. Prior to birth a *surfactant* is secreted, which acts rather like a detergent, and allows the sacs to be inflated when air is sucked in. Breathing can be difficult for premature babies because their lungs cannot inflate fully (a condition known as *respiratory distress syndrome*) until the surfactant is produced.

Clearly, at birth, or within hours of it, major changes in the circulatory system must occur to allow the baby to function in the outside world. The 'hole-in-the-heart' and the lung–bypass duct (foramen ovale and ductus arteriosus, Figure 3.8a) must close, so that blood returning to the heart from the body is routed through the lungs for re-oxygenation—incomplete closure is one of the causes of respiratory distress. Other changes in the circulatory system allow blood to perfuse the whole of the liver, instead of taking a 'fast track' through the middle, and the blood supply to the gut increases. This enables the products of digestion to be dealt with, now that the baby has to feed for itself.[18]

Let us now return to health care during birth.

[18]The television programme mentioned earlier, 'First steps to autonomy', is relevant here.

Care at birth

All the waiting through 9 months' pregnancy comes to a dramatic end in the process of labour and birth lasting just a matter of hours. This event involves a real and occasionally dangerous journey for the baby and a profound emotional journey for the mother—especially if it is her first baby. All cultures—including those of the Western world—surround birth with ritual observed by special attendants. Often birth will take place in a special area designated for that purpose. After looking at some aspects of the biology of birth, we will examine first the 'special area' and then some of the rituals developed by maternity care in the United Kingdom.

Place of birth

At first glance it may seem odd to devote much attention to the place of birth when, by 1991, just under 99 per cent of women in England and Wales were giving birth in hospital. The rise of hospital births has been meteoric: in 1927, 85 per cent of births were at home (Registrar-General, 1929, quoted in Campbell and Macfarlane, 1994, p. 13). The shift in place of birth is an important example of medical care influencing a normal and healthy part of human life, and it therefore has wider implications than the simple question of where birth should occur. We will examine the causes of this enormous change, the evidence used to support it, and its effects.

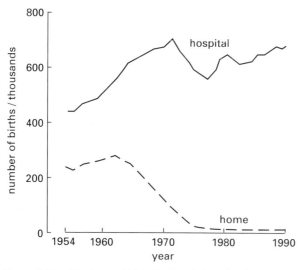

Figure 3.12 *Numbers of births in hospitals and at home, England and Wales 1954–90. (Data from annual OPCS Reports)*

Most of the shift to hospital births has occurred since World War II (Figure 3.12). As late as 1936 the British Medical Association said:

> All the available evidence demonstrates that normal confinements … can be more safely conducted at home than in hospital. (BMA, 1936)

But professional opinion was so altered by 1959 that the report of the Government's Maternity Service Committee chaired by Lord Cranbrook recommended:

> … sufficient hospital maternity beds to provide for 70 per cent of all confinements. (Ministry of Health, 1959)

and by 1970 a similar committee chaired by Sir John Peel recommended 100 per cent hospital delivery. By 1980 the back-bench House of Commons Social Services Committee, chaired by Renee Short, recommended that home delivery should be phased out further, and that deliveries in hospital should be centralised in larger maternity units. By 1984 the Maternity Services Advisory Committee chaired by Alison Munro felt confident in stating:

> The practice of delivering nearly all babies in hospital has contributed to the dramatic reduction in still births and neonatal deaths, and to the avoidance of many child handicaps. (Maternity Services Advisory Committee, 1984)

Soon after this report, by 1987, the percentage of home births had fallen to its lowest ever figure of 0.9 per cent in England and Wales; only about 6 000 babies per year were being born at home. Between 1987 and 1992 the perinatal mortality rate continued to fall, even though there was an increase in home births to 1.3 per cent (somewhat over 9 000 births per year).

The case for centralising birth care

In the early 1950s many women wanted to have their babies in hospital but could not. AIMS (the Association for Improvements in Maternity Services) was founded then to secure extra hospital beds. Medical science could claim some spectacular successes: penicillin could cure previously fatal infections, especially puerperal sepsis (infection of the birth canal after delivery). Anaesthesia and blood transfusion allowed safer caesarian section. Above all, the creation of the National Health Service (NHS) meant that women could obtain a hospital birth without charge and many wanted to do so, sometimes for medical reasons and sometimes for social reasons—they might get a rest, meals cooked for them and laundry done.

At first, only women who had certain 'risk factors' associated with their pregnancy were eligible for a hospital birth under the NHS—for example diabetes, high blood pressure, or carrying twins. However, this method of deciding eligibility did not detect all possible risks. Almost certainly there were women in the 1950s and 1960s having to have babies at home when they should have been delivered in hospital. In any case, birth is an uncertain business and not every risk is detectable in advance. Many obstetricians would know of a woman whose baby had died or who had herself died at home as a result of childbirth. After such a tragedy, it would have been natural to assume that the outcome would have been different had the woman delivered in a well-equipped hospital with specialist staff available. By the end of 1970 these tragic stories formed a mass of anecdotal evidence against home birth.

Furthermore, it was apparent that as the home birth rate fell, so also fell the overall maternal and perinatal mortality rates. Also, the perinatal mortality rate for home births stopped falling and began to rise, from 18.6 per thousand births in England and Wales in 1975 to 25.0 in 1980 (Campbell and Macfarlane, 1994). (The rate has since fallen again.)

☐ Does all this prove that hospital is safer than home?

■ It does not provide *proof*, though it certainly gives the proponents of home birth something to explain. The tragic stories do not tell us anything about how typical such events are. The fall in births at home may not have *caused* the fall in maternal and perinatal mortality and the rise in perinatal mortality for home births may not have occurred *because* the births were at home. In both cases what was observed was a relationship rather than a cause.

The above evidence on safety was, however, widely accepted as supporting centralisation, particularly by government and the specialist medical staff who advised government. However, associations can be misleading. The epidemiologist Archie Cochrane said in relation to policy on care at birth:

It is surprising how successive committees have been content to accept trends as something God-given which must be followed, instead of demanding a more rigorous analysis of causality. (Cochrane, 1972, p. 63)[19]

The case against centralising birth care

Women wish to feel safe during childbirth. Where a woman feels safest may not be where professionals believe she would be safest. Women who choose home birth do so for a variety of reasons. Most do so because they feel they are more likely to remain in control; that they will not have 'things done to them'. They feel they will be more likely also to exercise autonomy over their choice of positions in labour, where they labour, who is with them, whether they eat or drink, and so on. They will have a high chance of knowing the midwife (and sometimes doctor) who will look after them at home. These criteria have been summarised as the *3 Cs*: Control, Choice and Continuity of care(r). Of course, hospital care does not *have* to fall short on these criteria, but it often has.

Nevertheless, it remains true that the great majority of women in the United Kingdom choose hospital birth because they feel safest there. As you have seen, this view on safety was shared by influential professionals. If a case is to be made for continued centralisation of birth care on the grounds of safety, it would have to be supported by sound evidence from recent studies, showing worse outcomes for home births when confounding factors are taken into account. As we shall see, no such convincing evidence exists.

An early analysis of birth outcomes in relation to place of birth was performed by Marjorie Tew, a statistician working at Nottingham Medical School. In her large-scale and detailed study, she analysed data from the 1970 British Births Survey, a major observational study of birth in that year, and compared perinatal death rates in different places of birth. She recognised that one would expect more 'high-risk' deliveries in hospitals than at home. Tew attempted to control for this difference by using antenatal prediction scores and labour prediction scores to categorise expected risk. These scores had been measured as part of the 1970 survey, but had not been given in the published reports on it. Tew found that babies were more likely to survive if born in a GP unit or at home, rather than in hospital, at all levels of risk scores. (*GP units* are maternity units where the care is supervised by GPs with midwives.) Only at the very highest level of risk were

[19]Cochrane's book *Effectiveness and Efficiency* (1972) presents many criticisms of health care in the United Kingdom. It is discussed further in *Dilemmas in Health Care*, Chapter 4, and an extract about the role of randomised clinical trials is reprinted in *Health and Disease: A Reader*.

the better results for births in GP units and at home, compared with those in larger hospitals, not statistically significant (Tew, 1985).

Tew had great difficulty finding a medical journal that would publish these disturbing results. Some hospital specialists and statisticians still dispute Tew's interpretation of the figures from the 1970 British Births Survey. Such disputes can arise because it is always possible in an observational study like this that some confounding factor is confusing the results. Even though Tew allowed for this to some extent by taking the two risk prediction scores into account, it is not necessarily true that these scores took account of all possible confounding factors that might have been acting. Comparable data including risk predictions have not been collected on such a large scale since the 1970 survey, so it has not been possible to duplicate Tew's findings.

The rise in the perinatal mortality rate (PNMR) in home births during the late 1970s was explained by Iain Chalmers, then Director of the National Perinatal Epidemiology Unit. He, with others, analysed the Cardiff Births survey and showed that by 1979 *unplanned* home births in the study district outnumbered the planned deliveries, and that the outcome of delivery was very different between the two (Murphy *et al.*, 1984). A study of all 8 856 home births in England and Wales in 1979, carried out by Rona Campbell and others, showed how dramatic this difference was (Table 3.1).

The overall PNMR for all home births was substantially greater than the national average for all places of birth (14.6). But this figure was high because it included many unplanned home births, for which the PNMR was very high. For women *choosing* and booking home birth[20] the PNMR was remarkably low at 4.1. The implication of data such as these is that the rise in PNMR for all home births does not necessarily mean that *planned* home births are less safe than births in hospital.

One difficulty with both the Cardiff study and Campbell's study is that neither of them involved data about women who move during labour from home to hospital. Such women are moved usually because of a perceived problem in labour.

☐ Why might such 'transfers in labour' weaken the force of the arguments on the safety of planned home births in the studies just described?

[20]One should bear in mind, however, that at the time, because of the policies in favour of hospital birth, it was not straightforward for most women to obtain a booked home birth. Therefore those who were booked for home births may have been untypical in some way.

Table 3.1 Outcomes of home births in England and Wales in 1979, classified by where the birth was booked (planned) to occur.

Planned place of birth	Percentage of home births	PNMR
booked for home	67	4.1
booked for hospital but born at home	21	67.5
unbooked for either hospital or home	3	196.6
planned place of birth not known	9	45.2
all home births		24.1

Data from Campbell, R. *et al.* (1984) Home births in England and Wales, 1979: perinatal mortality according to intended place of delivery, *British Medical Journal*, **289**, p. 722.

■ In some 'problematic' labours, booked for home, a transfer to hospital will occur and the birth will actually take place in hospital. This might therefore increase the apparent safety of intending to deliver at home, and at the same time worsen the hospital PNMR figures.

The most persuasive data would come from a randomised controlled trial, but the obstetrician Richard Lilford has shown that such a trial would need to involve half a million women in order to achieve statistical significance (Lilford, 1987). Such a trial might perhaps have been possible in the 1960s, but numbers of home births are now too small and it is hard to believe many women would accept being randomly allocated to their intended place of delivery. Here is another cautionary tale: health policy ought not to be decided without firm evidence—after policy has changed it may be impossible to obtain such evidence. In this case, those who make decisions on maternity care must therefore make do with less robust data.

One source of relevant data comes from a slightly different comparison than that between home and hospital. In some areas, typically rural ones, some women deliver in small hospitals staffed by midwives and general practitioners. These are often called *isolated GP units*, in that they are distant from the specialist unit supervised by consultants. (Rural women may feel the *specialist* unit is 'isolated'.) Most of these rural units have few facilities beyond those available at home, though often it may be possible to carry out some simple kinds of intervention, such as assisted delivery with forceps. Nationally, there was pressure in the 1970s and 1980s to close rural units in line with the policy to centralise care in larger hospitals.

Bath Health District has seven rural units. A study of 'low-risk' births comparing women booked to deliver in the rural units with women booked to deliver in the specialist unit was published in 1990 (Sangala *et al.*, 1990). Altogether, more than 14 000 women were studied. This study overcame the distorting effect of transfers in labour by assigning perinatal death *after* labour began to the unit where the women began her labour. Considering only deaths after the onset of labour, the PNMR of the specialist unit was 0.6 per thousand births, compared with 1.5 per thousand births in the rural units—a difference which did not reach statistical significance.[21]

☐ How would you interpret this result?

■ To say that the difference did not reach statistical significance means that you cannot rule out the possibility that the true PNMR is the same in both specialist and rural units. This conclusion might be reached because in fact there is no difference. It might alternatively be reached because the study was not powerful enough to find a difference that did exist. For example, maybe the true PNMR really was higher in the rural units, but the study was too small to identify this securely.

It might seem strange to worry about the size of a study that included over 14 000 births, but you should bear in mind that this analysis is of perinatal deaths, which are rare events. An analysis of some other outcome measure may well have shown a very different picture. Nevertheless, the Bath study cannot be said to provide strong evidence in favour of centralising care at birth. In a further study covering three years (1988–90) an even smaller difference in PNMRs between rural and specialist units was found (Wiltshire Health Care Trust, 1991). Neither study provides evidence to support centralising birth care in specialist units on safety grounds.

However, studies such as those carried out in the Bath district do not compare like with like. Urban women living in Bath may be significantly different from rural women around Bath. The PNMR between different regions in the country shows a far greater difference than that found in the Bath studies. (For example, in 1990 regional PNMRs per 1 000 births ranged from 5.9 in East Anglia to 10.1 in West Midlands; OPCS, 1992b). It is likely that demographic factors have a greater impact on these variations in PNMR than do differences in the type of care given in different regions.

The Netherlands

The final evidence we shall consider here against the need to centralise care during birth comes from the Netherlands. The Dutch system of maternity care, unlike any other in the Western world, incorporates the belief that women with uncomplicated pregnancies can safely choose a home birth. Midwives are independent, self-employed and highly trained. (In rural areas the GPs undertake birth care themselves.) Approximately one-third of Dutch women deliver at home. The Dutch PNMR is very similar to that in the United Kingdom. We are not suggesting that a shift to the Dutch system would work in the United Kingdom—at present our midwifery and nursing structure is predominantly hospital-based—but it is further evidence that the policy of the United Kingdom and most other industrialised countries to centralise birth care was *not* based on scientific evidence that showed the alternative to be dangerous. (For a detailed study of the Dutch system see van Alten *et al.*,1989.)

Conclusions on place of birth

For women with uncomplicated pregnancies it remains uncertain whether they and their babies would be safer if they give birth in a large hospital, in an isolated GP unit or at home. Rona Campbell and Alison Macfarlane, of the National Perinatal Epidemiology Unit, after a review of all the available United Kingdom data, concluded their report:

> There is no evidence to support the claim that the safest policy is for all women to give birth in hospital. (Campbell and Macfarlane, 1994, p. 119)

and

> The policy of closing small obstetric units on the grounds of safety or cost is not supported by the available evidence. (Campbell and Macfarlane, 1994, p. 120)

The most recent government report stated:

> Whether a mother with an uncomplicated pregnancy is putting herself and her child at any greater risk by choosing to have her baby away

---

[21]The notion of *statistical significance* is discussed in *Studying Health and Disease*, Chapter 8.

from a general hospital maternity unit is a topic that has been argued with vehemence and emotion for decades. The inability to reach agreement after this length of time suggests that there is no clear answer. (Department of Health, 1993, p. 23)

It may seem strange, after the confident statements of earlier government reports, that the latest is unable to form an opinion. Is it better, when faced with a lack of data, to admit one doesn't know or to make a firm (but possibly wrong) recommendation? Ironically, this latest Department of Health report has been accused by some health professionals of not being based on evidence. This would not have been a surprise to Archie Cochrane:

> Midwifery is an unusually emotive subject so, *a priori*, a very high standard of statistical analysis or experimental approach would not be expected. (Cochrane, 1972, p. 63)

The subject of place of birth still arouses strong emotion. Yet it appears that, for women who *choose* (and book) to give birth away from specialist units, place of birth accounts for, at the most, a PNMR difference of less than 1 per 1 000 births and the data do not allow us to be sure in which direction the difference lies. Once again, this is not surprising. The majority of perinatal deaths are the result of unexplained deaths *before* labour, or pre-term birth, or congenital malformations (Table 3.2).[22] None of these would be affected by women choosing to deliver away from specialist units once they had completed 37 weeks of pregnancy.

That women and their babies can do as well away from big hospitals may at first seem contrary to common sense (which would suggest it *must* be safer where equipment and skilled personnel are available), but psycho–social factors affecting the woman, including the '3 Cs' already mentioned, may have a greater impact on the outcome of labour than is sometimes supposed.

Some hospital specialists, especially those who treat very ill women or very ill babies, find it very surprising that any woman should choose to give birth at home, and

Table 3.2 Cause of death in the 266 perinatal deaths in the Northern Region in 1983–1993 where the baby weighed 1 kg or more.

Cause of death	Number of deaths	Percentage of deaths (%)
congenital malformations	57	22
other deaths before labour began	131	49
lack of oxygen or injury during birth	35	13
problems of prematurity	16	6
other causes	23	9

There were 142 additional perinatal deaths where the baby's weight was below 1 kg; all of these are likely to be premature births. (Source: Northern Regional Health Authority, 1994, *Regional Maternity Survey Office Report*, Northern Regional Health Authority, Newcastle, p. 11.)

may claim that women do not understand the risks. Yet, as shown above, home may be as safe in uncomplicated pregnancies. Perhaps some women view 'the risks' differently. In any case, there is evidence from many sources that individual perceptions and choices involving risk are affected by much more than statistical measures of the chance of things going wrong.[23]

It is recognised by recent policy statements that the question of whether women should be able to give birth at home or whether they should be encouraged to give birth in hospital is not a matter to be decided by doctors. It is more a matter of personal freedom.

> The job of midwives and doctors, therefore, must be to provide the woman with as much accurate and objective information as possible, while avoiding personal bias or preference. (Department of Health, 1993, p. 23)

This task is far from easy when care during childbirth is such an emotive subject!

We have concentrated on place of birth because it illustrates important points about the interpretation of data and the exercising of professional power, and the effect of that power on personal freedom. However, you must remember that at present 99 per cent of women in the United Kingdom have their babies in hospital and

---

[22] It is not possible to provide national data for England and Wales about the proportion of perinatal deaths due to each of these causes. Since 1986, perinatal deaths have been certified in a way that does not allow them to be coded to a single underlying cause of death, in contrast to all deaths *after* one week of life. In 1991, for example, over one-third of the death certificates for stillbirths did not list a main cause of death (OPCS, 1993b).

[23] The question of perception of risk is covered briefly in *Dilemmas in Health Care*, Chapter 9.

about 90 per cent of these prefer to do so. It is, therefore, of more relevance for most women that the experience of birth in hospital should be improved. There have been many attempts based in several parts of the United Kingdom to make birth in hospital less of a medical activity and more like birth at home. One example is the 'home from home' scheme in Leicester. Such schemes often involve attempts to decrease the widespread and sometimes inappropriate use of interventions in childbirth.

Intervention in childbirth

All care can be considered intervention—even a cold flannel stroked over a hot brow in labour. Care during birth has come in for a great deal of criticism since the 1950s for intervening without benefit to mothers or babies, and sometimes to their detriment. There is a sound basis for this criticism. For example, *A Guide to Effective Care in Pregnancy and Childbirth* lists the

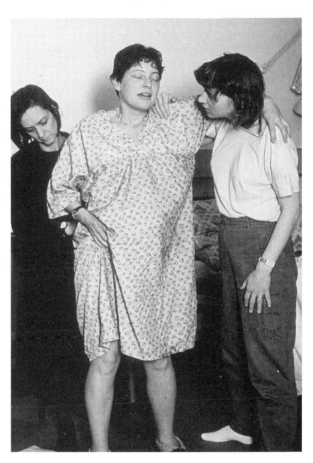

(a)   (b)

Birth at home (a) and birth in hospital (b) need not be as different as they typically have been in the past. (Photos: (a) Sally and Richard Greenhill; (b) Pam Isherwood/Format)

following among 'Forms of care unlikely to be beneficial' and 'Forms of care likely to be ineffective or harmful' :

- Routine pubic shaving

- Routine enema in labour

- Arbitrary limitation of the duration of the second stage of labour

- Requiring a supine (flat on back) position for second stage of labour

- Routine directed [maternal] pushing during the second stage of labour

- Routine or liberal episiotomy [making a cut at the entrance to the vagina]

(Enkin *et al.*, 1995, pp. 408 and 410)

Most of the above were routine in many United Kingdom hospitals in the 1960s. Some still are. It remains common to see staff directing the mother to hold her breath and push down hard until she can hold no longer, when in the pushing (second) stage of labour. Yet it is known that such enforced pushing raises the pressure in the womb high enough to prevent blood circulating in the placenta and the baby can suffer as a result. How the practice arose is uncertain, though it is likely it may have something to do with the anxiety of attending staff who felt the baby would be better out than in. Even today, rupturing the membranes in labour around the baby is often routine, yet it has almost no measurable effect on outcome—only a very small decrease in the overall length of labour. This in itself may or may not be beneficial.

Another cautionary tale

Let us examine in some detail the use of a particular technology—continuous **electronic fetal monitoring (EFM)** in labour. One of the biggest sadnesses in maternity care is for a baby to die late in labour or to be born brain-damaged. Researchers have tried to find ways of assessing how the baby is coping with labour. It is known that babies running short of oxygen (*hypoxia*) in the womb have lowered heart rates after a womb contraction and it takes many seconds for the rate to 'pick up' again. Electronic devices to allow a continuous recording of a baby's heartbeat and record womb contractions became widely available in the 1970s. The developers of such devices soon began to claim that such close surveillance could prevent babies dying in labour by allowing a hypoxic baby to be rescued by urgent caesarian section. Data from poorly-controlled trials soon convinced doctors that they should be using these machines. In part this was fuelled by a fear of very expensive litigation following the birth of a brain-damaged child.

From 1981 to 1984 the Dublin trial took place—over 13 000 women were randomised to have their labour assessed by continuous EFM or by the midwife listening periodically to the baby's heartbeat through a type of stethoscope (intermittent auscultation, or IA). (See Figure 3.13.) The trial showed no difference in PNMR. It did show double the number of neonatal fits within the first 24 hours after birth in the IA group (MacDonald *et al.*, 1985), though these fits were very uncommon in both groups. However, when all these babies were followed up to the age of 5, there were no measurable differences in rates of brain damage (as assessed by fits, learning, motor or behaviour disorders) (Grant, O'Brien *et al.*, 1989). This evidence of a very small and transient benefit of EFM is not enough on its own to encourage its widespread use. One must look at the other consequences. There may be negative effects which balance the small benefit. Some women find EFM uncomfortable or unnecessarily anxiety-provoking, and there is evidence that it increases medical intervention during labour without benefit to the baby (Enkin *et al.*, 1995).

In addition, EFM, like almost every other diagnostic method, is not infallible.

☐ What would be the consequences of a false-positive diagnosis of hypoxia from EFM?

■ There would be an unnecessary urgent caesarian.

The Dublin trial showed the very limited benefit of *routine* EFM. However, we cannot be sure that EFM does not have a useful role in selected high-risk labours. All the trials of EFM show a marked (about twofold) increase in the rate of caesarians for apparent hypoxia as assessed by alterations in the pattern of the fetal heartbeat. A very thorough study of the subject following a conference at the Royal College of Obstetricians and Gynaecologists in 1993 concluded that 'intermittent auscultation is the *method of choice* [our emphasis] for women at the normal end of the continuum of risk' (Spencer and Ward, 1993, p. 390).

The sociologist Jo Garcia, with colleagues, assessed women's views of EFM and IA in the Dublin trial and found that women having EFM were more likely (33 per cent) to feel left alone than those having IA (22 per cent) (Garcia *et al.*, 1985). It is probable that this is because they *were* left alone rather more, as the machine 'cared' instead of the midwife. The report of the Dublin EFM trial stated clearly:

In selecting from these and other policy options it will always remain important to take into account … the wishes of individual women in labor. (MacDonald *et al.*, 1985, p. 539)

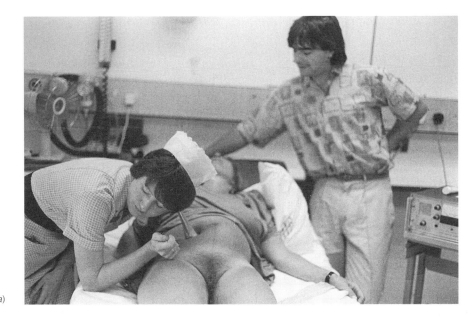

(a)

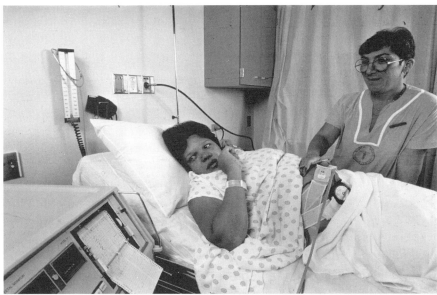

(b)

Figure 3.13 *A baby's heartbeat being monitored during labour by (a) a stethoscope, and (b) an electronic fetal monitor. This form of electronic fetal monitor is an ultrasound device. The Dublin trial instead used a small electrode attached to the baby's scalp. (Photos: (a) Sally and Richard Greenhill; (b) Science Photo Library)*

Yet it is not always clear how to obtain fully-informed consent. It seems unlikely that labour ward staff will say to women in labour, 'Would you like to wear this belt which won't increase your baby's chances of surviving or reduce the chance of lasting brain damage? The only benefit we know is that it cuts the rate of fits in the first 24 hours from 0.4 per cent to 0.2 per cent. It does mean you'll have to lie on the bed and stand more chance of a caesarian section—possibly an unnecessary one.'

More research needs to be done on the quality and quantity of information women need to make an informed decision, and on the optimum time for the information to be given.

Interventions chosen by women

It is not only professionals who choose to 'intervene'. Some women choose water births, though we have as yet no evidence of either benefit or harm (other than anecdote). The same could be said of homoeopathic remedies in childbirth. Furthermore, not all women wish to avoid intervention.

One such intervention often requested by women is *epidural anaesthesia* which can allow the woman a conscious, but pain-free, labour. An anaesthetic substance is introduced through a hollow needle into a specific location in the spinal canal in the woman's lower back. The pain signals from the lower part of the body to the brain are thereby blocked. This has some advantages over analgesic drugs taken by mouth or by injection elsewhere, which spread throughout the woman's body and into the baby, and which can thus make the woman drowsy and affect her baby's breathing after delivery. For caesarian section, epidural anaesthesia is safer for the mother than a general anaesthetic, as she remains awake and is much less likely to vomit and then inhale, which can be fatal (though it should be made clear that this consequence is very rare even for caesarians under general anaesthetic). However, as with most interventions in childbirth, epidural anaesthesia is not an unmixed blessing. First, it leads to a greater use of forceps and similar interventions. Second, there is some evidence that it decreases the sense of maternal satisfaction with the birth (Morgan *et al.*, 1982) and this in turn may have longer-term significance for the relationship between mother and baby.

Given the frequency of some interventions, such as breaking the waters around the baby during labour (rupturing the membranes) or giving an intravenous drip containing a hormone, oxytocin (both these interventions are used to speed up the course of labour), we need more research on their longer-term effects on both mother and baby. Management of childbirth may have long-term effects that go far beyond the period immediately after birth.

It is, of course, not only the mother who may be affected in the long term by professional care—so may her child.

Birth care and cerebral palsy

Can good birth care reduce perinatal morbidity? The major neonatal condition thought to be associated with poor birth care is cerebral palsy (though over a century ago, Freud suggested the damage done to the baby's brain occurred before labour and not during it). In a minority of cases, the condition can be caused by brain damage which is a consequence of lack of oxygen during labour and birth.

As you saw in the section on place of birth, Alison Munro's Maternity Services Advisory Committee of 1984 stated that increasing the hospital birth rate had led to 'the avoidance of many child handicaps'. This statement is astonishing because there was no evidence to make this connection at the time, nor had any been obtained a decade later. Indeed there has been no reduction in birth-related handicap. The rates of cerebral palsy in industrialised countries have not decreased during the twentieth century, despite obstetric advance. The false claim by obstetricians, that their expert care could prevent cerebral palsy, has been described in an editorial in the *Lancet* as a 'shot in the foot' (*Lancet*, 1989). Many mothers, lawyers and others assume, as a result, that cerebral palsy must be a consequence of medical negligence. It now seems highly likely that less than 10 per cent of cerebral palsy is a result of lack of oxygen during labour and birth (Nelson, 1988; Blair and Stanley, 1988). Even then, it is not clear how much of this 10 per cent is avoidable with the best care. The causes of the other 90 per cent of cases remain for the most part poorly understood.

We will now turn to the final section of this chapter: care given after the birth.

Postnatal care

Professional care of the newborn

Routine examination of the newborn baby can detect malformations, dislocated hips, undescended testes and congenital cataracts, to name but a few problems. Some of the above may be greatly improved by early treatment.

In the United Kingdom all babies are tested in the first few days of life, by taking a drop of blood from the heel, for two rare but important metabolic disorders—phenylketonuria (PKU; the build-up of an amino acid)[24] and hypothyroidism (inadequate production of thyroid hormone). Failure to detect and treat these conditions can lead to permanent brain damage and learning difficulties.

There have been huge advances in the care of very pre-term babies. These advances have allowed the survival of babies born as early as 24 weeks gestation. It is

---

[24]For further details of PKU see *Human Biology and Health: An Evolutionary Approach*, Chapters 4 and 9.

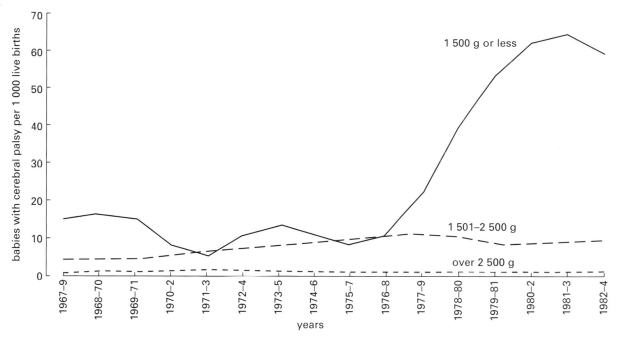

Figure 3.14 *Trends in the prevalence of cerebral palsy per 1 000 live births, for three different birthweight groups, 1967–84. These rates are estimated from data for the Mersey Health Region of the United Kingdom. Since the data for low birth weights are based on small numbers of births, fluctuations in prevalence have been smoothed by plotting average rates for groups of three years. (Source: redrawn from Pharaoh, P. O. D., et al., 1990, Birthweight specific trends in cerebral palsy,* Archives of Disease in Childhood, *65, pp. 602–6, Figure 1)*

beyond the limits of this chapter to describe these advances in care. However, they raise serious ethical issues about when a fetus can be considered viable and up to what stage abortion is justified. Part of the drop in perinatal mortality is due to very pre-term babies being kept alive.

☐ Describe the main patterns in the data shown in Figure 3.14.

■ For the heaviest group (over 2 500 g) the rate of cerebral palsy remained roughly constant over the period shown. There was a reasonably steady rise in the rate for the middle weight group (1 501–2 500 g), and a fairly dramatic rise over the latter part of the period shown for the lightest group (under 1 500 g).

☐ How might this pattern arise as a result of advances in the ability to keep very pre-term babies alive?

■ It may well be that very small, very pre-term babies who, before the late 1970s, would have died, are now surviving and living on with cerebral palsy.

There is evidence from other sources that the number of surviving, very pre-term babies with cerebral palsy is rising (Nicholson and Alberman, 1992).

Prompt resuscitation of full-term babies is a different issue. Getting oxygen into a newborn baby who is not breathing adequately can be life-saving and/or brain-saving.

Postnatal care for mothers

The main purpose of care up to and including birth is clear: a healthy mother and a healthy baby—in the broadest sense of healthy—physically and mentally well, confident and enriched by the experience. The purpose of postnatal care directed towards the new mother is far less clear. This aimlessness is exemplified by the activities undertaken by health workers which have not been shown to be effective—the routine taking of temperatures, routine enquiries about blood loss, measurement of the size of the womb as well as routine vaginal examination 6 weeks after birth (Chalmers *et al.*, 1989; Enkin *et al.*, 1995). Hospital birth, so common in most industrialised countries, suits the great majority of women, but hospitals are used to treating ill patients. Only a minority of United Kingdom midwives have 'direct entry' to mid-wifery schools, i.e. most were already nurses before they trained as midwives and are therefore used to caring for the sick as, of course, are all doctors. We will try to discover to what extent our present system of care helps the woman in her role as mother.

Care in hospital

Time spent in hospital after birth is very variable. In the nineteenth century 'lying-in' hospitals allowed (and, indeed, more or less forced) women to do just that, often for as long as 28 days. In the 1950s average length of stay was down to 12 days. This has since decreased and is now less than 5 days. Some women choose to go home just a few hours after giving birth. Others stay for some days and some may be discharged before they would choose. The justification now for 'early discharge' is pressure on hospital beds. It does not seem that the wishes of women were considered of paramount importance, nor that there was scientific evidence to indicate that any particular length of stay was better for the mother or her baby.

Until the 1970s (and later in some places) most postnatal wards were run much like other wards in hospital—with regular checks on temperature, blood pressure and bowels. Visiting was restricted and often still is, in terms of who may visit as well as when. One of the reasons put forward to limit the number of visitors was to control infection. Fear of infection led to a variety of measures being set up to avoid this threat to the newborn. Many of these measures—the wearing of gowns, hats and masks—are now known to be unnecessary when handling newborn babies.

The early separation of human mother and baby may not have quite the drastic consequences of rejection shown in some other mammals, but restriction of mother–baby contact has been shown in several well-controlled studies to be associated with less affectionate maternal behaviour and increased maternal feelings of incompetence and loss of confidence (Thomson and Westreich, 1989).

Breast-feeding

In human females the non-pregnant breast is large compared with mammary glands in other species, and under the hormonal regime of the third trimester of pregnancy (high oestrogen, high progesterone and the secretion by the pituitary gland of the hormone *prolactin*) the milk-producing parts of the breast increase enormously. The glands do not normally secrete actual milk, although they may produce small amounts of clear, protein-rich colostrum, the precursor of milk.

When the levels of progesterone and oestrogen fall at birth, the glands secrete large quantities of colostrum for several days, which later becomes 'transitional milk' and then normal or 'mature milk'. Milk secretion is initially dependent on the high level of prolactin at birth, but the level is only maintained if the breast is suckled. Sense organs in the nipple trigger reflex stimulation of the pituitary gland, causing the release of prolactin and another hormone, *oxytocin*. The oxytocin causes muscles around the ducts in the breast to contract and thus expel the milk, which is formed continuously between feeds. The colostrum contains little fat and milk sugar (lactose) compared with mature milk, but a high level of proteins, some of which are *immunoglobulins*, the proteins responsible for antibody activity of various types. These maternal antibodies are thought to confer local, passive immunity on the baby, giving it some protection against swallowed bacteria. The baby's main protection against infection in its first weeks will come from its mother's antibodies which crossed the placenta in the later stages of the pregnancy and circulate for a time in the baby's bloodstream.

Some of the benefits of breast-feeding for the first four months or so are clear: less gastroenteritis (in the Third World bottle-feeding can be a fatal choice, as sterilising water to dilute powdered milk may be impractical if not impossible) and fewer respiratory infections. Other benefits are possible but not yet proven—increased intelligence and a decreased incidence of atherosclerosis ('furring up' of the arteries) in later life have been suggested. Despite the evidence of benefit to the baby, the apparent convenience of instant ready-made meals and the financial savings, by 6 weeks after delivery fewer than half the mothers in the United Kingdom in the 1990s are breast-feeding. What makes women choose to bottle-feed is not always clear (though an early return to work and the ability to involve others in feeding are obvious reasons).

In a 1992 survey in Grampian, Scotland (Glazener et al., 1992), the most common complaints about postnatal care in relation to breast-feeding were: conflicting advice, staff who 'did it for them' and lack of staff time to help mothers establish breast-feeding. Staff commonly recommended bottle-feeding when problems arose.

Care after hospital

Nearly all women in the United Kingdom are home by 6 days after delivery, and many much earlier. There they will be cared for by community midwives. In the Grampian study, 33 per cent of the women had never met their community midwife before delivery. Usually the GP will visit, and the health visitor once the baby is 10 days old.

Does this care help the woman in her transition to motherhood? Does it help the baby? Unfortunately, as with antenatal care, much postnatal care has involved routine checks on all women, rarely tailored to individual need. Recently postnatal visiting by community midwives has become more selective, though this has largely been driven by the cost of visiting every woman at home at least daily up to 10 days after the birth.

However, women do value continuity of carers and this is more readily achieved in the community than in hospital, primarily because smaller numbers of staff are involved. (In the Grampian study 86 per cent of women in the large central unit rated their postnatal care as good, whereas in the small peripheral units 98 per cent of women rated it good. This probably reflects more personal, continuous care.)

Continuity could be much improved if the woman had the same midwife antenatally, in labour and postnatally; but midwives need time off duty and total continuity is an unattainable goal. However, the developing idea of midwives working in small groups could enable such care to become a possibility. The divide between community and hospital midwives is unlikely to be of benefit to women.

A further breakdown in continuity occurs when the midwife hands over to the health visitor at some time between 10 and 28 days. As mentioned above, breast-feeding is abandoned by many women. Whether prolonging midwifery input would overcome this is not known (nor is the effect of providing health visitor input from the moment of hospital discharge).

Postnatal depression

Many surveys in the United Kingdom show that 10 per cent or more of women giving birth experience a condition called **postnatal depression** (Cox *et al.*, 1987; Cooper *et al.*, 1988). This is not 'baby blues', a period of weepiness which commonly occurs a few days after birth, but a feeling of real misery and hopelessness, often accompanied by anxiety and feeling physically ill. Insomnia, guilt and tiredness are often present. The peak time for the onset of this illness is about 3 months after delivery. Many affected women feel guilty about being depressed as they believe people expect them to feel happy and fulfilled. Many cases are never reported to, or noticed by, health care workers.

There has been a mass of studies attempting to find factors associated with postnatal depression. Few are found consistently, but these include past psychiatric disorder, anxiety in pregnancy, marital conflict and adverse life events within the preceding year (Paykel *et al.*, 1980). Antenatal depression is commoner than postnatal depression though less notice is taken of it, perhaps because giving drugs in pregnancy is hazardous. A study by Jo Green showed depressed low antenatal mood is strongly associated with depressed postnatal mood (Green, 1990). There is conflicting evidence as to whether problems requiring medical intervention during pregnancy and childbirth can give rise to postnatal depression. The same study by Jo Green indicates that such problems do not lead to depression if the mother feels she is in control of what is being done to her, but passive recipients of medical intervention *may* become depressed. This appears to be especially so after caesarian section, particularly if it was done as an emergency.

Though breast-feeding is undoubtedly an advantage to babies, it is associated with greater tiredness in mothers and a higher incidence of late postnatal depression.

Many British mothers suffer a loss of status, income, support and friendship postnatally. Postnatal groups such as those run by the National Childbirth Trust fulfil an important need, as professional health care can do little to overcome these problems.

Severe, long-term postnatal depression is not a problem for the mother alone. There is a large number of research studies which consistently show poor developmental outcomes for the children of mothers who suffer from it. For example, children of clinically depressed mothers have been found to be at greater risk of poor health, psychiatric disorders, and other psychological and behavioural difficulties.

However, despite the recognition of the problem and its consequences, there is still a great deal of uncertainty about its causes and effects: for example, whether the conditions of both mother and child are a consequence of external factors such as social and economic circumstances, whether depressed mothers interact abnormally with their infants, or whether depression itself is precipitated by difficulties in the early stages of developing a relationship with the newborn infant.

A study by psychologist Lynne Murray (1992) of over 100 mothers identified as clinically depressed showed disruptions in infant intellectual development at 9 months of age, and effects on a range of psychological measures in the children when they were 18 months old. Attention is now focusing on infant–mother interaction as one of the links in this process. A further study by Murray

(1993a) has found evidence of consistent differences between the face-to-face interactions of depressed and non-depressed mothers with their infants. There is evidence from the same study that short-term psychotherapy can alleviate the condition and its effects on mother–infant interaction.[25]

Conclusion

Is maternity care effective?

Judged by the impressive decline in maternal mortality and perinatal mortality during this century (Figures 3.1 and 3.9), maternity care in the United Kingdom in the late twentieth century appears to have succeeded in its aims: healthy mothers and healthy babies in the vast majority of cases. But there are reasons for being cautious about praising the existing arrangements for maternity care too highly. Perinatal mortality rates show a close relationship to social class.[26] Improvements in maternal and child health may have had more to do with better food, better family planning and better housing than better care in pregnancy and birth. However, as we mentioned earlier, doctors and midwives can claim some credit for the improvement. Maternal mortality began to decline sharply in the 1930s, having been static before then. It is difficult to tie this in with any sudden and dramatic improvement in the standard of living.

Parts of the chapter have presented evidence that certain aspects of maternity care are not effective, which might lead one to conclude that professional care is much less useful than is claimed. One study which backs up the professional carers, however, is the following. Andrew Kaunitz and other American researchers studied members of the Faith Assembly in Indiana, USA, between 1975 and 1982 (Kaunitz *et al.*, 1984). This religious group does not accept any trained carers through pregnancy and childbirth (which takes place in the home). The group studied had, on average, achieved a higher educational status than the average in Indiana statewide. Higher percentages of Faith Assembly members were white, married and aged 20–34—all factors normally associated with better obstetric outcomes. Yet, in 355 births there were three maternal deaths—a rate of 872 per 100 000 births—nearly one hundred times higher than the rate in Indiana overall. Evidence like this, together with evidence on the timing and size of the decline in maternal mortality in countries like the United Kingdom, makes it likely that good health care from midwives and doctors has had a major impact on *maternal* mortality.

The effect on *perinatal* mortality seems to be less dramatic, though in the Faith Assembly study there were 17 perinatal deaths—a rate nearly three times higher than in Indiana generally. Most perinatal deaths in industrialised countries are due to one of four main groups of causes: pre-term birth, asphyxia, deaths before labour begins, and congenital malformations (Table 3.2). Very small, very pre-term babies are increasingly being kept alive by sophisticated (and expensive) neonatal care. The asphyxia group die from lack of oxygen during, or shortly before, birth; there is still no reliable way of ensuring this does not happen. The third group—deaths before labour—is least amenable to care and the number remains stubbornly high. The last group, as discussed earlier, is falling, possibly due to earlier detection and abortion (thus removing these fetuses from perinatal mortality data), but probably in part due to better diet and environmental conditions. The role of ultrasound scanning in detection of abnormalities is, as you have seen, not straightforward.

Future maternity care

Professional care in pregnancy and childbirth has made childbirth safer for the mother and, to a lesser extent, for her baby. However, these improvements have had their negative aspects. As we have already discussed, pre-term babies can be kept alive but the number of very pre-term babies with cerebral palsy is rising. Women have been subjected to a whole series of interventions, some of which have not been shown to be beneficial, and which reduce their autonomy in pregnancy and childbirth. The foreword to the most recent government report, *Changing Childbirth*, said that pregnant women have been cared for in a way

> ... more appropriate to states of ill-health than
> to a physiological process which, for the
> majority, results in a normal and uncomplicated
> outcome .... [a woman] should be able to feel
> that she is in control of what is happening to her
> and able to make decisions about her care.
> (Department of Health, 1993, pp. II and 9)

There is a hope that maternity care will become much more evidence-based and that it will become individually suited to each woman. If this can come about, maternity care may act as an example to other parts of health care. It will require considerable change in the way many doctors and midwives care for women, their unborn and newborn babies.

[25]Some of Lynne Murray's research is shown in the television programme 'First steps to autonomy', for Open University students studying this book.

[26]See *Studying Health and Disease*, Chapter 6.

OBJECTIVES FOR CHAPTER 3

When you have studied this chapter, you should be able to:

3.1 Distinguish the major stages of fetal development from conception to birth, explaining the underlying biological reasons for the most significant risk-points in the developmental process both in the womb and in the period immediately after birth.

3.2 Outline the standard provision of antenatal care to United Kingdom women, and summarise the evidence for and against the effectiveness of common antenatal procedures.

3.3 Summarise the main current influences on the decision on where a birth should take place, and comment critically on the evidence on safety grounds for and against the centralisation of place of birth.

3.4 Briefly describe and evaluate the evidence for and against routine electronic fetal monitoring in childbirth.

3.5 Discuss health issues affecting mothers and babies after childbirth, particularly those relating to breast-feeding and postnatal depression.

QUESTIONS FOR CHAPTER 3

Question 1 (*Objective 3.1*)

Look back at Figure 3.8. At birth, blood pressure rises sharply in the baby's aorta when the placenta detaches, but falls in the lungs as they inflate. What effect will this have on the ductus arteriosus?

Question 2 (*Objective 3.1*)

At what point from conception to birth is the developing baby most at risk?

Question 3 (*Objective 3.2*)

In this chapter it is stated that 'Ultrasound scanning is an example of a technology widely introduced before randomised controlled trials had defined its

value'. Outline the justification for this statement. What are the disadvantages of introducing an intervention like this before full evaluation has taken place? Might there be any advantages of such an introduction?

Question 4 (*Objectives 3.3 and 3.4*)

The following quote is from the Winterton Report (House of Commons Health Committee, 1991–2, pp. xxi and xxiii).[27]

> The choices of a home birth or birth in small maternity units are options which have been substantially withdrawn from the majority of women in this country. For most women there is no choice. This does not appear to be in accordance with their wishes … Until such time as there is more detailed and accurate research about such interventions as epidurals, episiotomies, caesarian sections, electronic fetal monitoring, instrumental delivery and induction of labour, women need to be given a choice on the basis of existing information rather than having to undergo such interventions as routine.'

(i)   Why is there 'no choice' for most women about place of birth?

(ii)   What changes in government policy on place of birth were there in the early 1990s?

(iii)   Why might it be particularly difficult to organise randomised, controlled clinical trials of interventions such as those listed in the quotation?

Question 5 (*Objective 3.5*)

The consequences for a baby of being breast-fed continue after the first few weeks of life. Briefly describe the continuing advantages and disadvantages for both child and mother.

[27]Also reproduced in *Health and Disease: A Reader* (second edition, 1995), pp. 339–40.

4 Child health and development

This chapter assumes some understanding of the influence of a person's genes on their physical growth and development, as discussed in another book in this series, Human Biology and Health: An Evolutionary Approach, *particularly Chapters 4 and 9.[1] In the present chapter, the focus widens to include psychological development and its relationship to health and illness in childhood. The television programme for Open University students, 'First steps to autonomy', is relevant to this chapter.*

The principal author, Jim Stevenson, is Reader in Psychology at the Institute of Child Health in London. His research has been concerned with the social and biological influences on abnormal development in children, initially through epidemiological analysis of behavioural disturbances and developmental delay, and more recently through genetic analysis of twins to estimate the relative significance of genetic and environmental influences on reading, hyperactivity and anti-social behaviour. John Oates, the second author, is Lecturer in Psychology in the School of Education at the Open University, and a member of the U205 Course Team; his research is into cognitive and social development in infants.

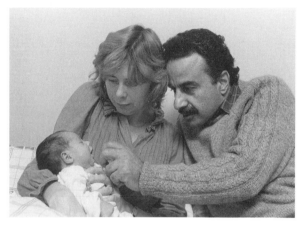

From high dependency ...   (Photo: Mike Levers)

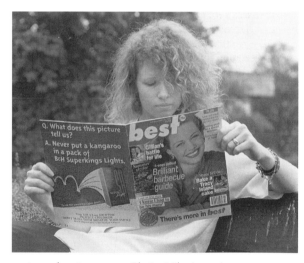

... towards autonomy.   (Photo: Mike Levers)

Introduction

Children's health from infancy to adolescence is strongly influenced by their transition during this period of life from high dependency towards autonomy in many

aspects of care and health-related behaviours. The chapter will describe some of the processes underlying this transition. Over time, the nature of the risks to health change from a passive vulnerability to the quality of care which the child's caregivers are able to provide, given

[1]*Human Biology and Health: An Evolutionary Approach* (1994).

their social circumstances, to an increasing degree of autonomy in which the child is more active in making health-related decisions. However, the child's health over this period is also vulnerable to the effects of experience before birth and during the early years, to the cumulative influence of experiences within and increasingly outside the family, and to the continuing influence of biological factors. The interplay between emergent self-determination and the social and biological constraints on development will be a recurring theme of this chapter.

Growth and development

In this chapter, the changes in children as they grow older are described under two headings: growth and development. **Growth** refers to the process of gaining in height and weight, and also the maturation of physiological processes, such as the hormonal changes associated with sexual maturation before and during puberty and the continuing structural changes that take place within the central nervous system long after birth. Although many people only think of these growth changes as taking place *after* birth, they are of course a continuation of a process that started at conception. Birth is only a transition point along the way; but it is nevertheless a particularly hazardous one since it faces the baby with having to cope with the switch to breathing air and to being physiologically independent of the mother. For this reason (as you saw in Chapter 3) much medical concern is directed towards maintaining the child in the uterus until it is sufficiently mature to manage this transition without undue risk.

The second type of change with age considered in this chapter is that of psychological **development**. This term is used to describe changes that are linked with the child's capacity to process information about the world—to see and hear, to act on the world and join the social world—to speak and to respond to other people's behaviour: in other words, changes due to *learning*. It is becoming increasingly clear how this developmental process is, like physical growth, strongly influenced by the child's genetic make-up and is also especially dependent on a responsive social environment within which this development can take place.

☐ What features of children's development do you think are dependent on a 'responsive social environment'?

■ To enumerate the possibilities in full would probably take another chapter, but among the more obvi-

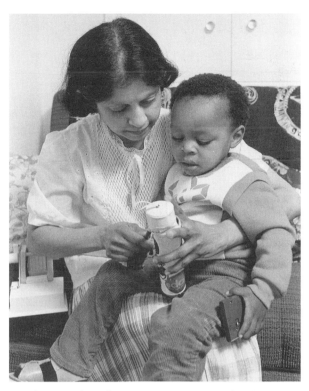

Development depends upon a responsive social environment. (Photo: Mike Levers)

ous are language and literacy, social relationships and emotional development, and self-care practices such as aspects of personal hygiene and choice of diet. Research in developmental psychology is also increasingly pointing to many aspects of intellectual development as needing supportive social conditions.

The maintenance of a normal progression of growth and development is the key to health in a child and, accordingly, many non-infectious illnesses in children can be seen as distortions or delays in these normal growth and developmental processes.

What is 'normal' development?

For most characteristics of physical and psychological development, it is possible to define a 'normal average' pattern: a *norm*. Such norms are identified by surveying large numbers of children of different ages and calculating the 'average for age' values of the characteristic

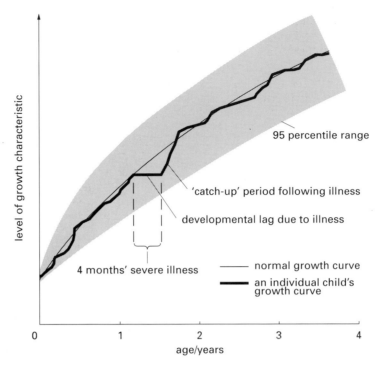

Figure 4.1 *A normal growth curve and a record of an individual child's growth.*

concerned. A universal feature of children's development, however, is that it varies. Thus most developmental norms need also to show the *extent* of variation in the characteristic. Figure 4.1 shows both of these; the **normal growth curve** in the figure shows the average value and the tinted area each side of the norm shows the range of variation within which the growth of 95 per cent of children falls. This is known as the *95 percentile range.*

Using such norms, it is possible to chart an individual child's development, as in Figure 4.1. This particular child's growth curve shows how it can be normal for a child's development to vary from time to time and also how the slowing-down of development, for example due to illness, is often (but not always) followed by a period of 'catch-up' growth that is more rapid than the norm.[2] However, as discussed later in this chapter, many psychological characteristics do not seem so 'resilient' as physical growth in that the effect of a

[2]See also Figure 11.1 and the related discussion in *World Health and Disease* (1993), Chapter 11.

developmental lag early in life does not necessarily recover when the cause of that lag is removed. The issue of assessing whether a particular child's growth is sufficiently different from the norm as to be considered 'abnormal' is discussed below.

Disorders of growth

We can think of an illness such as *insulin-dependent diabetes mellitus* as a **disorder of growth**. The cells in the pancreas fail to establish the required level of insulin production necessary for the body to maintain a stable level of blood glucose. The reasons for this failure are not well understood, but it is believed to be due to a genetic susceptibility to viral infection that leaves the cells in the pancreas vulnerable to attack by the body's immune system. The absence of a fully functioning pancreas leaves the child with an illness that may require life-long medication by insulin injections (in early childhood given by the parents, but later administered by the child). Note that an *environmental* change—the injection of insulin—can modify the impact of the genetic abnormality to such an extent that its effect on growth is avoided or reduced.

□ Can you think of another example of a childhood disorder caused by faulty gene expression, the effects of which can be greatly modified by a change in the child's environment?

■ Phenylketonuria (or PKU) is a genetic disorder which affects amino acid metabolism (amino acids are the 'building blocks' of proteins); a carefully-restricted diet from a very early age can greatly reduce the effects on growth and development.[3]

In the case of diabetes, in spite of the environmental change, the child will often remain more vulnerable in later life to other serious health problems such as blindness, kidney disease and heart disease.

Thinking of diabetes in this way illustrates the idea that *health* can be indicated by normal patterns of growth and development. This definition of health is a useful one in developmental psychology, and leads to a view of illness as the outcome of any circumstance that prevents this normal pattern of growth and development from taking place. Chronic illnesses such as diabetes are not usually considered as disorders of growth in this way.

Growth usually refers to changes in height and body mass. In this more familiar sense there are quite normal but marked variations in the rate at which children grow. In determining whether a child might be experiencing a disorder of growth it is necessary to identify a degree of growth retardation or acceleration that is unlikely to be due to normal variation. Typically this assessment will be made by comparing the child's current measurements (e.g. height or weight) against the normal average and range of variation for other children of the same age (as in Figure 4.1). A value outside the range within which most children fall (typically the 95 percentile range) will alert the clinician to a possible growth disorder. However, other factors will typically be taken into account, such as the stature of the parents (to identify a possible genetic component), and whether the child has recently had a significant illness (since illness often slows growth; the child may 'catch up' later, as in Figure 4.1). It has been found that children whose height places them in the shortest and tallest 3 per cent of children of the same age and sex are at significantly greater risk of having a condition that might require medical treatment. Children below the third centile for height may show delayed onset of puberty and retarded growth after puberty.

It has been suggested that disorders of prenatal growth and growth in the months immediately after birth are associated with differences in health in later life, in particular the incidence of hypertension (high blood pressure) and coronary heart disease. The research indicating such a link has been undertaken by a multidisciplinary team led by David Barker at the University of Southampton (see, for example, Barker *et al.*, 1990).[4]

Disorders of development

Like disorders of growth, **disorders of development** affect the child's ability to act on and react to the world. For example, children with *cerebral palsy* may have a profound inability to learn to regulate or control their muscular movements. This will limit their ability to express themselves in either spoken language or gesture. Although they may have unimpaired mental abilities, without an augmented communication system it may be difficult for them to demonstrate their normal cognitive (intellectual) abilities.

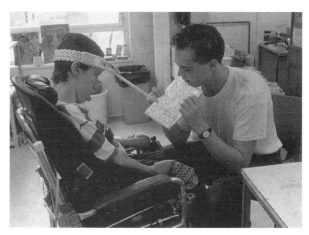

An augmented communication system can help a person to demonstrate their cognitive abilities. (Photo: Mike Levers)

Many other developmental abnormalities do involve impaired learning and may leave the child with severe psychological and social handicaps. Many such cases of learning difficulties are known to be associated with chromosomal defects such as *Down's syndrome* or single

---

[3]PKU is discussed extensively in *Human Biology and Health: An Evolutionary Approach*, particularly Chapter 4.

[4]This research has led to the so-called 'programming hypothesis', which broadly states that factors affecting the growth and development of the fetus and infant have long-term effects on health in later life. It is discussed in two other books in this series, *Studying Health and Disease* (revised edition, 1994), Chapter 10; and *World Health and Disease* (1993), Chapter 11.

major gene disorders such as *Fragile X syndrome*, which is now known to be a major cause of mental subnormality in children.[5] In both these cases the genetic origin of the disability is known but in many other cases the origin, whether it be genetic or not, has not been clearly established. Also in practically all cases where a gene defect does influence brain function the mechanism is not understood.

Classifying ill-health in children

One widely-used formal classification of childhood illness is that developed by the World Health Organisation (WHO). It is part of the more general framework for defining diseases called the **International Classification of Diseases (ICD)**. This framework has been developed and refined over the years and in 1994 reached its tenth version (World Health Organisation, 1994) and hence is referred to as ICD-10. A central feature of the logic behind this classification is that disease and related health problems can be classified into a set of categories based on:

- diagnoses,
- symptoms,
- abnormal laboratory findings,
- injuries and poisonings,
- external causes of mortality and morbidity, and
- other factors influencing health status.

On this basis each illness or disability is given a 3-character code, for example, P90—convulsions of the newborn; Q35—cleft palate.

☐ Can you think of any other categories which are important to assess in arriving at a full description of a child's health status?

■ Although the above are clearly important factors to consider, they do not include any assessment of the impact of the illness on a child's behaviour or their mental functioning. Neither is the child's immediate environment considered. This is significant, since, as suggested earlier, children's development is dependent in part on their psychological, social and material environment.

[5]Chromosomal disorders and single gene defects are explained and illustrated in *Human Biology and Health: An Evolutionary Approach*, Chapter 4.

It has been recognised that although *illnesses* may be classified in this way, it certainly does not represent an adequate description of an individual child's overall **health status**. An extension to the ICD code has thus been developed to include the physical and mental functioning of an individual. This has resulted in the development of a multi-axial (i.e. measured on several different axes) classification of disease where in every case the *person* is assessed in relation to their clinical state (as in the ICD categories above) plus an assessment of:

- the extent and quality of their social support,
- chronic social difficulties (such as poor housing, unemployment),
- social context, and
- the degree of handicap associated with the disease.

The approach to the classification of *adult* health is to identify the cause of biological malfunction in a previously normal, mature organ system (e.g. a normally functioning and fully grown kidney may become dysfunctional through infection). The same question can be raised in relation to some illnesses in children, although there is a major additional issue that must be considered. The child may never have had a normally functioning system; for example, their kidneys may have always been malformed—as in the condition called *polycystic kidneys*. Therefore in children there is a continual need to see childhood ill-health as often being a *failure* of normal development, whereas in adults the origins of dysfunction of *developed* biological systems are the main concern.

Being able to diagnose and classify illnesses is only one part of the formulation of the health status of a child. It is essential to take account of the impact of the child's state of health on their lives more generally—on their ability to attend school, to get around independently, to communicate with people, whether they are in pain or not, and so on. These features of a person's health status have come to be called *quality of life*.

Quality of life in children

The notion of **quality of life** for adults can be taken as something very broad—encompassing, for example, the degree of material wealth and individual happiness. In health terms the notion is somewhat narrower. Quality of life for a child is also significantly different in the features that contribute to it compared with some of the features that comprise quality of life for adults.

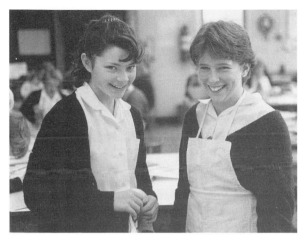

'Functioning in school' is a quality of life factor for young people but not for adults. (Photo: Mike Levers)

☐ In what respects does the assessment of quality of life have to take account of differences between adults and children?

■ There are certain aspects of daily life that are not relevant for young children, e.g. features associated with employment or sexual functioning. Equally there are features of children's lives that are less salient or absent for adults, e.g. functioning in school.

Donald Bailey and a research group from the University of North Carolina have shown (Bailey *et al.,* 1993) that parents, teachers and medical specialists can agree well on the extent to which the health of children attending a health centre is impaired. They did not include the child's perception of their functional limitations since the average age of the children they studied was 4.5 years. In attempting to provide a global assessment of a child's disability they used nine dimensions which formed the useful acronym—ABILITIES:

A   Audition (hearing acuity)

B   Behaviour and social skills

I   Intellectual functioning

L   Limbs (use of hands, arms and legs)

I   Intentional communication (comprehension and expression)

T   Tonicity of muscles (whether the muscles are strong or weak or rigid and inflexible)

I   Integrity of physical health (whether the child has an infection or a disorder of some aspect of normal physiological functioning)

E   Eyes (vision)

S   Structural status (shape, body form and structure)

This assessment is intended to describe the functioning of children across a wide range of disability.

☐ Is a measure of function such as ABILITIES all that is required to assess quality of life?

■ Of course it isn't, but there is the problem that if you start adding other components it is difficult to know where to stop. One essential additional dimension is the extent to which you are upset by your level of functioning, i.e. your *subjective* appraisal of the impact your level of functioning has on your life.

This subjective appraisal is of central importance to a quality of life assessment. Without it any system of assessment will inevitably apply values to forms and degrees of handicap that the person with the disability may not share. If an asthma sufferer insists that the periodic bouts of breathlessness do not detract from his or her quality of life then that appraisal must be respected. There is a specific problem here though, which comes to the fore where a child is concerned. What if other people in daily contact with the child see that by denying the adverse impact of their disability the child is being prevented from access to help and hence improvement in quality of life? To make this concrete, think of the child with cerebral palsy who has a profound speech handicap that prevents others from understanding him or her. That child may be satisfied with their limited level of communication, but a communication aid (for example, a machine that produces spoken messages from typing on a keyboard) would make it much easier for others to understand their communication and hence foster their development. Thus there is a need for the appraisal of quality of life to be based on a variety of sources as well as the child's own reports.

The quality of life has become a major concern in health care for children. This has traditionally been considered in terms of the impact of illness and disability. However, of more contemporary concern is the quality of life of children *after* experiencing treatment; for example, are the gains in life expectancy from heart/lung transplantation for children with cystic fibrosis sufficient to justify the pain, anxiety and vulnerability to infection? These

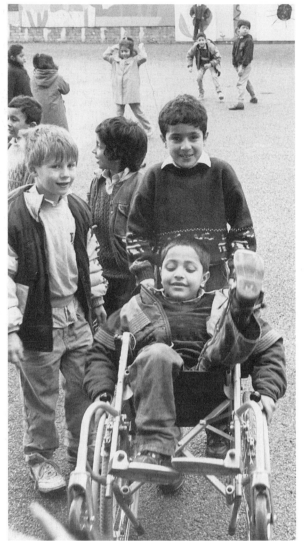

This child's subjective appraisal of his quality of life is of central importance to any professional assessment. (Photo: Mike Levers)

concerns are not limited to the impact of development in medical sciences on children; the same concerns are particularly pertinent to the care of elderly and terminally-ill people.[6]

The extent to which any particular illness impinges on a child's quality of life will change over time. This is

partly because the effectiveness of treatments and technologies constantly changes and also that the pattern of prevalence of illnesses changes both over time and across populations.

Patterns of physical illness and disability in children

There have been striking changes during this century in the patterns of physical illness in childhood, and prevalence rates have to be seen in relation to the particular population of children being studied; there are marked changes in prevalence over time within countries and also between countries. In Third World countries, infectious diseases and malnutrition are the two major influences on child health. As systems of medical care have developed in the industrialised world, medical science has provided effective treatment and preventive interventions for many previously fatal or debilitating illnesses in children. For example, Figure 4.2 shows the life expectancy of children born with *cystic fibrosis*, which has increased from less than 10 to over 40 years since 1960.

The risk to infants in the United Kingdom from infectious illnesses during early childhood has been substantially reduced during the twentieth century, with progress continuing even in recent years. For example, the introduction of *measles* vaccination in 1968 has reduced the rate of measles notifications from some 500 000 per year in the 1960s to less than 10 000 in 1991.[7] At the same time, techniques for the care of very premature and vulnerable infants have improved so that children who would have died in the perinatal period just 10 years or so ago are now surviving (as already discussed in Chapter 3); the infant mortality rate has fallen from 10 per 1 000 live births in 1980 to 7.5 per 1 000 in 1990 (the infant mortality rate or IMR is the number of deaths in the first year of life per 1 000 live births). This has meant that, as far as children in the United Kingdom are concerned, the main influences on morbidity (the level of illness in a population) in the 1990s are those stemming from biological

[6]Quality of life measurement is discussed more extensively in *Dilemmas in Health Care* (1993), Chapter 3, and in an article by Alan Williams, 'Priority setting in the NHS', in *Health and Disease: A Reader* (second edition, 1995).

[7]Throughout this chapter, where figures are quoted for prevalence or incidence rates, and are not otherwise attributed, they are taken from Woodroffe *et al.*, 1993. *Prevalence* refers to the number of cases of a disease in the population at a given *point* in time, divided by the number of people in the population who are at risk; *incidence* refers to the number of *new* cases of a disease during a given period, divided by the number of people in the population who are at risk. Both measures are discussed in *Studying Health and Disease* (1994), Chapter 7.

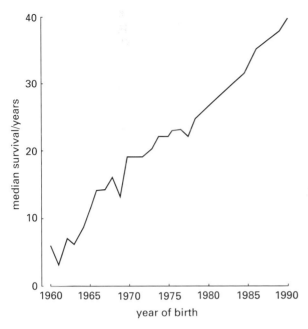

Figure 4.2 *Trend in predicted survival for children with cystic fibrosis by year of birth, England and Wales, 1959–90 (Source: Woodroffe C., Glikman, M. Barker, M. and Power, C., 1993,* Children, Teenagers and Health: The Key Data, *Open University Press, Buckingham, Figure 2.43, p. 52; data derived from Elborn, J. S., Shales, D. J. and Britton, J. R., 1992, Cystic fibrosis: current survival and population estimates to the year 2000,* Thorax, **46**, *pp. 881–5)*

deficits that are either genetically determined or are a consequence of adverse perinatal circumstances.

Because of improvements in diet and hygiene, in health and social care and medical treatment, the main sources of illness and disability in young children in Western nations are no longer infections. Instead several

genetically-based disorders have become predominant. The adverse effects of antenatal experiences during fetal development also make a contribution (as Chapter 3 described). This means that the rapid advances in medical genetics are likely to have a particular impact on child health.[8]

The prevalence or incidence of illness in children has to be considered in relation to the *age* of the child. There are substantial changes with age in the absolute level of the incidence of illnesses and there are also systematic changes in the *type* of illness that is more prevalent at different ages. In order to establish accurate prevalence and incidence figures it is essential to try to identify all children or a random sample of all children in an area of a certain age, rather than for example those attending health clinics or those seen by a doctor or health visitor.

☐ Why might prevalence and incidence figures based on the latter populations be unreliable?

■ Attendance at clinics, visits to doctors and visits by health visitors are likely to be affected by *social* and *psychological* variations; by caregivers' ease of access to health services, their attitudes towards illness and health care generally and, in older children and adolescents, by their own decisions about whether or not to seek medical examination or treatment.

Population prevalence rates for children with **congenital abnormalities** are given in Figure 4.3. These are abnormalities that are apparent at birth and which vary in severity and in their implications for the child's long-term

[8]Advances in medical genetics are discussed in *Human Biology and Health: An Evolutionary Approach*, Chapter 9.

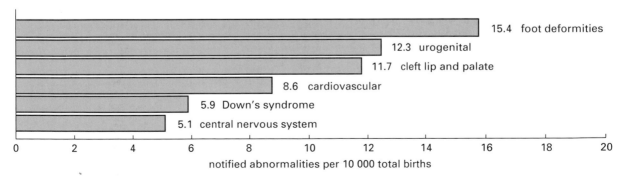

Figure 4.3 *The rate of selected congenital abnormalities per 10 000 total births, notified within 10 days of birth, England and Wales, 1990. (Source: Woodroffe et al., 1993, Figure 2.39, p. 49; data derived from OPCS MB3/6)*

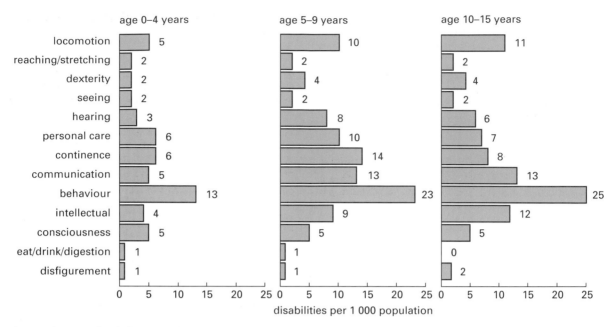

Figure 4.4 *Age-related changes in the rate of different disabilities in childhood (both sexes combined), per 1 000 population in each age-group, Great Britain, 1985–8. (Source: Woodroffe et al., 1993, Figure 2.28, p. 42; data derived from Bone, M. and Meltzer, H., 1989,* The Prevalence of Disability among Children, *OPCS Surveys of Disability in Great Britain, report 3, HMSO, London)*

health. It should also be noted that these categories are not independent, e.g. children with Down's syndrome are likely also to show cardiovascular problems.

The data in Figure 4.4 provide an age-related breakdown of the types of disability shown in children. There are age-related changes in certain types of disability; for example, locomotor disability and communication difficulties become more apparent after the pre-school period. There are also some areas where disability becomes less marked with age, e.g. continence is identified as a problem less frequently once the child enters adolescence. What Figure 4.4 does not reveal is that the overall rate of disability is about one and a half times higher in boys than it is in girls; this is a reflection of the consistently greater vulnerability of males at all stages of the lifespan.

Chronic illness

By far the main sources of **chronic illness** in children are those that concern the respiratory system. In Figure 4.5 the rate of long-standing *respiratory illnesses* is given as 78 per 1 000 (7.8 per cent) of children under the age of 15 years.

Possible influences on long-term illness in children may be identified from further research on the 'programming hypothesis' put forward by David Barker and

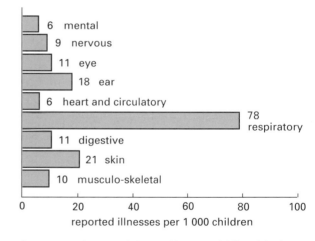

Figure 4.5 *The rate of chronic illness in childhood (both sexes combined), per 1 000 children aged 0–15 years, Great Britain, 1989. (Source: Woodroffe et al., 1993, Figure 2.26, p. 41; data derived from OPCS GHS 20)*

colleagues (mentioned earlier). Experiences in the womb (*in utero*) are thought to have long-term effects on health. This process is illustrated by findings from several other research groups on the long-term impact of maternal smoking during pregnancy. It has been found that babies born to mothers who smoke are on average 200 grams lighter than other babies. Mothers who smoke during pregnancy are twice as likely to enter into premature labour. This experience *in utero* often has long-term implications for health because of the increased risk associated with these adverse perinatal events.

Unfortunately the child of parents who smoke is also highly likely to have continuing adverse experiences after birth. It has been estimated that maternal smoking contributes to about one-third of sudden infant deaths (Royal College of Physicians, 1992). The same report calculated that 17 000 hospital admissions to children under the age of five years are attributable to parental smoking, especially for asthma and respiratory infections.

Current changes

There are new threats to child health in the 1990s in industrialised countries such as the United Kingdom. For example, an increasing level of atmospheric pollutants may be reflected in an increase in the prevalence of *asthma* in children.[9] Infection with the *Human Immunodeficiency Virus* (HIV) is likely to become of increasing concern in child health. To date, the majority of children with HIV in the United Kingdom became infected via blood factor transfusions to treat haemophilia. However, a very small number of babies is being born each year with HIV transmitted from their mothers; if a pregnant woman is infected with HIV there is a 15 per cent chance that her baby will be born with the infection. The transmission of HIV in the general population through heterosexual intercourse is now established, although its prevalence in mothers is still very low. In February 1994, an editorial in the *British Medical Journal* recommended that HIV should be considered as a possible diagnosis in any child presenting with unexplained severe illness, at least in areas with high HIV prevalence, such as parts of Edinburgh and London (*British Medical Journal*, 1994).

The picture of health, illness and disability in children in the United Kingdom is one where the pattern of morbidity and mortality has changed radically during the last 50 years. No longer are infections the major cause of death in infants and young children. This means that other threats to the health and quality of life of children have become proportionately more significant.

---

[9]Reasons for the increase in the prevalence of childhood asthma are discussed in *Experiencing and Explaining Disease* (revised edition, 1995); they include pollution and changes in diagnostic criteria.

Psychiatric and psychological disorders in childhood

Public concerns about child health are usually centred on life-threatening acute illnesses (e.g. meningitis), those that represent profound physical disability (e.g. cerebral palsy) or create chronic illness (e.g. cystic fibrosis). The significance of psychiatric and psychological disorders in children is often overlooked. It has been found in epidemiological studies in both urban and non-urban settings within the United Kingdom that the largest source of morbidity in children is **psychiatric disorders**, that is, disorders recognised as distinct diagnostic categories within medical psychiatry. **Psychological disorders** are also of great importance: these include behavioural problems that fall outside psychiatric diagnoses, learning difficulties, reading disabilities and so on. Their prevalence was illustrated earlier (Figure 4.4), which shows that at all ages the most common form of disability was that associated with behaviour problems: the rate per 1 000 children was 13, 23 and 25 at ages 0–4, 5–9 and 10–15 years respectively. This was more than twice the rate at each age for locomotor disabilities such as cerebral palsy.

Often the treatment of psychiatric and psychological disorders is thought of as less significant than the maintenance of physical health. A commonly-held view is that such disorders in children are not primary, but rather represent normal children's responses to stressful events in the family or school. There are two fallacies in this line of argument.

First, many behaviours are not simply a child's reaction to *current* stressful events and circumstances; once the stress is reduced, the child's behaviour does not always improve. (This is in contrast to aspects of physical development, which often show good recovery from temporary stresses.) In a study published in 1982 of several hundred children followed from their third to their eighth birthday, a team from the Institute of Child Health, University of London (Naomi Richman, Jim Stevenson and Philip Graham), were able to show that *adverse family factors*, such as a marriage with low mutual support, or maternal depression, were related to whether the child showed behaviour problems at three years, e.g. sleep disturbance, challenging behaviour, temper tantrums. The presence of these adverse features in families of children *not* showing behaviour problems at three years was related to the *subsequent* onset of behaviour problems. However, such behaviour problems did not disappear if the adverse factors subsequently improved. It appears that although children's behavioural and emotional disturbances are influenced by stresses within the family, they cannot be remedied simply by taking away the adverse factors that caused them.

Second, many of the behavioural and emotional disturbances shown by children have been found to be influenced by biological (often genetic) factors. For example, look at Table 4.1, which is taken from a review of genetic influences on psychiatric and psychological disorders in children by LaBuda *et al.* (1993). This review was based on studies that compared the similarity of *monozygotic* (genetically identical) twin pairs with that of *dizygotic* (non-identical) twin pairs, who share in common 50 per cent of the genes that vary between unrelated people. Data from studies of twin pairs can be used to estimate **heritability**, that is, the extent to which, within a particular population, the condition is influenced by genetic difference between children: a heritability value of 1.00 indicates that the condition is completely determined by genetic factors and a value of zero indicates that no genetic factors are involved.[10]

Findings such as those in Table 4.1 suggest that for a number of childhood psychiatric disorders genetic factors are paramount: for example, *autism*—a profound disorder of normal social relationships and language ability which is often accompanied by low intelligence, and *attention deficit hyperactivity disorder*—an inability to sustain concentration on a task as part of a generally disorganised and chaotic behavioural style often accompanied by restlessness and inability to sit still. For other conditions, variation in the nature and quality of the environment experienced by the child is primary: for example, *conduct disorder*—an anti-social behavioural style often associated with physical or verbal aggression and rule breaking, such as destruction of property.

The experience of psychological disturbances can be just as profoundly handicapping for the child as a physical disability or illness; these are not self-limiting conditions from which a child can recover unaided. Note, however, that even if there are indications that a certain psychiatric disorder is highly heritable, it does not follow that intervention is thus unlikely to be effective. Just as in the cases of the growth disorders of diabetes and phenylketonuria, environmental manipulations can drastically change the impact of the genetic problem.

[10]Heritability estimates based on twin studies are discussed further in *Human Biology and Health: An Evolutionary Approach*, Chapter 4.

Table 4.1 Selected twin heritabilities for psychiatric and psychological disorders with childhood onset

Psychiatric/psychological disorder	Heritability value
autism	1.00
anorexia nervosa	0.78
obsessive compulsive disorder	0.68
hyperactivity	0.64
Tourette's syndrome	0.64
reading disability	0.48

Data derived from LaBuda *et al.* (1993) Usefulness of twin studies for exploring the etiology of childhood and adolescent psychiatric disorders, *American Journal of Medical Genetics*, **48**(1), pp. 47–59.

□ What does this tell us about the meaning and limits of heritability statistics?

■ It shows that heritability statistics are only valid insofar as they relate to the environments within which the studied individuals grew up; radically different environments *might* generate very different heritability estimates if the gene expression is hence modified. A high heritability figure associated with a particular aspect of development shows a strong genetic component, but does not *necessarily* mean that nothing can be done to ameliorate the impact of the genetic factor.

The development of autonomy

A feature of child development that is central to issues of health is the gradual move from high dependency on parental care to one of increasing **autonomy** in children's decisions about aspects of behaviour and lifestyle that influence health, as well as many other aspects of children's lives such as their friendships and recreation. In this concluding section of the chapter, we have drawn primarily on data from research studies carried out on children in the USA, where investigation of key concepts in the development of autonomy (such as 'locus of control' and compliance with medical treatment, both discussed later) has a longer and more established history than in the United Kingdom. However, the findings from American studies can be applied—with due caution—to the children of other Western industrialised nations.

The first major transition was described in Chapter 3, namely, the switch at birth from a physiological dependency on the mother's body to one of independent respiration and excretion, and a degree of control over the intake of nutrients. Later childhood developmental transitions are more subtle and less immediately life-threatening. They concern the regulation of diet, patterns of activity and sleep, risk taking in relation to lifestyle (accidents in childhood are the subject of Chapter 5 of this book; alcohol, drug-use and sexual activity in adolescence are discussed in Chapter 6), and decisions about when to consult for medical advice and whether to comply with the advice given. These changes involve caregivers and health professionals in considerations about the cognitive (i.e. intellectual) development of children—do they have sufficient understanding of the issues involved to be able to make an informed choice? For example, a 4-year-old would not be expected to understand the implications of a prolonged fever and therefore be able to decide when to seek medical assistance. There are also concerns about the child being sufficiently mature to carry the 'emotional load' associated with decision making in relation to health care. It is inappropriate to expect children as young as 5

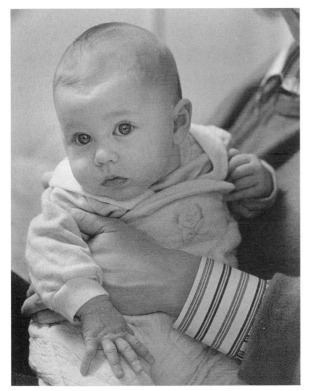

While still dependent in some ways, the young baby has already gone through the major transition at birth from physiological dependence to relative autonomy.
(Photo: Mike Levers)

or 6 to make choices between alternative treatments (e.g. request antibiotics or allow the immune system to fight an infection unaided).

☐ What factors should be taken into account when deciding how far to involve a child in choices about his or her treatment?

■ One key factor is the level of a child's understanding of the illness, its causes and treatment. Such understandings form part of the child's general cognitive development, which undergoes radical changes before adolescence. An assessment of a child's level of cognitive function is thus relevant to decisions about the extent of the child's involvement in key treatment choices.

Children aged 3 to 5 years often cannot provide a clear account of the origins of illness; by 6 to 7 years they tend to attribute illness to infection, and by 8 to 9 years they identify 'germs' as the agents producing ill-health; finally, by 11 to 12 years they are able to appreciate that illnesses can have a range of multiple causes. In addition, some young children interpret illness as a punishment for their own bad behaviour (an interpretation which they can also apply to accidental injury, as you will see in Chapter 5).

Locus of control

Attitudes towards and beliefs about health change through childhood and adolescence. One facet of health beliefs concerns what is called **locus of control**. In relation to health, this indicates whether you see your health as something you can determine (*internal* locus of control) or as something largely controlled by others or by fate (*external* locus of control). Adults seem to differ from one another in their position on a continuum between these two extremes, but there is also a complicated set of changes with age. For example, in 1990, Rita Yopp Cohen and other psychologists from the University of Delaware found that in a sample of nearly 4 000 children aged 9 to 17 years, the younger boys were more likely to show an internal locus of control than young girls. In the adolescents on the other hand the sex difference was reversed. The findings from this large study indicated that 11 and 12 are crucial ages for health education since it is at this age that health behaviour and attitudes tend to become fixed.

Autonomy in health decisions

Children themselves expect and are expected by others to take increasing responsibility for their own health care as they get older. These expectations from others should be based on knowledge of children's emergent understandings of the nature of illness. With adults, those responsible for health care can misunderstand the situation, but with children the sources for confusion are more complex. Take the following example involving a 13-year-old boy with cancer:

> Jim was referred for psychiatric consultation with the question of psychotic behaviour. There was nothing in the history of his 13 years to suggest psychosis. Talking with the nurse who asked for the consultation revealed that Jim refused loudly to have an IV [intravenous drip] placed which was necessary for the delivery of the antimetabolite [drug]. It was not conceivable at the time to the nurse that anyone would refuse potential life-giving treatment. This created such disbelief and anxiety that the mental health consultant was called. After a brief interview with Jim, who clearly needed to feel that he had some control over his own destiny, control that was taken away by his cancer, management suggestions were discussed with the nurse to allow for such control. By allowing Jim to choose the time (medicine had to be given once a day), the site of the IV, and to keep track of the flow (reporting to the nurse if any deviation occurred), the nurse found that no further difficulties arose. (O'Malley and Koocher, 1977, p. 55)

□ On the basis of the above case, and with reference back to the discussion of the ICD-10 classification system, can you explain why a simple analysis of the illness itself is inadequate in planning the details of treatment?

■ The management of the difficulty in the treatment of this boy illustrates a general principle: that it is essential to supplement the disorder diagnosis with a careful assessment of the feelings and thoughts of the child, as well as their level of understanding of the issues involved, before implementing decisions on care. Often these will be specific to the individual concerned and will require individually-tailored care plans to be made.

Compliance with treatment

One condition where extensive research on **compliance** with medical treatment and advice has been carried out is insulin-dependent diabetes mellitus (IDDM). A research group at the University of Florida led by Suzanne Bennett Johnson have undertaken an extensive examination of the factors associated with compliance amongst children and adolescents with IDDM (Johnson *et al.*, 1990). They have shown that compliance is complex in that young

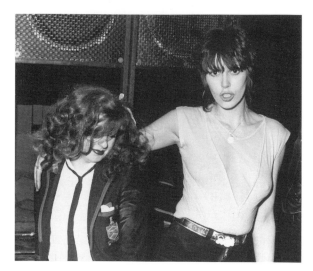

Adolescents tend to be less conforming than young children. (Photo: Mike Levers)

people who are diligent about one aspect of their care, e.g. regulating diet, are not necessarily those who are most careful in other aspects, e.g. monitoring blood glucose levels. In general, adolescents were *less* compliant than younger children with IDDM.

This illustrates a broader tendency that accompanies increased self-regulation in adolescents, namely a greater tendency towards unconventionality (this is discussed further in Chapter 6); even healthy adolescents tend to be less conforming than younger children. However, it has also been found that those adolescents and young people who are more generally unconventional in their behaviour and attitudes are also less likely to follow guidelines on health-related behaviours concerning diet, exercise, substance use and so on (Donovan *et al.*, 1991).

Autonomy and genetic influences

At the same time as the child achieves greater autonomy in health care, this very feature of self-determination may be contributing to an *increase* in the extent to which the child's development is influenced by genetic factors. Figure 4.6 is taken from a paper published in 1983 by Ron Wilson, who directed the Louisville Twin Study. The closer the correlation is to 1.00, the greater the similarity in IQ (intelligence quotient) between a pair of twins.

□ Describe the trend over time in Figure 4.6.

■ The IQ of genetically identical twins gradually becomes more similar as they get older and at the same time the IQ of non-identical twins becomes less similar.

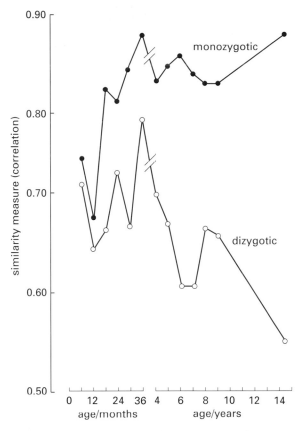

Figure 4.6 *Similarity in IQ (intelligence quotient) between members of monozygotic or dizygotic twin pairs, studied from 6 months to 15 years (Data derived from Wilson, R., 1983, The Louisville Twin Study: developmental synchronies in behavior,* Child Development, ***54**(2), pp. 298–316, Table 2)*

for example in terms of influences on sensation seeking, on substance use and on diet. Developmental psychologists such as Robert Plomin have begun to argue that conventional thinking about the ways that nature and nurture interact will have to be radically altered (Plomin and Bergeman, 1991).

The sorts of models that developmental psychologists are finding increasingly useful in describing such interactions are **transactional models**. In such models, development is seen as the outcome of complex multidirectional effects between child and environment. For example, a child's behavioural style may evoke particular child-rearing behaviours from the child's parents (the child producing a change in the social environment) which then evoke particular behaviours in the child and lead to particular sorts of child learning occurring (the environment producing a change in the child). In such *transactions*, both child and environment are seen as co-determining development and a simple partitioning of effects into either 'nature' or 'nurture' is not meaningful.

Conclusions

This chapter has shown how health in children can be viewed from a developmental perspective. This orientation sees health in children as the maintenance of growth and development within normal limits. Illness is then considered as a departure from this normal sequence of changes. This view of health is only appropriate while the child is maturing physically and is developing new abilities. The maintenance of normal growth and development is dependent on individual children's biological make-up, the quality of their psychological, social and material environment, and the experiences they encounter.

During the course of development, children become more able to determine the type of environment they wish to experience—given prevailing socio-economic and cultural constraints. This relative autonomy in terms of lifestyle has very significant life-long implications for health, for example in terms of deciding on whether to smoke cigarettes, what type of diet to eat and how much exercise to take. At the same time that the child/adolescent is becoming more autonomous, genetic differences between individuals may come to exert an increasing influence over the nature of the environment the child will choose and experience.

Although similar results have been found for aggressive and anti-social behaviour, at present there is a lack of information on possible parallel findings in other aspects of development. It is thought that the phenomenon illustrated in Figure 4.6 is produced by the child and adolescent gradually becoming more able to select their own activities as they become older. This means that any *genetic* tendency to behave in certain ways or to seek out specific types of environment or experiences will become *more* marked as the child gets older. Most people would expect that as you get older genetic factors become *less* significant, as accumulated experiences gradually form your personality. Instead the reverse seems to be true. The implications of these influences for health have only just begun to be explored in the 1990s,

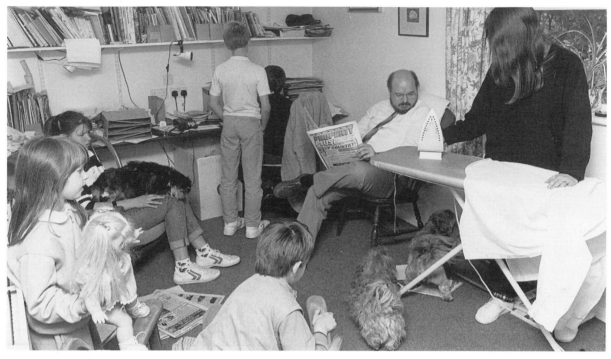

Development is the outcome of complex multi-directional effects between child and environment. (Photo: Mike Levers)

OBJECTIVES FOR CHAPTER 4

When you have studied this chapter, you should be able to:

4.1 Give examples to illustrate a concept of health and illness in children based on normal and abnormal growth and development, and discuss the interaction of genetic and environmental factors in children's health.

4.2 Summarise the most prevalent forms of morbidity (both physical and psychological) in children up to adolescence, noting the sources of difficulty in and the value of assessing a child's overall health status and quality of life.

4.3 Describe the main features of the development of increasing autonomy in health-related behaviour during childhood and early adolescence, and comment on the likely implications for children's health.

QUESTIONS FOR CHAPTER 4

Question 1 (*Objective 4.1*)

What are the strengths and limitations of defining health in children as the maintenance of normal growth and development? How usefully could such a definition be applied to later stages of the lifespan?

Question 2 (*Objective 4.2*)

How has the level and type of childhood illness changed during the twentieth century in the United Kingdom?

Question 3 (*Objectives 4.1 and 4.3*)

Do children simply become more competent at looking after their own health as they get older? Give reasons for your answer which refer both to social and biological development.

5 Children and accidents

During your study of this chapter you will be asked to read an article entitled 'Prevention is better ...' by Helen Roberts, Susan Smith and Carol Bryce, which appears in the Reader.[1] The television programme, 'First steps to autonomy', is relevant to this chapter. The principal author, Judith Green, is a Senior Lecturer in Sociology in the Department of Legal, Political and Social Sciences at South Bank University in London; she has published widely on her research into primary care, the organisation of hospital emergency services, and accidents. Basiro Davey, from the U205 Course Team, developed the distance-teaching aspects of this chapter.

Introduction

Childhood accidents are so common they can be described as endemic in all sections of society and in all regions of the United Kingdom, but the scale and severity of the problem is often underestimated. When researchers in South Glamorgan studied the records of hospital Accident and Emergency (A&E) departments in their area, they concluded that accidental injury to children was an 'endemic of epidemic proportions' (Sibert *et al.*, 1981). Childhood accidents are a major cause of premature death, acquired disability, morbidity and distress. The 1991 Green Paper *The Health of the Nation*, published by the Department of Health, noted that accidents were the most common cause of death under the age of 30 and estimated that they accounted for 13 per cent of all years of life lost under the age of 65, and for 7 per cent of NHS expenditure. An accident can happen to anyone but, in an environment designed by adults, children and young people are particularly vulnerable. Reducing the impact of accidental injury on children is an important task for Britain's public health services.

[1] *Health and Disease: A Reader* (second edition, 1995).

The epidemiology of childhood accidents

Mortality

Although the accident mortality rate is falling in the United Kingdom, accidents remain the major cause of death for children and young people aged between 1 and 30 (Table 5.1).

Table 5.1 Leading causes of death under the age of 30 years in the United Kingdom in 1987 (numbers of deaths in that year are given in brackets)

Age-group/ years	First ranked cause	Second	Third
under 1	sudden infant death syndrome (1 489)	congenital abnormalities (687)	respiratory diseases (364)
1–4	accidents (269)	congenital abnormalities (250)	cancer (122)
5–9	accidents (214)	cancer (131)	congenital abnormalities (73)
10–14	accidents (271)	cancer (131)	congenital abnormalities (57)
15–19	accidents (1 018)	cancer (210)	congenital abnormalities (83)
20–24	accidents (1 123)	cancer (280)	congenital abnormalities (80)
25–29	accidents (770)	cancer (418)	heart disease (107)

Source: NAHA/RoSPA Strategy Group (1990) *Action on Accidents*, NAHA/RoSPA, Birmingham, p. 8.

☐ What relationship between the number of accidental deaths and age-group is revealed by Table 5.1?

■ The number of accidental deaths is more or less the same for the age-groups listed between 1 and 14 years, but rises very sharply to roughly four times that number for the age-groups between 15 and 24 years, with some decline between 25 and 29.

In this chapter we are primarily concerned with the younger age-groups; the contribution of risk-taking behaviour to mortality among older teenagers is discussed in Chapter 6.

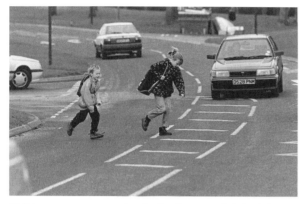

Children may not recognise the inadequacy of their ability to judge speed and distance when crossing busy roads, particularly when bad weather makes visibility poor. (Photo: Mike Levers)

Data collected by the Office of Public Censuses and Surveys (OPCS, 1993d) shows that, in 1991, 425 boys and 226 girls aged under 14 died from accidental injuries: this represents 10 per cent of all deaths for this age-group.[2] About half of these deaths were due to road traffic accidents. Although the numbers of deaths are not large, the social cost is enormous. As Chapter 12 will indicate, most people in the United Kingdom now die in their old age and the deaths of children and young adults are experienced as particularly distressing. Mortality from causes such as infectious disease is generally low in industrialised countries, and accidents therefore represent a relatively large proportion of the mortality for children and young people. As accidents disproportionately affect children and young people, this represents a significant number of years of potential life lost.[3]

[2]This figure includes deaths for which it was unknown whether the injuries were accidentally or purposefully inflicted.

[3]Years of life lost as a method of representing mortality data is discussed in *World Health and Disease*, Chapter 3.

Accidents cause the unexpected deaths of previously healthy children and many of these deaths could have been prevented.

☐ Look at the causes of fatal accidents to children, shown in Table 5.2. What do you notice about where they happen?

■ Most fatal accidents happen on the road, where pedestrians are the most vulnerable. The next most dangerous place for children is the home, where the most common cause of accidental death is fire.

Table 5.2 Leading causes of fatal accidents to children under 15 in the United Kingdom in 1987

Type of accident	Number of deaths	Percentage of total
pedestrians	260	31
burns and fires (mainly home)	119	14
vehicle occupants	96	11
pedal cyclists ·	73	9
drownings (home and elsewhere)	63	7
choking on food	50	6
falls (home and elsewhere)	40	5
suffocation (home)	34	4
others (includes electrocution, falling object, poisoning)	107	14

Source: NAHA/RoSPA Strategy Group (1990) *Action on Accidents*, NAHA/RoSPA, Birmingham, p. 9.

Morbidity

Fatal accidents may be the major cause of childhood deaths but, as childhood mortality is generally low in the United Kingdom, they are still a relatively rare occurrence. However, non-fatal accidents needing some medical treatment are very common and minor accidental injuries are experienced by almost all children. Serious accidents can cause physical disabilities, psychological damage and incalculable suffering. It has been estimated by the Child Accident Prevention Trust (CAPT, 1989) that about 10 000 children annually are permanently disabled by accidents. For every child who suffers a serious accident, many more need medical treatment: one in five children visits a hospital A&E department with an injury each year (Sibert *et al.*, 1981). Studies from general practice report similar estimates for the numbers of children needing some medical attention (Carter and Jones, 1993). Many more accidents are unreported, but nevertheless result in pain or distress to the child and anxiety for parents.

The causes of non-fatal accidents are distributed rather differently from those of fatal accidents. Many examples can be found in a comprehensive review entitled *Children, Teenagers and Health: The Key Data*, by epidemiologist Caroline Woodroffe and her colleagues from the Wolfson Child Health Monitoring Unit (Woodroffe *et al.*, 1993). For instance, although poisoning accounts for few deaths of those under 15 years old, it causes considerable distress and necessitated the hospital admission of about 12 000 children in this age-group in 1985. Similarly, fires are a major cause of fatal home accidents, but account for only a small proportion of non-fatal home accidents requiring medical treatment. Looking only at the major causes of fatal accidents would give a misleading picture of the injury and trauma caused by all accidents. As the general practitioner is often the first contact for treatment for minor injuries, general practice records can help identify the range of common accidents affecting children. Although the data in Table 5.3 are based only on the under-5s, they illustrate some of these causes.

□ Compare the causes of fatal accidents shown earlier in Table 5.2 with those of the non-fatal accidents seen by general practitioners (GPs) in Table 5.3. How do they differ?

■ A much larger proportion of these non-fatal accidents to young children happen in the home. Although the road is the site of about one-third of fatal accidents to the under-5s, few non-fatal road accidents are reported to GPs. Fires and burns account for a large proportion of deaths, but relatively few of the non-fatal accidents. Falls are the major cause of injuries (often serious) needing medical attention, although they are not a leading cause of fatal accidents and might be ignored if we were to focus just on the leading causes of fatal accidents.

Interpreting the statistics: definitions and implications

The statistics given so far in this chapter provide a useful profile of accidental death and morbidity in childhood, which helps to identify some of the hazards for children, but we need to treat them with some caution.

First, there is some ambiguity in the meaning given to the term 'accident'. All definitions of an **accident** agree that it denotes a *non-intentional* injury, but in everyday speech this tends to imply an event that was 'no one's fault', a random chance occurrence that could not be prevented. This notion of an accident is one that has been criticised by epidemiologists and experts in accident prevention, who argue that it encourages the view that nothing can be done about accidents—'they just happen'. They point to the fact that the distribution of accidental injuries and deaths is not random, so accidents cannot be due to chance alone: there are specific hazards and some groups of children are more likely to be injured or die than others. It has been argued that we could use a more objective word (such as 'injury'), which would not imply that they are unpreventable misfortunes. However, the word 'accident' is commonly used to differentiate injuries that were *not* intentionally caused from those that were, and it is unlikely that it will disappear from everyday usage.

Table 5.3 Causes of accidents among 100 children aged under 5 years in a north Staffordshire general practice survey conducted in 1991

Cause	Number of accidents (N = 120)	(percentage of total in brackets)
falls		
on the same level	28	(23.3)
from one level to another	23	(19.2)
stairs	14	(11.7)
from buildings	1	(0.8)
other	1	(0.8)
bumping into objects	11	(9.2)
pulling/twisting	7	(5.8)
foreign body (swallowed/in nose)	7	(5.8)
jamming/crushing	6	(5.0)
ingestion of poisons	6	(5.0)
bicycle	5	(4.2)
fires and heat	4	(3.3)
cuts by sharp object	2	(1.7)
road traffic accidents (other than bicycles)	2	(1.7)
scalds	2	(1.7)
stings	1	(0.8)

Source: Carter, Y. H. and Jones, P. W. (1993) Accidents among children under five years old: a general practice based study in north Staffordshire, *British Journal of General Practice*, **43**, p. 161.

Second, there is a further problem in defining 'intentional' injuries. In recent years, 'non-accidental injury' or **child abuse** has been more widely recognised as a cause of childhood injury, and so has become more readily diagnosed. Many injuries that were classified as 'accidental' in the past are now recognised as intentional, and apparent reductions in accident rates may reflect changes in the ways we define various causes of death. What counts as an 'accident' may change over time, making it difficult to interpret historical statistics on accident mortality rates, even for recent decades. Like other statistics, accident rates are not an objective measure, but reflect in part the beliefs and concerns of those people who produce them.

Third, deaths are attributed to accidents when there is no natural cause for the death and the death was not intentional. It is difficult to know how reliable judgements about 'natural causes' and 'intention' are, as they can both be contested, as research by the author of this chapter has shown (Green, 1992). After a coroner's verdict of 'accidental death', for example, it is not uncommon to read reports in the media that disagree that the death was 'an accident' because someone could be blamed for it. An example of changing ideas about 'natural causes' is Sudden Infant Death Syndrome, now the major cause of death for children under one year (see Table 5.1). These deaths were only assigned to a separate category in the mortality statistics in 1971: before then many were classified as 'accidental suffocation' or as deaths from unknown cause (OPCS, 1982).

We also need to be cautious about the reliability of morbidity data. There are no national databases of non-fatal accidents, and many different agencies are responsible for collecting these data: the Department of Trade and Industry collects information about home accidents from its surveys of A&E departments; the Department of Transport is responsible for collating road accident statistics. Although these statistics are based on much larger numbers than is the case for mortality data, there are sources of potential bias.

◻ What sources of bias can you think of in using the number of people seeking treatment at A&E departments as a measure of morbidity from accidents?

■ A&E attendance figures can only show the number of people who decide to attend for treatment. This decision is likely to be affected by a number of factors, such as how far away the hospital is, how serious the injury is perceived to be and past experience of health care for similar injuries.

Similarly, many injuries from road accidents, particularly if they only involve injuries to pedal cyclists (those most likely to happen to children), are never reported to the police and so do not appear in traffic accident statistics (Department of Transport, 1993).

Inequalities in the risk of accident

So far, we have looked at the overall patterns of childhood mortality and morbidity based on aggregated data for the whole population. When we examine these data in more detail, we can begin to see how accidents are not randomly distributed throughout the childhood population, but are distributed unequally by social factors such as age, gender and social class. Studying these patterns gives important insights into potential causes of children's accidents.

Age

The major causes of injury and death from accidents change as children get older. In the first year of life, suffocation and choking are the most common cause of accidental death. For the under-5s, the home is the site of most accidental deaths, where the major causes are fires, drowning, choking and suffocation, poisoning and scalds. Figure 5.1 shows that as children get older, road traffic accidents become increasingly important: between 1987 and 1990 they accounted for 35 per cent of accidental deaths for 1–4 year olds, but 81 per cent of accidental deaths of 15–19 year olds. Other research has shown that, in 1990, two-thirds of the under-15s killed or seriously injured in road traffic accidents were pedestrians, whereas those aged 15 and over were more likely to be car occupants or motorcycle riders (Woodroffe et al., 1993, pp. 121–2, based on data from the Department of Transport's Casualty Report, 1992).

◻ How can these age differences be explained?

■ As children develop biologically and psychologically, and move from close dependency on their parents to increasing autonomy, they are exposed to different environmental hazards. Infants are less mobile, so the major risks are from suffocation. As children get older, they spend more time playing outside the home and are more likely to face hazards on the roads before they have developed the necessary abilities to judge traffic speed and distance adequately. The high mortality rate of adolescents aged 15–19 is accounted for by the high rate of road traffic accidents in this group, who are learning to face the additional risks of motorcycle and car driving.

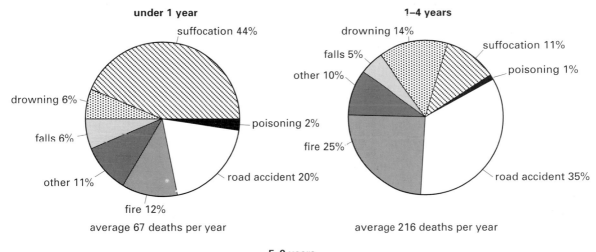

under 1 year

suffocation 44%

drowning 6%

falls 6%

other 11%

fire 12%

poisoning 2%

road accident 20%

average 67 deaths per year

1–4 years

drowning 14%

falls 5%

other 10%

suffocation 11%

poisoning 1%

fire 25%

road accident 35%

average 216 deaths per year

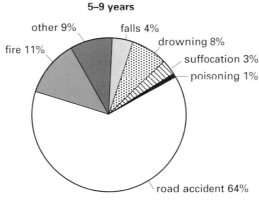

5–9 years

other 9%

fire 11%

falls 4%

drowning 8%

suffocation 3%

poisoning 1%

road accident 64%

average 188 deaths per year

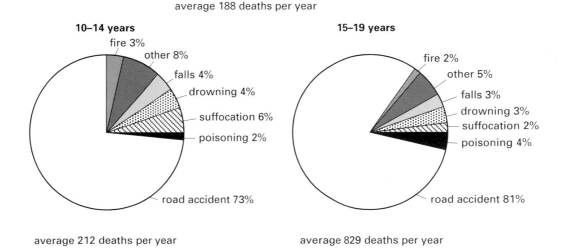

10–14 years

fire 3%

other 8%

falls 4%

drowning 4%

suffocation 6%

poisoning 2%

road accident 73%

average 212 deaths per year

15–19 years

fire 2%

other 5%

falls 3%

drowning 3%

suffocation 2%

poisoning 4%

road accident 81%

average 829 deaths per year

Figure 5.1 *Types of fatal accident to children at different ages in England and Wales between 1987 and 1990 (Source: Woodroffe et al., 1993, p.115, based on data from OPCS/DH2)*

ISLE COLLEGE
RESOURCES CENTRE

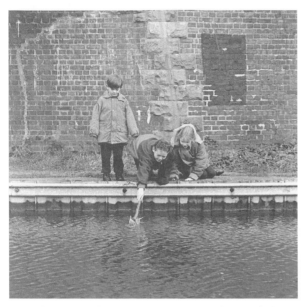

As children get older, they face increasing risks outside the home and parents have the difficult task of balancing their safety against their needs for outdoor exercise and independent play. (Photo: Mike Levers)

Broad categories of accidental death also obscure age differences which reflect these different environmental risks. For example, a study of all child deaths from drowning in the United Kingdom in 1988–9 by two doctors, Alison Kemp and J. R. Sibert, showed that the mean age of children who drowned in the bath was just over a year, whereas it was around two years for those who drowned in garden ponds or domestic swimming pools, and around seven years for children who died in rivers, canals, lakes and the sea (Kemp and Sibert, 1992).

Gender

There are also gender differences in the rates and causes of accident mortality, which have not been adequately explained as yet. At all ages, boys are more likely to die from accidental injury than girls.

The gender difference is most obvious in the 16–19 age-group, when road traffic accidents account for the largest proportion of fatal accidents. According to the Department of Transport's *Casualty Report*, 477 males aged 16–19 years died from accidents in 1992 (Department of Transport, 1993). Of these, 378 (79 per cent) were road accident deaths. In comparison, 149 females in the same age-group died from accidents, with 115 (77 per cent) killed in road accidents. Such differences are likely to reflect different gender roles and the expectations we have of young adults: young men may be more likely to

own motorcycles and to drive cars, and thus risk more road accidents. In the younger age-groups, we may encourage girls to be more aware of physical risks, whereas boys are expected to engage in more 'rough and tumble' play which inevitably exposes them to higher risk of accidental injury. There is some evidence to support this view in a survey carried out by the Policy Studies Institute, which found that parents were more likely to allow boys aged 7–11 to cross roads on their own and to cycle on main roads than they would girls of the same age (Hillman *et al.*, 1990).

There has been much debate about whether some children are 'accident prone', and if so, whether there are specific psychological traits such as high levels of aggression or hyperactivity that might contribute to this tendency. Although common sense might suggest that some children do seem to have more accidents than others, it is difficult to demonstrate this in research. A child who appears to be accident prone may be a child who is exposed to a more hazardous environment than others: it is difficult to separate psychological attributes from social factors. An American study which did attempt to control for social factors such as crowding in the home and material possessions, suggested that traits like aggression and over-activity were related to how many accidents children had, and how serious those accidents were, particularly for boys (Bijur *et al.*, 1988). If there is a relationship between gender, individual psychology and

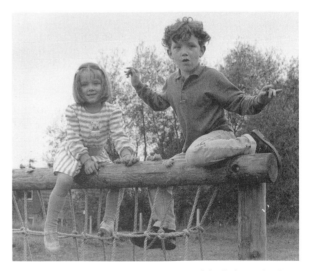

Girls may be socialised to be more careful of physical risks, whereas boys are encouraged to be more physically daring and thus risk more accidents. (Photo: Mike Levers)

accidental injury it will be difficult to tease out. We return to this issue later in the chapter.

Social class

In 1980, the 'Black Report' (Department of Health and Social Security, 1980) which examined social-class inequalities in health, reported that the social-class gradient for accidental injury in childhood was more pronounced than for any other cause of death. As Table 5.4 shows, in the early 1970s fatal accidents disproportionately affected children from lower social classes: for example, girls aged 1–14 years with a father from social class V had a risk of fatal accident three times that of girls with a father in social class I. For boys, the risk was five times greater.

Table 5.4 Fatal accidents in children aged 1–14 years in Britain in 1970–2, by sex and social class (mortality rates per 100 000 population)

Children	Social class of father					
	I	II	IIIN	IIIM	IV	V
boys	25.8	39.0	44.5	56.3	66.2	122
girls	18.8	19.0	21.4	24.4	35.1	63.1

Data derived from Office of Population Censuses and Surveys (OPCS), *Occupational Mortality 1970–72*, quoted in the 'Black Report', Department of Health and Social Security (1980) Table 6.7, p. 175. Social class is based on the Registrar-General's classification of father's occupation.

Although the data in Table 5.4 are over two decades old, they are the most recent national statistics available. childhood deaths from *specific causes* (such as accidents) distributed by social class, have not been made publicly available since the 1970s. Table 5.4 must be interpreted with caution: the mortality rates for accidental deaths have fallen sharply since the 1970s, and we cannot tell how this change has affected the 'gap' between the social classes. However, it is reasonable to suggest that a social-class gradient still exists for childhood accidents in the 1990s, for two reasons. First, most causes of death in *adult* age-groups, including accidents, continue to be published nationally by social class and are more prevalent in lower than in higher social classes[4] it is unlikely that children have become exempt from this persistent trend.

[4]See *World Health and Disease*, Chapter 9, for details of social-class gradients in mortality and morbidity in the United Kingdom, and Chapter 10 for a discussion of whether these differences are real or an artefact of the way the data are collected.

Second, national data *are* published on social class and childhood mortality from *all causes combined* (Table 5.5) and these show a very marked social-class gradient. Since accidents are the largest contributor to these deaths, the data strongly suggest that children from lower social classes remain more likely to die in accidents than their middle-class counterparts, and that the effect of social class on mortality is particularly evident among boys.

More recent research into the relationship between social class and children's accidents has been based on small local studies, but all studies face particular difficulties in investigating what aspects of a child's social class have an influence on their risk of accidents.

Table 5.5 Mortality of children under 16 years in England and Wales; combined data from 1979–80 and 1982–3, rates per 100 000 population by age, sex and social class

Sex and social class	Age at death/years		
	1–4	5–9	10–14
males			
I	33.04	24.19	20.52
II	34.20	19.04	21.88
IIIN	41.28	22.93	20.26
IIIM	52.70	25.88	26.30
IV	63.84	31.65	30.47
V	111.54	50.14	36.23
I : V ratio	3.38	2.07	1.77
females			
I	33.12	16.53	15.11
II	31.22	15.12	15.44
IIIN	35.84	17.54	14.02
IIIM	41.96	18.34	19.05
IV	52.18	22.56	17.35
V	85.55	30.55	23.94
I : V ratio	2.58	1.85	1.58

Data derived from Office of Population Censuses and Surveys (OPCS) (1988) *Occupational Mortality: Childhood Supplement*, Series DS no. 8, HMSO, London, Table 2.6, p. 20.

□ Briefly explain the main source of difficulty.

■ Father's occupation is the commonest criterion on which the social class of other family members is assessed, but this ignores many other aspects that might have an influence on the risk of accidents: for example, household income, maternal employment, number in the household, crowding, type of accommodation (flat, house, caravan, etc.), use of a car, local environment, presence of adults who smoke, and so on. These confounding factors must be taken into account.[5]

Investigating the relationship between social class and *non-fatal* accidents can be even more problematic, given the additional difficulty (discussed earlier) of measuring the occurrence of morbidity from accidents. For example, one study in west London, by Rafi Alwash and Mark McCarthy (1988), found that children whose father came from social class V were four times more likely to attend hospital with an accident sustained at home than those from social class I (see Table 5.6). The authors also reported that:

> We found a clear trend of greater severity of injuries to children of working class parents. Thus not only do these children have accidents more commonly but their injuries are more severe. (Alwash and McCarthy, 1988, p. 1 453)

Alwash and McCarthy's study identified other factors that increased the risk of a young child having an accident at home, including overcrowded housing and living in accommodation rented from the council. Their data supported other findings which suggest that ethnicity (here indicated by parent's country of birth) is *not* related to accident risk. It seems that relative deprivation, rather than cultural difference, is most important. Interestingly, although the employment status of the father was not related to accident risk, the children whose mothers did *not* have any paid employment were *more* likely to have accidents.

□ Can you suggest any explanations of this finding?

■ Several speculative explanations could be offered: perhaps those who care for children while mothers work are better at protecting children from accidents; or mothers in paid employment may be able to afford more safety equipment; or there could be some connection between mothers' increased

[5]Confounding factors in epidemiological research are discussed in *Studying Health and Disease*, Chapter 8.

Table 5.6 Rates of attendance for treatment, following an accident in a house or garden, of 402 children at a hospital A&E department in west London in a 12-month period (1983–4), by socio-demographic indicators

Socio-demographic indicators	Attendance rates per 1 000 children*
social class	
I and II	19.9
III non-manual	35.3
III manual	35.4
IV	51.3
V	83.8
inadequately described	73.4
parent's country of birth	
British Isles	38.2
Asian	37.0
Caribbean	36.8
other	40.2
father's employment status	
employed	37.7
unemployed	40.1
mother's employment status	
employed	20.7
unemployed	58.9
people per room	
1.5 or under	30.5
more than 1.5	86.8
housing tenure	
owner	30.3
private rent	30.1
council rent	67.0
housing association	61.4

*Adjusted to take distance from hospital into account. Social class was based on father's occupation according to the Registrar-General's classification. (Source: Alwash, R. and McCarthy, M., 1988, Accidents in the home among children under five: ethnic differences or social disadvantage?, *British Medical Journal*, **296**, Table 1, p. 1 452)

self-esteem from going out to work and the risk of accidents to children in the home. Alternatively, the study may be confounding unemployment with material deprivation, since women in the poorest circumstances are the most likely to be unemployed.

Possible explanations for the social-class gradient in childhood accidents have variously focused on possible differences between the social classes in attitudes to accidents, in levels of supervision of children, or in knowledge about safety and risks; in relative access to material resources and the quality of local physical environments; or in individual psychology.

We will look at each of these explanations in more detail.

Attitudes and knowledge

It has sometimes been argued that working-class parents might be more 'fatalistic' about accidents, and might therefore not take so many actions to prevent accidents happening. However, there has been little research that would support this view, and recent work suggests that fatalistic ideas are no more common among working-class people than among other groups. 'Parenting skills', such as level of supervision, are difficult to measure but as factors such as employment rates of mothers, which might affect supervision levels, are similar in working-class and middle-class families, it seems unlikely that these could explain much of the difference.

At this point, please read the article 'Prevention is better …' by Helen Roberts, Susan Smith and Carol Bryce, which you can find in the *Reader*. It deals with a study of childhood accidents on the Corkerhill housing estate in Glasgow, which is also featured in the television programme 'First steps to autonomy'. Then answer the following question.

☐ What do the findings of Helen Roberts and her co-workers suggest about the Corkerhill parents' knowledge of risks?

■ The parents interviewed in this study were very knowledgeable about risks to safety. In terms of local environmental hazards, they were often more knowledgeable than professionals and took considerable action, both individually and as campaigners, to keep their children safe most of the time. Although professionals involved with accident prevention on the estate proposed that what was needed was more education for parents, parents were actually well aware of the risks their children faced. They were not 'fatalistic' about accidents: they shared to a large extent the concerns of the professionals.

Social explanations

If attitudes and knowledge explain little of the social inequalities in accident mortality and morbidity, there is perhaps better evidence for a link between material factors and accidents. The Corkerhill study suggests several ways in which material factors can influence the social distribution of accident risks. The first is the physical environment in which children are brought up. Working-class children may be more likely to live in areas where there are fewer safe places to play and in homes which have more hazards.

☐ What hazards that might lead to accidents did parents and teenagers living in Corkerhill describe?

■ Outside the home, hazards included a main road, broken fencing around the railway track, broken glass on the play areas, road works and building works. Many hazards in the homes were identified as due to bad design: gaps in the balconies big enough for toddlers to crawl through, inadequate window fastenings and electric sockets with no 'off' switches.

An additional material consideration, noted elsewhere by Roberts and her co-workers, is the prohibitive cost of much safety equipment for parents on low income or on benefits. Parents do feel responsible for their children's safety. Given that it is difficult for individual parents to improve dangerous environments, and that the costs of making the home safer can be high, education aimed at increasing knowledge of risks may merely increase maternal anxiety (Roberts *et al.*, 1992)

Psychological explanations

Explaining in general why working-class children have more accidents than those from middle-class homes does not of course explain why individual children suffer them. As well as the social factors that have been correlated with accident risk, there are a wealth of psychological factors. A WHO report (1981) on accidents involving children and adolescents suggested that psychological and environmental factors interact to increase vulnerability to a 'risk situation', and to the likelihood of this risk situation leading to an accident. The factors that predisposed children and adolescents to accidents included such psychological attributes as unbalanced personality, excessive aggressiveness or passivity, and risk-taking behaviour. Attributes of the family, such as size, marital discord and parental substance abuse, were mentioned as factors that have been linked to an increased risk of accidents among the children. This range of contributory factors is very broad, and is perhaps not very informative in explaining the links between social environments and individual accidents.

There is some evidence that psychological *stress* may be one factor that links material deprivation and accident rates. George Brown and Sue Davidson (1978) found that psychiatric disorder interacted with social class to increase the risk of accidents to children: working-class mothers suffered stressful 'life events' more often than middle-class mothers. The researchers found that children of working-class mothers with a psychiatric disorder had an accident rate of 19.6 per 100 children per year, compared with a rate of 9.6 accidents per 100 children for working-class mothers with no psychiatric disorder. The rates of accidents among children of middle-class mothers were lower: 5.3 per 100 when the mother did have a psychiatric disorder and 1.5 per 100 when she did not. Brown and Davidson suggested that the mechanism linking psychiatric disorder to accident rates could be the mothers' increased anxiety, which might lead to higher levels of activity in the children.

Making sense of accidents

Almost all children will have some experience of accidental injury, even if relatively trivial. Understanding how they make sense of these accidents is important if we are to provide safety messages that are meaningful.

In the 1930s Jean Piaget, a Swiss psychologist, published some influential work on children's psychological development. He suggested that children up to the age of seven may have limited notions of chance events such as accidents (Piaget, 1930), because they ascribe motivation (such as malevolence) to inanimate objects and they may have a weak understanding of direct cause and effect relationships. Although Piaget's theories of child development have been contested, recent research on children's perceptions of accidents supports some of his views. In her study of what parents and children thought about accidents and accident prevention, Gill Combes found that children sometimes attributed malevolence to inanimate objects such as toys and cars: 'the naughty car knocked the man over' (Combes, 1991).

As young children may not understand the rational causes of accidents, they may use a concept Piaget described as 'immanent justice' to explain why an accident happened to them. Immanent justice involves interpreting the injury as a punishment for a misdemeanour, rather than as the rational and predictable outcome of risk-taking behaviour. This tendency makes providing appropriate safety messages for young children very difficult. Children under seven may not be able to interpret road safety information in a meaningful way.

Apart from being unable to make the accurate judgements about speed and distance needed to cross roads safely, children may see what adults call 'safe places to cross the road' as magical places which are safe whatever they do. Adult messages that roads are dangerous may be translated into unsafe behaviour, such as running quickly across to minimise the time spent in a dangerous area. If we give children messages such as 'don't play with matches because it's dangerous', children may interpret a resulting accident as being caused not by the risk of fire, but directly by their disobedience.

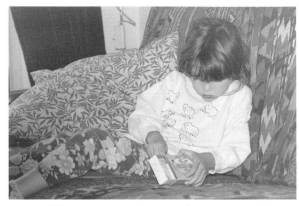

Young children may not understand why certain activities are dangerous; keeping them safe involves removing the hazard rather than relying on changing their behaviour. (Photo: James McCarthy)

It would be misleading to think that only children have non-rational ideas about accident causation. Ideas about fate, luck and chance are important to most adults as well in understanding why misfortunes happen at a particular time. However sophisticated our understanding of risk factors becomes, it will not help make sense of why individual accidents happen to particular individuals at particular times. It is often only in hindsight that parents can see how an accident could have been prevented, but they may still have complex feelings of guilt and responsibility for their children's accidents. Gill Combes found that parents felt responsible even for accidents they could not have prevented, and sometimes felt that professionals such as health visitors did not believe that an injury really was accidental.

Prevention

In Charles Dickens' novel *David Copperfield*, Mr Micawber says: 'Accidents will occur in the best regulated families and in families not regulated ... they may be expected with confidence and borne with philosophy'.

Professionals involved with accident prevention are no longer so resigned: the basic premise of much accident prevention work is that because the distribution of accidents is well known, we can describe the risk factors.

> It is vital to counter the view of accidents as random events due to bad luck … RoSPA [the Royal Society for the Prevention of Accidents] recommends that all health authorities adopt a positive approach to accident prevention based on the premise that the majority of serious accidents could be avoided or prevented and that the risks of serious injuries can also be reduced. (Henwood, 1992, p. 26)

As the epidemiological data suggest, the reduction of risks to children may not be an easy task. Many diseases are caused by one identifiable agent, but there are an infinite number of hazards which can potentially cause accidents. An individual accident results from a combination of social, environmental and personal factors, including the biological and psychological development of the child. Many of the risks (such as broken glass on playgrounds, or busy roads) are outside the traditional remit of the health services. Accident prevention involves identifying the major risks that can be changed, agreeing a policy that risks should be reduced and developing strategies to reduce them, or at least to make people more aware of them.

Policy

Accident prevention is becoming recognised as a high priority, and there are a wide range of initiatives concerning childhood accidents. In the United Kingdom, the 1992 Department of Health White Paper *The Health of the Nation* identified accident prevention as a key issue for public health. It recommended an inter-agency approach which utilises the experience of government departments, health authorities and the voluntary sector to develop accident prevention strategies. Two of the three targets set for accident prevention concern children and young people:

> To reduce the death rate for accidents among children under 15 by at least 33% by the year 2005 (from 6.6 per 100 000 in 1990 to no more than 4.4 per 100 000).

> To reduce the death rate for accidents among young people aged 15–24 by at least 25% by the year 2005 (from 24 per 100 000 to no more than 18 per 100 000). (Department of Health, 1992a, p. 104)

Strategies

Like other health promotion activities,[6] accident prevention measures can aim to reduce the impact of accidents at three levels:

> **primary accident prevention**: prevents the accident happening at all;

> **secondary accident prevention**: minimises or reduces the effect of the accident if it does happen;

> **tertiary accident prevention**: minimises the outcome of the injury resulting from the accident.

These levels are all important, but some are more relevant in different situations than others. For infants under one year, for instance, who are more vulnerable to injury, primary prevention to stop the accident happening at all is the major priority. In some activities, such as dangerous sports or driving on the roads, it may not be possible (or even desirable, in the case of sports) to eliminate completely the risk of an accident happening. In these circumstances it will be important to look at ways of reducing the damage accidents cause, for example by improving standards of equipment or medical care for those who do suffer an accident. Strategies for accident prevention at all these levels can be divided into what are known as the '**three 'E's of accident prevention**': *education* to increase awareness of possible risks and ways to avoid them, *engineering* to make the environment safer, and *enforcement* to provide legal sanctions against risk-taking behaviour (see Cliff, 1984, for a fuller discussion).

> ☐ Think of some education, engineering and enforcement strategies for preventing accidents. In each case, identify whether your example is operating at the primary, secondary or tertiary level of prevention.

> ■ We cannot know what examples you chose, but here are three of ours. An education strategy is first-aid training for parents; this belongs to the tertiary level of prevention because it may reduce the adverse outcome of an accidental injury. An engineering strategy is the supply of child-resistant caps for drug bottles; this works at the primary level, by stopping accidental poisoning from occurring. An enforcement strategy is the compulsory use of

---

[6]Health promotion and disease prevention are discussed in more detail in *Dilemmas in Health Care*, Chapter 9.

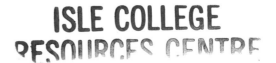

seat belts in cars: this is secondary prevention because it reduces the risk of injury if an accident happens.

But how effective can such preventive measures be? The range of initiatives that could be directed at reducing childhood mortality from accidents may include such diverse activities as discussion groups for mothers about hazards in the home, safety equipment loan schemes, campaigns to improve public playgrounds, and fitting thermostats on water heaters to prevent scalds from hot water. Resources are needed for any intervention and, as there may be unforeseen disadvantages to such programmes, it is important to evaluate their effectiveness.

Effectiveness

As most accidents are multifactorial in cause, it is difficult to recommend single preventive strategies that will have a demonstrable impact on accident rates. One enforcement strategy that has had an effect is the law passed in February 1983 requiring car drivers and front seat passengers to wear seat belts: according to the Department of Transport, in the period following the new legislation, the proportion wearing seat belts increased from 30 per cent to 95 per cent and the proportion of front seat passengers killed or seriously injured was reduced by 30 per cent (Department of Transport, 1985). Engineering strategies have also been successful: measures to separate pedestrians from motorised traffic can successfully reduce childhood accident rates (Sutherland, 1992); the introduction of flameproof nightdresses and child-resistant medicine containers have reduced burns and accidental poisonings respectively (Croft and Sibert, 1992).

However, there is less evidence for the success of education strategies (Croft and Sibert, 1992). Indeed some studies have suggested that education on its own may have little benefit, given that there are few demonstrable links between knowledge of safety and actual behaviour. Although the focus of much accident prevention is on improving knowledge about risks, two studies suggest that knowledge about risk factors for home accidents is *not* related to the risk of an accident occurring. The first was carried out by health visitors who followed up accidents to children attending their local A&E department (Melia *et al.*, 1989). The second involved an examination of visits to the general practitioner as well as to the hospital (Carter and Jones, 1993). Both studies compared children who had suffered an accident with

similar children who had not, and found no significant differences in either the parent's knowledge of risks or presence of safety equipment in the children's homes.

Despite the relative lack of evidence for the success of education strategies compared with engineering and enforcement ones, it appears that these are the most common (as in the Corkerhill estate featured in the television programme, 'First steps to autonomy'). A review edited by Jennie Popay and Angela Young of accident-prevention interventions undertaken in Britain and Scandinavia found that the majority were 'educational': they were designed to increase knowledge or raise awareness of safety issues, rather than to make the environment safer or bring about changes in the law (Popay and Young, 1993).

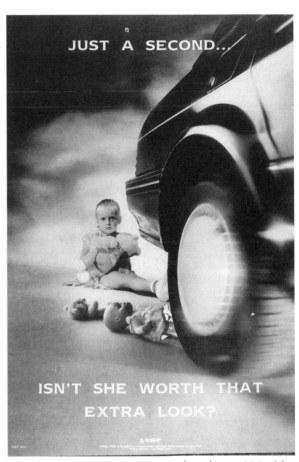

Some accident prevention campaigns have been criticised for 'victim blaming' because they seem to suggest that careless parents are to blame for road accidents to children. (Reproduced by kind permission of the Royal Society for the Prevention of Accidents)

☐ Given the evidence on causes of inequalities in accident rates, which strategies are likely to have the most impact on childhood accidents in the home?

■ Changes in the physical environment. Education may have limited value if risks are already well known or are unavoidable.

☐ Can you think of any possible negative effects of prevention strategies based solely on education for parents?

■ Although parents generally do accept responsibility for their children's safety, information campaigns may increase anxiety if little can be done to reduce risks such as busy local traffic. They may reinforce a 'victim blaming' ideology, which holds individuals responsible for their children's safety and ignores the wider social influences.

There may also be unforeseen disadvantages, even when accident prevention campaigns appear to be successful. One example is hidden in the reduction in child pedestrian deaths. Between 1968 and 1987, the child pedestrian death rates in England and Wales fell by 67 per cent for 0–4 year olds, and by 39 per cent for 5–14 year olds (Roberts, 1993). Ian Roberts has analysed the data on road accidents and argued that this does not represent the success of road-safety training for children or their parents, but is the result of their reduced exposure to traffic as pedestrians. Car driving has become more common: in 1961, for instance, 80 per cent of children walked to school but by 1981, 80 per cent of children were driven to school (Sutherland, 1992). Paradoxically, making our roads *unsafe* for children may mean they have *fewer* traffic accidents, but only because their parents are less likely to allow them to play outdoors than was the case when today's parents were young. This restriction on children's independent travel and outdoor play may have other consequences for their health.

☐ Can you suggest some adverse consequences of this trend?

■ A reduction in outdoor play and in walking to school, to shops or to visit friends, may lead to inadequate exercise for good health. Children may

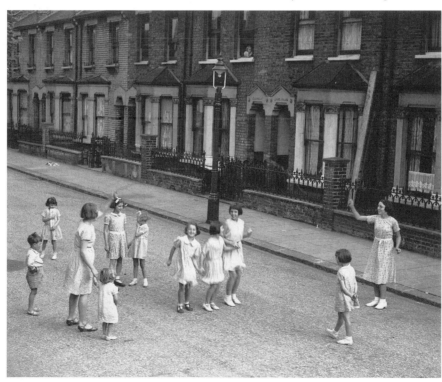

The increasing volume of traffic on Britain's roads means that children's opportunities for outdoor play and walking unescorted to school have reduced sharply since this photograph was taken in London in the 1950s. (Source: The Hulton-Deutsch Collection)

remain dependent on parents for transport until well into their teens, reducing their opportunities for developing responsible independence.

It has been suggested that a separate domain away from home and school that is specifically child-controlled may be very important for children, because it is where they develop their ideas of control and negotiation (Mayall, 1993). Increasing the amount of time children spend in the home to keep them away from dangers outside may restrict their psychological development. Ian Roberts (1993) notes that not only does the increase in car driving reduce children's mobility, but that it also reinforces social inequalities. One-third of British households do not have a car, and so do not have a choice about driving children to school. These are also the children least likely to have any alternative to playing or walking in the now dangerous streets. Parents have a difficult task in balancing the risks of road traffic accidents with the risks of limiting time spent outdoors.

A success story

One project that successfully combined education and engineering strategies was the New York 'Children can't fly' programme (Spiegel and Lindaman, 1977). This was an attempt to reduce the number of falls from heights, which accounted for 12 per cent of all accidental deaths in New York City. The programme involved a media campaign highlighting the dangers of open unguarded windows, door-to-door visits by outreach workers who counselled parents on prevention, and the distribution of free easy-to-install window guards for families with pre-school children living in tenements in high-risk areas. Between 1973 and 1975, the programme recorded a 50 per cent reduction in all reported falls from windows and a significant reduction in fatal falls. No falls were reported from windows where guards had been installed. This project demonstrates that it is possible to reduce childhood accidents from specific causes with appropriate strategies. However, many of the risks children face may be more difficult to reduce.

☐ What problems would be faced in *evaluating* a strategy aimed at reducing local accident mortality rates?

■ Accidents have multifactorial causes, so it may be difficult to separate out the impact of the strategy from other variables, such as a change in risk-taking behaviour.

☐ As an example, consider how the introduction of safer surfaces in playgrounds might affect the behaviour of children and parents.

■ It may encourage children to take greater risks in their play, thereby increasing the chance of an accident happening. It may also sensitise parents to the hazards of playgrounds and alter their attitudes to children's use of them or their willingness to report accidents.

Changes such as these make it difficult to evaluate the success of the intervention.

Conclusions

Accidental injury is a major threat to the health of children and young adults. Although some accidents do 'just happen', the distribution of fatal accidents and injuries suggests that many are amenable to prevention. Many people and organisations have a responsibility for children's safety, including parents, the health services, local authorities and manufacturers. This chapter has focused on children's accidents as a consequence of these external factors, but as children get older and more able to control their environment, the responsibility for assessing risks and preventing accidents moves from parents to the children themselves. The next chapter will look specifically at adolescents and the view that a limited degree of risk taking may be part of normal development in this stage in the life course.

OBJECTIVES FOR CHAPTER 5

When you have studied this chapter, you should be able to:

5.1 Distinguish between the major causes of accidental death and non-fatal accidents in childhood and offer some explanations for these differences.

5.2 Summarise common difficulties encountered in research into the causes of childhood accidents.

5.3 Assess alternative explanations for inequalities in the distribution of childhood accidents by age, gender and social class.

5.4 Explain what is meant by the 'three E's' of accident prevention and distinguish between primary, secondary and tertiary prevention strategies; within this framework, critically evaluate the likely success of specific prevention strategies.

QUESTIONS FOR CHAPTER 5

Question 1 (*Objectives 5.1 and 5.3*)

> Britain has one of the lowest road accident death rates in Europe, but conversely one of the highest child pedestrian accident rates. (Henwood, 1992, p. 17)

Which children are most at risk of dying as pedestrians in a road traffic accident? What explanations have been offered, even tentatively, for the patterns you have identified? Finally, you are invited to speculate about possible reasons for the differences in accident rates in Britain and the rest of Europe.

Question 2 (*Objective 5.2*)

Look back at Table 5.3, which shows the causes of accidents to children under 5 years who attended a north Staffordshire general practice in 1991. What reasons are there for being cautious in interpreting data such as these as indicating the causes of minor accidental injury to young children *in general* in the United Kingdom? What is the main conclusion we can draw from Carter and Jones' study and why is this information important?

Question 3 (*Objective 5.4*)

The White Paper *The Health of the Nation* suggested that in achieving target reductions in fatal accident rates

> ... the Government will rely primarily on information and education and will avoid the imposition of unnecessary regulations on business and individuals. (Department of Health, 1992a, p. 106)

Comment on the likely success of this policy as the major strategy for reducing childhood accidents. What is the evidence that greater regulation might be necessary in specific cases if accidents to children are to be reduced?

6 Adolescent development and risk taking

This chapter builds on the discussion of puberty as a unique phase of human biological development, which occurred in *Human Biology and Health: An Evolutionary Approach, Chapter 2, and includes revision of the associated Reader article 'Why must I be a teenager at all?' by Barry Bogin.[1] During your study of this chapter, you will be asked to listen to an audiotape entitled 'Exploring adolescent development'. Viviane Green, the principal author of this chapter, is a Senior Child Psychotherapist, and works and teaches in London at the Anna Freud Centre and at the Marlborough Family Service. She takes a psychodynamic view (defined below) of adolescence and has drawn on her professional experience in illustrating the chapter. The second author, Basiro Davey, chairs the U205 Course Team, and is a Lecturer in Health Studies in the Biology Department at the Open University.*

The psychodynamic perspective

In this chapter, adolescence is described in developmental terms as a period of transition from childhood to adulthood, which takes place somewhere between the ages of approximately 10 and 19 years. The age-range cannot be defined in precise terms and indeed the phase of life that we commonly refer to as 'adolescence' was only distinguished as different from either childhood or adulthood during the late nineteenth century. Adolescence is a phase marked by a series of physical changes brought about by changes in the person's biological state,

[1] *Human Biology and Health: An Evolutionary Approach* (1994), Chapter 2; *Health and Disease: A Reader* (second edition, 1995).

which underpin shifts at a psychological level. The biological changes are referred to as *puberty* and, coupled with cultural expectations about the adolescent age-group, are seen as giving rise to specific psychological tasks. In negotiating these tasks, adolescents have to reshape their view of themselves to incorporate the sense of an adult sexual male or female body. Adolescents also have to continue the process (begun in childhood) of separation from their actual parents/caretakers and of forming an 'internal picture' of themselves as separate beings with increasing levels of autonomy and responsibility for their own lives. These changes can bring in their wake diverse feelings, which commonly include confusion, a sense of empowerment, excitement, anxiety and fear.

The idea that there are internal conscious and unconscious psychological processes at work in adolescent development comes from a **psychodynamic** point of view, in which the *psyche*—the internal emotional world of the individual—is of central importance. The psychodynamic view

> ... assumes that mental processes are dynamic as opposed to static: they involve movement and force, that an individual's behaviour and subjective experience are the outcome of a conflict, largely unconscious, between opposing forces in the mind. (Fabricius, 1993, p. 45)

In this model, the individual psyche is conceived of as structured and made up of different parts, which can either work harmoniously together or at other times find themselves in conflict. For example, part of the psyche may exert pressure on an individual to follow a particular impulse, wish or desire, but may find itself in conflict with the voice of a forbidding conscience. This would produce an internal conflict. The balance between wishes and restrictions is particularly important for adolescents who need to find an acceptable way of accommodating their growing sexual demands without giving rise to too much anxiety.

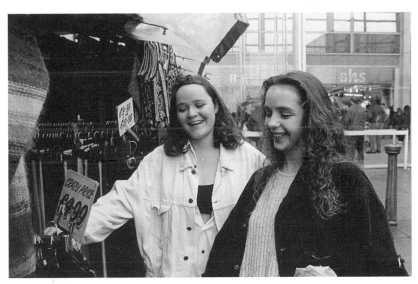

Physical changes in adolescence often promote an upsurge of interest in appearance.
(Photo: Mike Levers)

When an individual has an unconscious wish that gives rise to anxiety, the anxiety has to be kept at bay. Internal defence mechanisms come into play to prevent the person from being overwhelmed by their feelings. One such defence is the *repression* or banishment of anxiety-provoking thoughts and feelings from the conscious mind; another common mechanism is *denial* that the feelings exist. In everyday experience we are recognising denial at work when we say someone is 'protesting too much'; we suspect that the real feeling is the very opposite of what they are so insistently disclaiming. These defence mechanisms are part of ordinary mental functioning and only become problematic if they begin to interfere with an individual's life. For example, this occurred in the case of a young adolescent boy referred for therapy because he continued to deny his feelings of loss, grief and anger when his father left home unexpectedly, but would erupt in rages against his mother.

For many adolescents, anxiety is kept at a manageable level through the use of defences or by active mastery of their feelings. This is often closely linked to the ways in which their parents can help them manage their emotions. In some instances there can be a failure to experience sufficient anxiety and, as a consequence, the person can put themselves at great risk. For some adolescents, the experience of anxiety is unbearable and they will seek to discharge any internal conflict through activity, some of which may also involve risk taking.

In the course of development there are both progressive and regressive internal forces at work. The progressive push propels an individual into actively wanting to grow up and take more responsibility for their life. The regressive undertow may make an individual hanker after the safety and comforts of childhood. In adolescence there is usually an oscillation between the two, but with progressive wishes prevailing. Another source of conflict can be between competing progressive and regressive wishes that make it hard for the adolescent to move forward.

This is the ideal point in the chapter to listen to the audiotape 'Exploring adolescent development'.[2] It will reinforce and illustrate the main points we have made about the psychodynamic view of adolescent development. When you have listened to the tape, consider the following questions.

□ Can you identify the point at which one of the adolescents talks about experiences that would fit our description of an 'internal conflict'?

■ Susan seems to be in conflict over her sexual fantasies and wishes, particularly when she feels attracted to other young women; she describes feeling both excited and humiliated.

[2]The audiotape has been recorded for students of the Open University course, of which this book is a part. Students should consult the Audiocassette Notes before listening to the tape.

□ Well-managed anxiety may have a protective function. Identify the situation in which a lack of realistic anxiety resulted in damage to the speaker.

■ Jeremy describes vividly how, instead of anxiety, there was only excitement when he rode his motor-bike at great speed while under the influence of hallucinogenic drugs or sat on the roof of his friend's speeding car—he was injured on both occasions.

□ Which adolescent most obviously illustrates the expression of strong progressive wishes towards independence, tempered to some extent by an age-appropriate regressive attachment to the safety of childhood?

■ Laura enjoys the freedoms she is granted but makes it clear that she needs to feel a continuing background of safety provided by her parents; she would turn to her parents if she had a problem to sort out.

To sum up, adolescents must successfully negotiate the psychological tasks of constructing an inner picture of themselves as a sexual male or female, resolving inner conflicts and managing the anxiety the transition to adult-hood generates, and balancing progressive and regressive impulses. The extent to which these tasks are achieved has an impact on physical and mental health.

In the next section of the chapter, we review the general health profile of adolescents in the United King-dom, before considering the profound biological developments known as puberty which drive adolescent development forward. Then we return to the psychologi-cal arena to ask whether adolescence is necessarily an emotionally turbulent or problematic phase of the life course. The psychological tasks inherent in adolescent development are then considered within a family con-text. Towards the end of the chapter, we present a view of *risk taking* as part of the normal process of adolescent development; in this model, a high degree of risk taking is seen as a consequence of the individual's difficulties in resolving their internal conflicts. Finally, mention is made of some of the societal attitudes and socio-economic forces that facilitate or disrupt the passage from adoles-cence into adulthood.

Health in adolescence

Adolescence presents its own distinctive set of health, social and psychological problems. Young people are the future and everyone hopes and expects that they will grow into adulthood. Where that hope is curtailed

because of death through illness, accident or self-harm we usually feel a sense of shock and waste. In 1990, in the whole of the United Kingdom, the deaths were recorded of 679 young adolescents aged 10–14 years and 2 021 older adolescents aged 15–19 years. The major causes of these deaths are shown in Table 6.1. Note that in the older age-group deaths from cancers have fallen and congeni-tal abnormalities have disappeared as a cause of mortal-ity, whereas deaths from injuries and poisoning have risen and cardiovascular disorders and drug abuse have begun to claim lives.

Table 6.1 Causes of death among adolescents aged 10–14 (679 deaths) and 15–19 years (2 021 deaths) in the United Kingdom in 1990

Cause of death	10–14 years/ per cent of total	15–19 years/ per cent of total
injury or poisoning	39	60
cancers	18	9
nervous system disorders	9	8
congenital abnor-malities	6	–
respiratory disorders	5	4
cardiovascular disorders (heart and circulation)	–	4
drug abuse	–	4
other causes	22	11

Data compiled by Woodroffe *et al.* (1993), Figures 2.12 and 2.13, p. 32, based on OPCS DH2/17, DH6/4; RG Scotland 1990; RG Northern Ireland 1991.

Table 6.1 conceals the fact that deaths from injury are far higher among boys than girls: in 1987–90, on average, the mortality rate from injuries for boys aged 15–19 was 46 per 100 000 population in that age-group, compared with 13 per 100 000 for girls of the same age (Woodroffe *et al.*, 1993, p. 57). Road traffic accidents are the major contributor to fatal injuries and, as you already know from Chapter 5, this cause of death is particularly com-mon among 15–19-year-old boys.

The second most prevalent cause of fatal injury in this age-group is *suicide*, which is relatively rare before the age of 14 but begins to rise thereafter. The number of teenagers who kill themselves is small in absolute terms (around 15 a year in 1987–90), but about the same num-ber of deaths were given 'open verdicts' by coroners and some of these were probably due to suicide. Of great concern is the sharply rising trend in suicides among young males in recent years, as shown in Figure 6.1. By contrast, the prevalence of non-fatal self-inflicted injury is much commoner among teenage girls than among boys, and the incidence has also been increasing in recent years (Brooksbank, 1985). According to the charity Action for Sick Children (Kurtz, 1992, p. 7), the annual suicide rate among all 15–19-year-olds is 3 per 100 000 and a further 400 per 100 000 are believed to attempt suicide each year.

In countries such as the United Kingdom, where infectious diseases have almost ceased to be a cause of death among teenagers,[3] attention has focused largely on those causes of death and chronic illness that have persisted, despite medical advances in other areas, or (like suicide and drug abuse) have even increased. The General Household Surveys, government-sponsored annual surveys of 12 000 households, show that the prevalence of chronic illness reported among 5–15-year-olds was 16 per cent in 1991, and 20 per cent among those aged 16–19 (Woodroffe *et al.*, 1993, pp. 39–40). Respiratory diseases such as *asthma* have contributed the largest proportion of the increase in chronic illness in recent years and there is evidence that among 15–19-year-olds (though not among younger age-groups) there has been a sharply-rising trend in deaths from asthma, which account for roughly 40 deaths a year in older teenagers (Anderson and Strachan, 1991).[4] *Diabetes* is another cause of chronic illness that has been increasing in younger children in recent decades and is becoming more prominent in adolescents as diabetic children now usually survive.

Trends in suicide and drug abuse have focused concern on mental health problems among young people. There are no reliable *national* data on rates of psychiatric illness among adolescents, but there is a general belief among practitioners that depression and anxiety are more common among teenage girls than among boys. Estimates of sex differences in these emotional disorders based on medical diagnoses or hospital admission rates have to be interpreted cautiously.

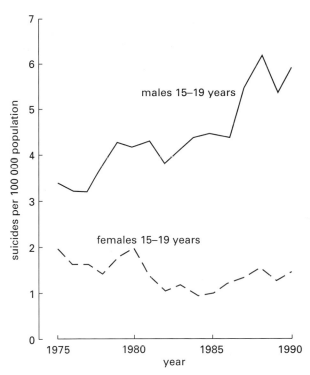

Figure 6.1 *Trend in suicide among young people aged 15–19 years in England and Wales, 1975–90. (Source: Woodroffe* et al. *(1993), Figure 2.65, p. 68; data derived from OPCS DH2)*

☐ Can you suggest why?

■ Different rates of diagnosis may reflect a tendency among practitioners to withhold diagnostic labels such as 'depression' from distressed young males and a willingness to assign them to females; and/or cultural expectations about gender roles may enable girls to disclose their feelings of depression and anxiety but discourage boys from doing so.

Evidence that girls do experience higher rates of mental disorder than boys has been emerging from a study of around 1 000 Scottish teenagers (West, 1994), which we will discuss later in the chapter, when we return to the subject of mental health in adolescence and assess the prevalence and severity of emotional problems. There is no dispute that the eating disorder *anorexia nervosa* is about 12 times more common among girls than boys, or that the peak age of onset is 16–17 years. A report by the Office of Health Economics (1994) estimates that in the United Kingdom about 70 000 girls and young women (in the age-range 15–29 years) may be affected.

---

[3] It remains to be seen whether the arrival of HIV (the human immunodeficiency virus) and AIDS (acquired immune deficiency syndrome) will change this situation.

[4] The vexed question of whether reported increases in asthma attacks are due to increased air pollution or to changes in diagnostic criteria is discussed in a case study on asthma in *Experiencing and Explaining Disease* (revised edition, 1996).

This brief examination of the strikingly different health profiles of adolescent girls and boys leads us to consider the very different biological changes that take place for the two sexes during puberty. These give us some clues about the underlying psychic tasks that males and females have to undertake in reshaping their inner identity as adult sexual beings.

Puberty: biological changes in adolescence

The characteristic and visible changes in body size, shape and hair growth that indicate the onset of **puberty** are external signs of underlying biological changes in the reproductive organs, which ultimately enable most individuals to produce fertile eggs or sperm and, in girls, become pregnant and carry a baby to full term. These outward physical changes are commonly held to be a sign of 'growing up' in a wider sense—adolescence as a socially-recognised phase cannot begin without them. They include the development of breasts in girls and facial hair in boys, and enlargement of the genitals and growth of pubic hair in both sexes. These physical changes are referred to as **secondary sexual characteristics** and they start to appear about two years earlier in girls than in boys.

The underlying biological triggers for the onset of puberty are sharp increases in the concentration in the bloodstream of various **sex hormones** secreted by the reproductive organs: the testes in males and the ovaries in females. The principal male sex hormone is *testosterone*, which also occurs at a much lower level in females. The principal female sex hormones are the *oestrogens*, which also occur at much lower levels in males, and *progesterone*. In both sexes, the release of these hormones is under the control of another group of hormones (the gonadotropins) secreted by the pituitary gland at the base of the brain. There is still considerable uncertainty about what starts this cascade of hormone release in the first place: certainly there must be a genetic component unique to each individual, but the state of an individual's general health, nutrition, body weight and exposure to daylight also seem to be important. For example, as nutrition has improved during the last century, so the age at *menarche* (the first menstrual period) has reduced in all developed countries.

Once the process of developing secondary sexual characteristics is under way, adolescents enter a phase of very rapid growth in height and weight (the adolescent 'growth spurt'), which has no equivalent in any other species. It occurs about two years later in boys than in girls and is due primarily to increased output of *growth hormone* from the pituitary gland. All parts of the body are affected, but the relative growth of muscle size and

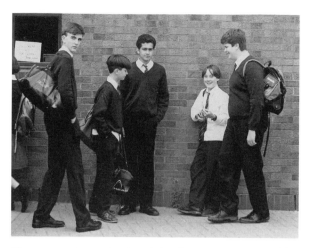

The onset and rate of pubertal development can vary widely, as seen in this group of 11-year-old boys. (Photo: James Dickson)

shoulder width is greatest in boys, whereas girls develop wider hips.

In boys, the development of adult male physical characteristics coincides closely with the achievement of male **reproductive maturity**, the capacity to produce and ejaculate fertile sperm. By contrast, in girls there is a delay of several years between breast 'bud' development and the menarche, and a further delay before full reproductive maturity is achieved. About 50 per cent of the menstrual cycles in the first two years after the menarche do not produce a fertile egg and even after five years about 20 per cent of cycles are infertile; the aperture of the pelvis does not enlarge to its full extent until about the age of 18. In a *Reader* article, 'Why must I be a teenager at all?',[5] an evolutionary biologist—Barry Bogin—offers a tentative explanation for this difference between the sexes in the development of secondary sexual characteristics and reproductive maturity.

☐ Can you recall Bogin's hypothesis about why these differences may have evolved?

■ He suggests that in our evolutionary past, adolescent girls began to look like 'women' and experience sexual and maternal feelings before they were fertile because this was advantageous to the species as a whole: pubescent girls are invited into adult female society, where they learn essential child-rearing skills before they are capable of having a child of their own. Boys develop sexually and become fertile

[5]See *Human Biology and Health: An Evolutionary Approach*, Chapter 2, and *Health and Disease: A Reader* (second edition, 1995).

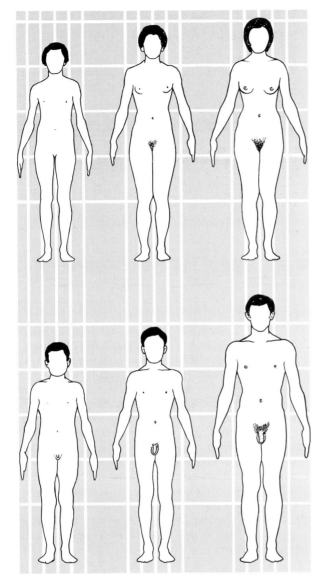

Figure 6.2 *The age at which the external physical signs of puberty appear can vary greatly between individuals, as shown in these drawings (based on actual photographs taken in the 1970s) of three girls aged 12 years 9 months and three boys aged 14 years 9 months. The girl and boy on the left have not yet begun puberty, whereas those on the right have already completed most of the physical changes associated with adulthood. (Based on Tanner, 1992, p. 103)*

several years before their bodies resemble those of adult males; this may have enabled them to practise the physical skills needed to fend for their future dependents, without being perceived as 'competition' by mature men.

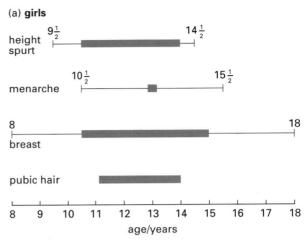

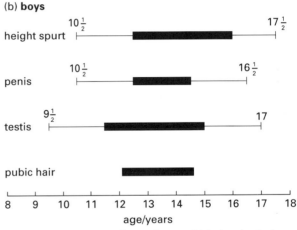

Figure 6.3 *The range of ages during which the physical changes of puberty occur, on average, in girls and boys. The solid bars represent the average period in which development of that characteristic occurs; the thin lines at either end of the solid bars represent the maximum extent of the ages at which this characteristic can begin and end pubertal development. (Based on Tanner, 1992, p. 102)*

The secondary sexual characteristics are powerful markers of the transition from childhood to adulthood. They appear in very much the same *sequence* in all individuals of the same sex, but they can start at very different ages and proceed at different rates from one individual to another, as Figures 6.2 and 6.3 illustrate.

The extreme variation in the age at onset of these physical changes (Figure 6.3) and in the speed at which a given adolescent progresses through puberty is well recognised in such terms as 'early' or 'late developer'.

The distress experienced by young people whose development is out of step with their peers can be recalled by most adults and may contribute to the perception that adolescence is a time of turbulent emotions. We return to the psychological arena to consider the differing views of academic researchers and health professionals about whether adolescence is necessarily a turbulent phase of the lifespan.

Calm or turbulent waters?

The very term 'adolescence' evokes the notion of a troublesome, difficult or wayward phase. Media representations of this age-group frequently depict adolescents engaged in dubious activities. In popular music these attitudes are parodied and the activities embraced, as in Ian Dury's song: 'sex 'n drugs 'n rock 'n roll, that's all my body needs'. Cultural media such as literature, cinema, theatre, television, magazines and pop songs offer us numerous ways in which adolescent experience is constructed that are both a reflection of and a contribution to **stereotyping**, the formation of fixed and oversimplified mental images. Thus, there is the angst-ridden lovelorn teenager of magazines, pop songs and Sue Townsend's creation 'Adrian Mole', and the alienated, self-conscious but witty hero of J. D. Salinger's novel *The Catcher in the Rye*. Whether viewed sympathetically or critically, the transition to adulthood is often represented as problematic.

According to many authors in the psychoanalytic tradition, the major and rapid changes that take place in adolescence create a period of turbulence, which is viewed as both an extensive and expected part of *normal* development. Adolescence is understood as a necessarily problematic phase in which some form of rebellion is needed to loosen the ties to the self of childhood and the family of origin, in order to emerge with a greater degree of independence. Anna Freud describes adolescence as

> ... by its nature an interruption of peaceful growth and ... the upholding of a steady equilibrium during the process is by itself abnormal. (Freud, 1958, quoted in Rutter, *et al.*, 1976, p. 35)

A contrasting view is that most adolescents experience a relatively trouble-free and healthy transition to adult life and the difficulties have been grossly exaggerated. Conflict either within the individual or with parents or other authority figures is minimal and the more serious problems of a few are not characteristic of the group as a whole. This was the conclusion of an in-depth study of 24 people published in 1981 by two British sociologists, Frank Musgrove and Roger Middleton. One of their interviewees, a male teacher, made this typical comment:

> I had a very happy home life ... we didn't really have any major conflicts. Well there were some differences, of course. Smoking and drinking, that sort of thing. But adolescence was not the traumatic experience for me that it may be for others. (Musgrove and Middleton, 1981, p. 43).

□ In recollecting your own adolescence or through observing adolescents you have known, does your experience match that of this teacher?

■ If it did not, some common anxieties in adolescence are bewilderment at mood changes, lack of confidence, worries about physical appearance, feelings of not belonging to a group, fears about relationships with the opposite sex, and unhappiness because of rows in the family.

There are several difficulties in establishing a firm view on the degree of turbulence in adolescence. Research has often been conducted on unrepresentative samples, such as Musgrove and Middleton's cited above, or adolescents who have sought therapeutic help. However, the in-depth insights gained from adolescents in psychotherapy offer the clinician an unusual degree of access to an individual's innermost thoughts, wishes, feelings and fantasies, which can provide a rich picture of the anxieties that beset adolescents. Another difficulty stems from variability in the criteria employed for evaluating 'inner turmoil', and another is that academics and clinicians tend to employ different methods to collect their data and they are not comparable. Thus, a view of adolescence based on the memories of adults in their thirties in response to questionnaires is very different to the experience conveyed by an individual in a clinical setting while in the throes of adolescence, which is subsequently recorded by the clinician.

An important large-scale study was conducted in the 1970s by Michael Rutter, a British academic and child psychiatrist, and his colleagues. They used three methods to study all the 14–15-year-olds on the Isle of Wight: extensive questionnaires filled in by parents and teachers, designed to build up a total picture of individual youngsters' lives; psychological assessments of adolescents; and psychiatric evaluation of a sub-sample. The researchers were able to draw several conclusions:

> ... there can be no doubt from these findings that many 14–15-year-olds experience quite marked feelings of affective disturbance which could well be described as 'inner turmoil'. Although only a small minority appear clinically depressed, many reported feelings of misery which were often accompanied by self depreciation. (Rutter *et al.*, 1976, p. 42)

These feelings caused suffering to the individual but were often unnoticed by the adults. The authors suggested that it remained uncertain if feelings of inner turmoil constituted indicators or portents of psychiatric disorder. Conclusions about the true prevalence of psychiatric disorder in adolescence remained tentative, although it was thought to be 'probably somewhat commoner than in childhood' (Rutter *et al.*, p. 46). More recently, a picture of the prevalence of mental health problems amongst adolescents has been put forward in a report, *With Health in Mind*, published in 1992 by the charity Action for Sick Children in association with the South West Thames Regional Health Authority.

> The overall prevalence [of mental health problems] in the child population is estimated at up to 20% with 7–10% having moderate to severe problems. Emotional or behavioural problems sufficiently severe to be disabling were found in 2.1% of all children (aged up to 16) in Great Britain, according to a survey carried out in 1988. In a population of 250,000 one might expect between 5,000 and 15,000 children with mental health problems at any one time. (Kurtz, 1992, p. 6)

The report estimated that approximately 20 per cent of adolescents have mental health problems, with higher rates in inner cities than in rural situations, particularly where the young person's family suffered serious economic hardship. A study in Scotland by Peter West and Helen Sweeting has revealed even higher levels of emotional or psychological problems among a cohort of about 1 000 teenagers from Central Clydeside (West, 1994). Their mental health was assessed using a standard rating scale (the General Health Questionnaire, or GHQ). Among the 15-year-olds, over 10 per cent of the boys and 18 per cent of the girls had psychological or emotional problems of possible psychiatric significance; by the age of 18, the proportions had leapt to a staggering 33 per cent of males and almost 42 per cent of females. The most common problems in this age-group are depression, anxiety states, phobias, psychosomatic physical symptoms, aggression, persistent delinquency and (among teenage girls) eating disorders such as anorexia nervosa (Kurtz, 1992, p. 7). The intensity of distress can be gauged by the rates of suicide, attempted suicide and self-inflicted injury discussed earlier.

Mental health professionals are cautious about making definitive diagnostic pronouncements on the status of an adolescent's mental health because they recognise that this phase is one of fluidity, experimentation and sometimes turbulent change. In this sense, periods of inner turmoil and uncertainty are part and parcel of adolescence and usually diminish with time. The distinction between what is a disturbing but transient aspect of a normal developmental phase and what is the onset of a more serious mental illness can be hard to make. However, there are certain psychiatric difficulties with more clearly definable symptoms. Adolescence can be the time when, for a very small number of people, the visible onset of a schizophrenic illness occurs, marked by a break with reality; the adolescent withdraws from peer and family contact into his/her own world and is overwhelmed by delusional beliefs.[6]

If we consider the steps an adolescent must take in developing an adult identity, it may become clearer why this part of the life course can bring with it periods of inner turmoil.

Developing autonomy

The period from infancy to adulthood sees the unfolding of three interlinked processes: *sexual* development, *separation* from the family of origin, and *individuation*—the formation of a unique and stable sense of 'self'. Chapter 4 described the child's steps towards autonomy in terms of a gradual growth in the capacity for self-regulation, which leads children to take increasing responsibility for their own bodies. We expect adolescents to take over the care of their own bodies and become responsible for their health. They are faced with numerous choices: what to eat, whether or not to diet or take part in sports or potentially risky activities such as driving at speed, drinking alcohol, smoking, drug-taking, or having unprotected sex.

Adolescence is also the time when individuals have to begin to make decisions about other aspects of their lives, such as which exams to take, whether to stay on at school for further study, or how to earn their living. The adolescent also exerts a far greater degree of social autonomy as he or she moves away from the family of origin and forms stronger ties with their peer-group and more intimate sexual relationships.

In taking these steps towards independence, the individual has to carve out a sense of their future social, professional and personal identity. The road is often marked by the question 'Who am I?' and preoccupations with emerging sexuality.

Sexual awakening

One of the major psychological tasks for the adolescent is to accommodate a new sense of themselves as sexual beings. Hormonal changes give rise to growing sexual desires and at the psychological level there is an

[6]Schizophrenia is the subject of a case study in *Experiencing and Explaining Disease* (revised edition, 1996).

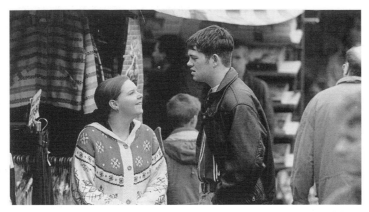

One of the major psychological tasks for adolescents is to accommodate new sense of themselves as sexual beings. (Photo: Mike Levers)

alteration to a fantasy life which reflects a range of sexual preoccupations. There is a need to find a balance between relaxing internal controls sufficiently to make room for the expression of sexual feelings, and controlling what may at times feel like unmanageable desires. Puberty brings a disruption of the familiar body of childhood and the individual has to incorporate an altered internal picture of their more adult male or female sexual body. For some adolescents the physical changes are alarming and they may wish to repudiate what is happening. In anorexia nervosa, the adolescent girl's starvation can, in part, be understood as a desperate attempt to fight against the development of her womanly body and to restore her childhood body. For most adolescents, if there is worry about awakening sexuality and a sense of mourning for childhood, it can also be mixed with a feeling of pleasure and anticipation, as illustrated in the following account.

> An 18-year-old girl referred herself for psychotherapeutic help because she felt worried and confused by her sexual fantasies and unconfident about her female body. After she had slept with her boyfriend for the first time, she remarked that although she had enjoyed the experience she had cried and kept repeating to herself, 'I am no longer a virgin'. Her therapist took up with her how this experience signalled her departure from childhood and entry into adulthood and that this hatching of an altered self might feel both pleasurable and scary. The girl replied that she supposed it was a bit like a baby being born and that it took a while to learn to stand on your own feet. (Author's example)

Separating from the family

An equally important psychological task is that of loosening the ties to the family of origin. This process can feel very confusing, not only for individual adolescents but also for the adults around them, as the young person makes seemingly conflicting demands. Adolescents may vacillate rapidly between independence and dependence, as they attempt to regulate the distance in their ties to their caretakers. On the one hand, they are *progressing* by making bids for more freedom, but on the other, they have periods of *regressing*, that is reverting back to more childlike modes of demanding, dependent behaviour. For example, a 12-year-old boy orders his mother to get out of his room and stop telling him to tidy it, as it is *his* territory, but follows this outburst with 'And mum, when will dinner be ready?'

Adolescents still need their parents or caretakers to confirm and approve of them and at the same time to provide boundaries which they can question.

> A 16-year-old girl told her therapist that she enjoyed having battles with her father, but got very frustrated if he refused to fight back. 'I just want him to go through the necessary procedure,' she complained. (Author's example)

The role of caretaking adults is a difficult balancing act, demanding flexibility in providing a 'safe-enough' family environment with 'firm-enough' boundaries, while at the same time yielding enough freedom for the adolescent to explore new roles and relationships.

> ☐ Can you give an example of 'freedom within limits' from the audiotape you listened to earlier?

■ Laura describes being allowed to travel around London on her own and to go out to parties, but her father set limits by suggesting it would be unsafe to go to a local fair. Laura acknowledges the sense of safety this offers.

An adolescent who grows up in a safe family context, where the adults are firm in their limit-setting without being too rigid, is less likely to take serious risks. There is evidence from several studies that the severity of risk taking correlates with family history; the lowest risk takers tend to come from intact families (Plant and Plant, 1992, p. 118).

Adolescence is also the time when, in the service of separation and individuation, parental and social authority can be questioned. The beliefs and prohibitions inculcated during childhood need to be reshaped as the individual attempts to form their own sense of what is or is not acceptable. The adolescent may kick against certain social and parental values, preferring to identify with the views and beliefs of a peer group, who can sometimes give licence to behaviours that the individual would not undertake alone.

It should be remembered that the optimal period for attaining new levels of independence is culturally specific. In this chapter, the assumption has been made that a move away from the family of origin—negotiated through struggles—is a sign of health. However, in a multicultural society such as the United Kingdom, there are large variations amongst the different ethnic groups in determining the optimal period and manner in which separation occurs. This can set up conflicting expectations for an adolescent who has to juggle with competing cultural norms. All adolescents, whatever their ethnic origins, have to chart their own course through the values and wishes of several different groups—their family, peer group, the wider society in which they live, and for some, a religious community—each of which exerts a powerful and often competing influence on a young person as he or she negotiates greater independence. There are practical pressures too: for example, socio-economic forces determine the availability of jobs, financial support for further education, and social benefits—all of which affect the ability of an adolescent to take essential steps towards autonomy and independent adult status.

We return to these socio-economic issues at the end of this chapter. First, we consider difficulties with separation and individuation that can arise within the family and within the individual.

Family context: conflict and compromise

The ways in which individual adolescents will deal with their anxiety about sexuality, separation and individua-

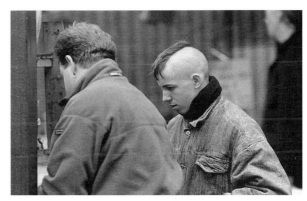

The task of building a separate identity may be aided by adopting peer-group fashions that are distinctively different from those of one's parents. (Photo: Mike Levers)

tion will, in large measure, be a recapitulation of their childhood experiences. Resilience (except where a severe mental illness interferes with overall functioning) is afforded by what psychoanalysts call *ego strength*. This term refers to the whole range of psychological and emotional capacities that an adolescent can use to regulate their internal states of mind and feelings, manage decision-making and develop a variety of interests and abilities. Where earlier childhood experience has led to the development of a resilient ego, then the strains of adolescence will be easier to withstand. Where earlier experience has been marked by trauma or inadequate parenting, then the upheavals of adolescence can be hard to manage.

For some adolescents the task of separation can be made doubly difficult because one or both of their parents finds it hard to facilitate their movement towards independence. The manner in which parents react to their adolescent offspring is affected by their own experiences of this phase of their lives. Parental attitudes towards, for example, sexuality and aggression will play an important part in how far they can tolerate these aspects of their adolescent children's behaviour.

A parent may wish to disavow the fact that their child is growing up and curb their moves into adolescence by exerting too much control. One (of several possible) types of explanation for anorexia nervosa locates the difficulty in the parents' wish to keep their daughter a child. She may then feel angry, trapped and engulfed within the parent/child relationship and caught between the competing wishes to grow up and to remain a child. In turn, she may try to exert control over her parents by arousing their anxiety by endangering herself through starvation. Her fight is for separation and autonomy by showing that her body is hers and hers alone to control.

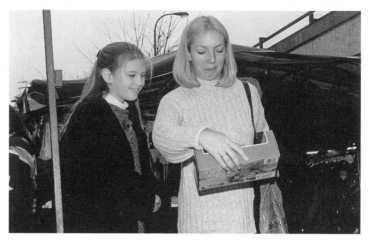

Manageable disagreement between adolescents and their parents is an inevitable and often fruitful arena for identity formation, but parents who cannot tolerate any disagreement make it doubly difficult for children to separate constructively from their family. (Photo: Mike Levers)

Paradoxically, her actions may reduce her chance of separation by generating anxiety in her parents, thus ensuring that they are kept intimately involved. There are other ways in which adolescents can feel driven to attempt a sense of independence or to manage conflictual internal states through the use of their bodies.

> In a group run for teenage mothers, a 21-year-old told the therapists that she became pregnant at 19 because her body and fertility was the one area that no one else could have control over. Another teenage mother spoke of her despair throughout adolescence and how becoming pregnant ensured that she would not be tempted to make a suicide attempt. (Author's example)

Conversely, some adolescents may be granted more freedom than they can manage, or they may have experienced rejection and abandonment earlier on in life. Without a previous or ongoing background of safety and anchoring in a family, they may feel psychologically 'unheld' and adrift, that there are no caring adults who hold their well-being in mind. Separation is hard to bear if it generates intolerable feelings of anxiety when alone.

> A 14-year-old boy whose early life had been marked by a series of separations from his biological mother, prior to adoption at the age of 3, told his therapist that he would be flooded by feelings of disorientation when he was alone in his room, despite now having caring adoptive parents. A 14-year-old girl who had been brought up in a children's home for several years told her therapist that whenever she felt her mother had abandoned her she was overcome with the urge to run away from the home. (Author's example)

Internal conflicts

The rapid physiological changes associated with puberty, and inner conflicts over the psychological tasks the adolescent must face, often give rise to anxiety and bewildering mood swings ranging from depression to elation. At one end of the spectrum of coping with these feelings is the individual who can bear their distress and excitement and perhaps reflect on them; at the other is the individual who finds their feelings intolerable and resorts to strategies that seek to disguise or discharge them. Adolescents who find other feeling states too conflictual or unmanageable may simply 'switch off' their feelings and go numb. There may be a feeling of emptiness and protracted bouts of depression which mask underlying conflicts. For some adolescents, who have not amassed a sufficient fund of earlier experiences enabling them to feel vitally connected to caring adults, a sense of unmitigated aloneness can prevail.

An alternative strategy is adopted by some adolescents who immediately seek to discharge their unmanageable feelings by 'acting out'. This term is used by mental health professionals to describe behaviours that *have* to be enacted to discharge anxieties that cannot be thought about or communicated. For example, on the audiotape, Susan describes how she would 'get stoned' (smoke cannabis) when her confused feelings about her sexuality got too much to bear. For many adolescents, a degree of acting out is a normal part of adolescence, which carries relatively low risk to themselves and others and may only occur for a short period, while more constructive ways are being sought for managing their feelings.

However, young people with pervasive difficulties stemming from childhood and inadequate current support often express their distress and attempt to resolve their internal conflicts by using or abusing their own bodies. This may take many forms: a pseudo-maturity and flight into promiscuity, eating disorders, persistent drug-taking, self-harming behaviours such as cutting and attempted suicide. Sometimes they attack others.

> A 17-year-old boy told his therapist that he linked his attacks on his girlfriend to his low self-esteem. Any criticism by his girlfriend was experienced as humiliatingly undermining and gave rise to uncontainable anger. (Author's example)

There has been considerable interest in establishing whether males and females choose to retreat from or discharge their unmanageable feelings in different ways. Between 1983 and 1985, M. Choquet, a French epidemiologist, and H. Menke, a clinical psychologist, set up a study of 327 French high-school students. They concluded that a degree of distress is common amongst adolescents, but there were clear differences between the sexes in how they reacted to it. Behaviours related to drug consumption, drinking and violence were more prevalent amongst boys, whereas sleep disorders, headaches and depressive symptoms were more common amongst girls (Choquet and Menke, 1987, p. 303). This echoes our earlier discussion: boys were more likely to act out their feelings and girls were more likely to turn their feelings against themselves or express them in bodily terms.

A spectrum of risk taking

The term **risk taking** encompasses actions that might lead to misfortune, loss or harm even though the individuals concerned do not perceive themselves to be at risk, and to deliberate self-exposure to something that is potentially or actually dangerous. It has been suggested that a degree of risk taking in the first sense of the term is a 'normal transitional behaviour during adolescence' (Irwin, 1989, p. 124). In middle and late adolescence it serves the developmental need to establish autonomy by encountering and developing mastery of new unexplored activities, which contain the possibility of loss or misfortune. The pursuit of new activities and taking the initiative, fuelled by curiosity, could be viewed as positive attributes that may have positive or negative outcomes. As part of normal adolescence there may be a need to walk an emotional tightrope between apprehension and excitement. For many adolescents, this form of risk taking is expressed in a transient flirtation and experimentation with drugs, drink and changing sexual partners. This can be differentiated from risk taking that has a dangerous or self-destructive component, or that exposes others to harm. Risk taking falls outside the realm of 'normal' development if there is a compulsive element in behaviour that drives individuals into repeating inherently self-destructive activities, contrary to their conscious wishes and ideals.

Risk taking is a complex phenomenon, which is neither easy to explain nor reducible to one type of explanation. There are several difficulties in thinking about risk taking (whatever the age-group): for example, in determining the kind of activity that can be deemed 'risky', the degree of participation that constitutes a risk, and what is perceived to be an *acceptable* level of risk. In their study, *Risktakers: Alcohol, Drugs, Sex and Youth*, Martin and Moira Plant note that a difference often exists between 'objective' criteria for determining the level of risk associated with a certain behaviour, and the individual's own perception of what that risk might be and of their personal vulnerability to it (Plant and Plant, 1992, p. 114).

A further difficulty is that behaviours deemed usual in one cultural group may be judged deviant in another. For example, there are widely differing attitudes to alcohol consumption based on religious beliefs between (say) fundamentalist Muslims or Plymouth Brethren and a non-devout population. Similarly, the use of ganga (cannabis) amongst Rastafarians is acceptable and inextricably linked to an ideology, whereas at a wider social level, as reflected in legislation, it is considered a 'soft' but still illegal drug. In the United Kingdom, there are marked regional differences in patterns of high alcohol consumption, based on complex socio-economic and cultural factors: data from the General Household Survey reveal that 'heavy' drinking is least prevalent in Scotland, East Anglia and the South West, and most prevalent in the North and North West of England (Foster *et al.*, 1990). In addition there are differences in consumption based on gender, which are particularly marked among young people, as Figure 6.4 (*p. 105*) shows.

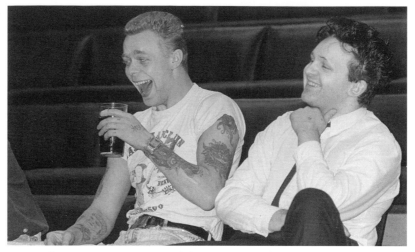

'Heavy' drinking may be more prevalent among young men partly because getting drunk is more readily excused for men than it is for women—particularly after the age of 18. (Photo: Mike Levers)

☐ Look at Figure 6.4. Can you suggest possible reasons for the difference in alcohol consumption between males and females, and the trends with age?

■ You may have suggested differences in 'acceptable' behaviour associated with gender roles: getting drunk is more readily excused for men, particularly after the age of 18, than it is for women. Heavy drinking may reflect modelling on parents, whose attitudes to alcohol may be even more strongly 'gender-biased' than those of the present generation.

The consumption of large amounts of alcohol is commonplace among young men; Figure 6.4 shows that a third of males in the 18–24 age-group are regularly drinking at least the equivalent of 10.5 pints of beer a week, an amount matched by more than one in ten 16–17-year-old boys. It is doubtful that this level of alcohol use is seen as risk taking by the drinkers themselves, though it may be by older adults. This echoes the difference in attitude between different generations to the use of 'recreational' drugs by teenagers; adults tend to see this behaviour as reckless or deviant, in contrast to the young people themselves who inhabit a youth culture in which such drugs are commonplace. Several studies have shown that the use of certain illegal drugs, particularly cannabis, has become relatively common among young people. A government consultation document, published in October 1994, gave the following statistics on drug misuse among adolescents and young adults in the United Kingdom:

- Among school children, 3 per cent of 12–13-year-olds and 14 per cent of 14–15-year-olds admit to taking an illegal drug.

- Drug misuse is more prevalent among men: one third of male survey respondents aged 16–29 report use of an illegal drug in the past.

- Of young people living in inner city areas, some 42 per cent of 16–19-year-olds and 44 per cent of 20–24-year-olds have taken drugs at some time, with between 20–30 per cent of the 16–29 age-group using a drug in the last year.

- 24 per cent of people aged 16–29 report long-term cannabis use … Among 16–19-year-olds, 11 per cent have tried amphetamines, 9 per cent Ecstasy and 8 per cent LSD … under 1 per cent report ever using heroin, cocaine and crack.

- Rates of reported use of solvents for young people are: 12–13-year-olds (3 per cent); 14–15-year-olds (7 per cent), and 15–16-year-olds (6 per cent). (*Tackling Drugs Together*, 1994, pp. 83–4)

Plant and Plant put studies such as these on alcohol and drug use among young people into a wider context:

There are, of course, different levels of risk. Some activities are inherently more dangerous than others. It is possible to indulge to a modest, and relatively safe extent or to take repeated and major risks … most of those who use alcohol, tobacco and illicit drugs do not become chronic or problem users. Most young adults do not drink heavily and use neither tobacco nor illicit drugs. (Plant and Plant, 1992, p. 114)

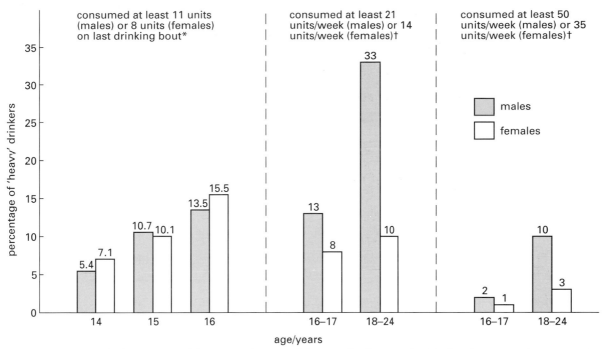

Figure 6.4 *'Heavy' drinking among adolescents and young adults in England* (or England and Wales†) in the late 1980s. A 'unit' of alcohol is equivalent to half a pint of beer, or a glass of wine, or a 'single' measure of spirits. (Data derived from two large-scale studies: *Plant, M. A., Bagnall, G., Foster, J. and Sales, J., 1990, Young people and drinking: results of an English national survey, Alcohol and Alcoholism, **25**, p. 688; †Goddard, E., 1991, Drinking in England and Wales in the Late 1980s, HMSO, London.)*

The question as to whether certain behaviours are even perceived as risks is pertinent to adolescence. Certain activities that are deemed hazardous by adults may not be felt to be risky by the adolescent. In this sense, risk taking is not necessarily perceived by the adolescent as a flight from distress or the deliberate seeking of feelings of excitement, but simply something that is done because it is enjoyable and thought to be without personal consequences.

There are certain internal mental mechanisms at work that enable adolescents to sustain the belief that they are untouchable. This sense of invulnerability is a feature of adolescent development. Health campaigns aimed at this age-group come up against the difficulty that teenagers imagine themselves to be magically protected from harm. This 'personal fable' as it has been termed (Elkind, cited in Plant and Plant, 1992, p. 114), is linked to the feeling of unfolding possibilities, which can provide adolescents with a feeling of inner strength or potency. It may also be in the service of reaching for exceptional goals. On the negative side it can lead to failures in self protection, for example, failure to use contraception or 'safe-sex' practices. Attitudes to sexual risk taking among young people have been researched largely in the context of HIV infection and AIDS: Dominic Abrams and colleagues concluded their study of 16–19-year-olds in Scotland by stating that:

> Young people's response to AIDS appears to be mixed. On the one hand they are concerned about the presence and spread of the disease in the community at large, but on the other they have a strong sense of AIDS invulnerability, which seems to involve a perception that they have control over the risk at which they place themselves. (Abrams, Abraham, Spears and Marks, 1990, p. 49)

Another example of failure in self-protection is revealed by the prevalence of drink–driving deaths among young road-users, who fail to recognise the dangers. In summary:

> Available evidence sustains two broad conclusions … Firstly, risk taking is natural, commonplace and in some form or another, inevitable. Secondly while most young people can be expected to take some risks, a variety of potent

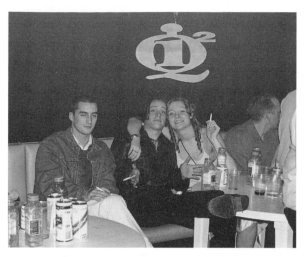

Young people enjoying a 'night out' are unlikely to consider their use of alcohol, tobacco or other drugs as exposing them to serious risk. (Photo: James McCarthy)

> factors foster and perpetuate risky or problem behaviours. On the basis of current information it appears that there is considerable overlap between one form of risk taking and others. Risks are often interconnected. (Plant and Plant, 1992, p. 120)

But if most adolescents engage in 'normal' risk taking, Plant and Plant point to a considerable body of evidence that a minority of individuals are liable to engage in a wide range of risky or problem behaviours, moving from one to another in a 'lifelong career'. Where risk taking is no longer a one-off or occasional experience, but involves a compulsive repetition of potentially destructive or self-destructive activities, then it can indicate more severe underlying developmental difficulties. For example, some young people seek sensation because it creates a state that is preferable to underlying feelings of numbness, depression or emptiness. On the audiotape associated with this chapter, Jeremy describes his flight from boredom into exhilaration, where the 'kick' was part and parcel of taking life-threatening risks. This suggests that his adolescence took a more 'pathological' course up until the time he allowed himself to become more aware of the possibility of losing his life.

What are the factors that feed persistent, serious risk taking? In an article on the causes of anti-social behaviour in adolescence, J. Coleman (1979) suggested that the influences leading to a specific behaviour may be both direct and indirect. Thus, although the peer group may appear to exert a prime direct influence (as Plant and Plant suggest is the case with first-time drug or drink

experiences), there is unequivocal evidence that the great majority of teenagers start their drinking careers in the home. Teenagers who drink heavily frequently come from homes where excessive alcohol is common, which suggests that adolescent identification with a significant adult is also a potent factor. This was confirmed by an influential large-scale study in the USA, published in 1978 by Kandel and her colleagues. They focused on the social and psychological antecedents of entry into the different stages of alcohol and drug use, and distinguished between peer influence, parent influence, the adolescent's attitudes, and his or her involvement in other activities. Parental behaviour was the most fundamental determinant in leading the young person into early experiments with alcohol. However, no single factor stood out in relation to drug taking.

It seems that peer group pressure to conform can only be exercised under certain circumstances. Vulnerability to peer group pressure, writes Coleman:

> ... occurs in circumstances where parents leave a vacuum by showing little concern or interest, or where they themselves provide models for anti-social behaviour. (Coleman, 1979, p. 185)

The work of Kandel and her colleagues also suggested that there was a difference between *initiation* into an activity and the factors that *sustained* the activity. Various socio-cultural forces (school, peer group, family support, etc.) played a part during the stage at which the individual was likely to be initiated into drug-taking activity. However, what Kandel identified as individual personality traits, states and feelings, seemed to be more important in determining whether the adolescent would *continue* their involvement with drugs.

With the arrival of AIDS, sexual risk taking has become a crucial area of concern. Current research points to the complexities of the social and personal processes involved when adolescents have to make a decision about whether or not to use condoms. As Marina Barnard and Neil McKeganey highlight in their study of 14–16-year-olds:

> Our findings suggest that for many adolescents the whole issue of sex is negotiated with awkwardness and embarrassment. (Barnard and McKeganey, 1990, p. 113)

In common with other researchers they found that although girls are most likely to encourage the use of condoms, they were markedly reluctant to buy and carry them because of the negative comments they felt they would attract. Janet Holland and her co-workers, drawing on feminist social theory, argue that although girls

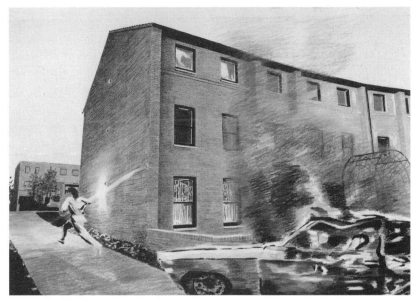

The excitement of risk taking can have damaging outcomes. (Centrepiece of a tryptych, 'The news comes to town', by Milton Keynes artists Boyd and Evans, gouache, 1985, in the collection of The Open University, courtesy Flowers East)

need to be able to negotiate and control sexual practice, they do not enter into negotiations with boys as 'equal partners' and may thus succumb to pressure to take a risk (Holland *et al.*, 1990).

In conclusion, although a degree of risk taking is a normal part of adolescent experience, persistent risk taking, where the individual is repeatedly endangering his or her health and safety, could be viewed as a curtailment of the developmental process. Adolescents who behave in this way may be finding their internal feelings, conflicts, pressures and anxieties too hard to think about or manage; risk-taking activities offer a solution of sorts, but the underlying difficulties remain unresolved, thus hampering the young person's ability to make further forward moves towards adult adjustment. However, the processes of adjustment do not occur in a social vacuum; they have to be negotiated not only within the personal world of family and peer-group but within a wider socio-economic and political framework, which shapes the actual or perceived 'forward moves' that a young person can make. We end this chapter with a brief commentary on adolescence from the social perspective.

Whose disturbance is it, anyway?

Adolescent development takes place not only in a family context but a social one. There are those who suggest that the phase we identify as 'adolescence' is a social construction. From this perspective, contemporary society has brought the adolescence 'problem' on itself by segregating young people from the adult world.

□ Can you think of some examples of how this segregation occurs in the United Kingdom?

■ We place adolescents in rigidly age-stratified compulsory education until the age of 16 and govern the transition to adulthood by imposing several legally-enforced restrictions on, for example, the age at which a person can marry, have sex, buy alcohol, vote, leave school, get a mortgage and so on.

As we said earlier, adolescents have to carve out an internal sense of their sexual identity, a sense of themselves as male or female. However, the characteristics of what are deemed to be appropriate male or female behaviours are also part and parcel of socially-constructed gender roles, which can exert considerable pressure on young people.

□ Can you list some of the social expectations that are linked to gender roles and their possible consequences for risk-taking behaviour?

■ Ideas about typical 'manly' behaviour may be linked to reckless driving, football hooliganism and high levels of alcohol consumption, with its attendant problems of dependency, drunken-driving and drink-related crime. Young women suffer from relatively few problems associated with alcohol, perhaps because drunken behaviour is deemed unfeminine; conversely, the current 'feminine ideal' may exert a pressure to be slim and hence partly explain the prevalence of anorexia nervosa. Difficulty in fulfilling the gender roles 'offered' to young people can in itself add considerable stress and anxiety, which may contribute to risk-taking behaviours.

Others argue that problems associated with adolescence are located not in the adolescents themselves but in the political and socio-economic structures of our society. It is less a question of locating difficulties in *either* the individual *or* society, but of considering their relative contribution. If adolescence is defined as the time when an individual is carving out their current and future professional, personal and sexual identity, then the relative ease or difficulty with which they achieve these tasks, and the forms their identity will take, depend not only on individual psychological factors but also on external conditions in society. Particularly in a period of economic recession, unemployment is a stark social reality, not a developmental failure of individuals.

There is also a complex inter-related set of factors based on social class, ethnic group, education and culture, which ensures that not all adolescents are granted equal access to further education and the job market. Lack of opportunities can have an important negative impact on development. Job and educational opportunities lead to economic independence, with attendant feelings of self-esteem. Where these openings are unavailable or in short supply, this can lead to feelings of frustration, a forced continued dependency on parents and lack of self-worth. Peter West, whose research into

teenage health in Scotland we mentioned earlier, sums up these interactions:

> In this complex web of influences, a perception of what the future holds in store may matter for your present health, your current identity and what that identity means for your current lifestyle ... If perceptions of the future do matter for health now, it may explain the high levels of psychological malaise experienced by so many young people. The spectre of low-paid jobs, no jobs and dependency on parents now extends to traditionally protected groups such as graduates ... Some of the appeal of rave culture, for example, may reside in its very immediacy and its capacity to postpone future concerns. (West, 1994, p. 40)

Conclusion

In this chapter we have described the biological changes occurring during puberty and explored the psychological demands that these physical developments give rise to. We have considered the major psychological tasks adolescents have to negotiate both in relation to themselves and to their families, and discussed possible reasons underlying poor adjustment to a new adult identity. This will have given you a framework in which to understand risk-taking activities, both as a part of normal development and as a form of 'acting out' to discharge unmanageable feelings or to compensate for feelings of emptiness. In the last section, adolescence was viewed in a broader social context—a focus continued in Chapter 7, which analyses the influence of social values in shaping sexual and reproductive behaviour.

OBJECTIVES FOR CHAPTER 6

When you have studied this chapter, you should be able to:

6.1 Outline the major features of mental functioning according to the psychodynamic perspective, and use this model to describe the major psychological tasks that adolescents have to negotiate in making the transition to adulthood.

6.2 Describe the physical and mental health of adolescents in the United Kingdom in the 1990s, pointing to gender differences in the major causes of morbidity and mortality; discuss the evidence on

whether adolescence is generally a period of serious psychological distress.

6.3 Summarise the major physiological changes that occur during puberty, noting their relationship to psychological changes in the same period.

6.4 Distinguish age-appropriate behaviours and anxieties during adolescence from what might be considered signs of greater difficulties, using risk taking to illustrate the discussion.

6.5 Discuss a range of influences on adolescents, arising from within their family or from the wider social environment, which may be supportive or provoke inner conflict.

QUESTIONS FOR CHAPTER 6

Question 1 (*Objective 6.1*)

What are the major psychological tasks that adolescents have to attempt to negotiate in making the transition to adulthood?

Question 2 (*Objective 6.2*)

Briefly summarise the evidence on physical and mental health in adolescence which supports the view that this phase of the life course is a time of severe, often unresolved, psychological conflict. What arguments could be used to challenge this view?

Question 3 (*Objective 6.3*)

Figure 6.5 shows the trend over time in the age at which girls have their first menstrual period (menarche) in six industrialised countries. Briefly describe the patterns in these data. Reflect on the

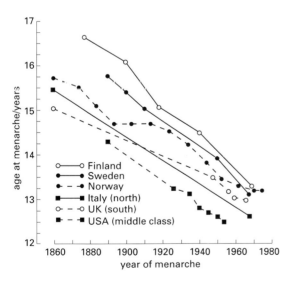

Figure 6.5 *The trend in age at menarche in six Western industrialised countries, 1860–1980 (Source: Marshall, W. A. and Tanner, J. M. (1986) Figure 12 in Falkner, F. and Tanner, J. M. (eds) Human Growth, Volume 2, 2nd edition, Plenum Press, London)*

possible reasons for this trend and its possible impact on the psychological tasks that adolescent girls must negotiate in the later twentieth century compared with earlier decades.

Question 4 (*Objective 6.4*)

What do the findings of the studies reported in (a) and (b) below tell us about the perception of risks associated with drug use or sexual activity among young people? How might adolescent perceptions of these risks differ from those of adults?

(a) A study of 1 929 teenagers aged 13–18 years at schools in Haringay in North London showed that approximately 25 per cent had used solvents or illicit drugs at least once; if legal drugs (tobacco and alcohol) were included, then only 15.4 per cent of the young people surveyed had never used drugs (Abdulrahim *et al.*, 1994). 'Curiosity' and the fact that 'it was exciting' were given as the most important motives for taking drugs for the first time.

(b) A study of sexual behaviour, knowledge and attitudes among 2 000 14–15-year-olds in schools in the North of England revealed that a third claimed they had already experienced sexual intercourse, but only 55 per cent of these sexually-active adolescents had used contraception during their first intercourse (Miller, 1994). The reasons given for having unprotected sex were the belief that a girl cannot become pregnant 'the first time' (19 per cent), no time or nowhere to get contraception (18 per cent), 'I did not think it was necessary' (12 per cent), 'I didn't want to' (8 per cent), too embarrassed to get or use it (6.5 per cent), lack of knowledge about what was available (3 per cent).

Question 5 (*Objective 6.5*)

The study of teenagers in Scotland by Peter West and colleagues (discussed earlier) contains the following tentative statement:

> One of the key issues we are currently exploring which may link these pieces of the jigsaw relates to identity, and specifically self-esteem. (West, 1994, pp. 39–40)

What do you consider might be the most important influences on self-esteem for an adolescent and how might self-esteem have an impact on health?

7 Sex, fertility and adulthood

While you are studying this chapter you will be asked to read the article 'The stigma of infertility' by Naomi Pfeffer, which appears in the Reader.[1] Naomi Pfeffer is also the author of this chapter; she is a social historian and Senior Lecturer in Health Studies at the University of North London, who has written and published widely on population policies and on infertility. Basiro Davey, from the U205 Course Team, developed the distance-teaching aspects of this chapter.

Shifting boundaries

During the transition to adulthood, young women and men are assumed to gain the maturity thought necessary to engage in sexual relationships and become parents. Indeed, sex and fertility are central preoccupations in adult life. It is almost impossible to discuss individual concerns about sex and fertility without considering society's attitudes to them. This is because these intimate aspects of our private lives are ineluctably connected to the public sphere. Differences in opinion about sex and fertility are fought over on moral and political battlefields. Throughout the twentieth century, skirmishes have been provoked by controversial developments in science, medicine, political and social policy, which have unsettled hitherto fixed points in apparently natural processes.

Despite or perhaps because of a century of unprecedented scientific, social and medical exploration, we approach the millennium with few certainties about the limits on our capacity to be sexual and fertile human beings. Boundaries are constantly shifting, both backwards and forwards. All over the world, many women and men are struggling both in favour of and against the extension of hard-won rights to make individual choices about sexual relationships; similar struggles are being fought over access to an appropriate means of regulating fertility. This chapter explores some of the issues raised by the tension in the realm of sex and fertility, between individuals' decisions to do what we choose with our own bodies, and the social conventions and legal regulations that govern us.

☐ 'Sex' is an ambiguous word; can you think of three different meanings?

■ **Sex** can refer to a set of physical characteristics indicative of biological maleness or femaleness, a person's gender identity, and certain acts in which people engage.

The issue is further complicated by the tendency of people to attach a variety of different meanings to 'having sex'. In a recent survey, for example, heterosexual respondents equated the term 'having sex' with vaginal intercourse, whereas homosexual respondents described a broader repertoire of sexual acts (Wellings *et al.*, 1994, p. 19; the survey is discussed in more detail below). In this chapter, 'having sex' refers to penetrative intercourse unless we state otherwise. The definition of **fertility** also changes according to who is using the term. For example, demographers define fertility as reproductive performance, and measure it in terms of live births. Doctors and probably the majority of the general public take fertility to mean the physical capacity to bear a child, whether or not one is actually born. The medical definition is the one adopted in this chapter.

[1]'Health and Disease: A Reader (second edition, 1995)

Sexual identity and sexual behaviour

The publication of the results of the 'British National Survey of Sexual Attitudes and Lifestyle' (summarised in *Sexual Behaviour in Britain*, Wellings *et al.*, 1994) has provided us with considerable information on the sexual behaviour of people aged between 16 and 59 years, based on a sample of around 20 000 men and women across Great Britain.[2] It found that most of the population in the early 1990s are heterosexual, responsible with contraception, stick to one partner, and don't have sex more than ten times a month.

The survey also provides details of a repertoire of heterosexual and homosexual sex acts with respect to age, gender, ethnicity, social class, education, marital status, and place of residence. It is the second large-scale empirical investigation into sexual experience carried out during the twentieth century. Other surveys have been on a much smaller scale.

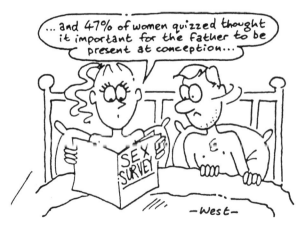

From the Journal of the National Association of Family Planning Nurses, *early 1990s. (Source: First Response to Pregnancy Planning Experts)*

[2]This age-range was chosen because the study's principle aim was to provide data on sexual behaviour to inform the development of strategies to combat the spread of AIDS; people below 16 and over 60 were not considered to be significantly at risk from sexually-transmitted diseases. Attitudes to sexual behaviour among older people are discussed in Chapter 10 of this book; Open University students studying this course in 1995 will receive a supplement on AIDS, which will be incorporated in *Experiencing and Explaining Disease* (revised edition, 1996).

The first large-scale investigation into sexual behaviour was carried out by Alfred Kinsey and his team of investigators in the USA from the late 1930s to the mid 1950s. A zoologist by training, Kinsey began to collect empirical data on sexual behaviour when he was appointed coordinator of a course set up by Indiana University in 1938, in order to educate young people for successful marriage. By the 1930s, many influential people had come to accept the idea that mutual sexual satisfaction is crucial to a happy marriage. Although initially Kinsey sought data for teaching purposes, his investigations into sexual behaviour attracted considerable financial resources from the powerful US Rockefeller Foundation. The Foundation was keen to find ways of encouraging stability in marriage, which it believed formed both the bedrock of social stability and an essential bulwark against the threat of communism, which was then notorious in the USA for, amongst other things, its promotion of 'free love', challenging the desirability of monogamy.

The concern that inspired the 'British National Survey of Sexual Attitudes and Lifestyle' in the 1980s was AIDS, a predominantly sexually-acquired infection, caused by the human immunodeficiency virus (HIV). Data available on current sexual behaviour were insufficient for the purposes of predicting the spread of HIV, and for mounting an appropriate and effective health education campaign to prevent its further spread. Initially the survey attracted the support of official bodies such as the Health Education Authority, the Economic and Social Research Council, and the Medical Research Council. However, in 1989, at the last moment, instructed by Margaret Thatcher, then Prime Minister of the Conservative government, the Department of Health declined to fund the full investigation, on the grounds that it was an excessive intrusion into people's private lives. Investigators in other countries have suffered similar fates; in both the USA and Sweden, governments have frustrated attempts to conduct national surveys into sexual behaviour. The Wellcome Trust stepped into the breach and funded the British survey; that organisation derives some of its income from Wellcome Foundation plc, a pharmaceutical company which manufactures Zidovudine (also known as AZT), one of the few drugs prescribed by doctors to people who are HIV-positive or have AIDS-related illnesses, in an attempt to delay the progress of the disease.

Figure 7.1 (*overleaf*) shows some of the data on age and heterosexual sex from the 'British National Survey of Sexual Attitudes and Lifestyle'.

☐ Briefly summarise the main patterns in these data.

■ Experience of vaginal intercourse at some time is almost universal among heterosexuals aged 25–59 years, and over 90 per cent of 25–44-year-olds reported it in the last year; the lower prevalence in older and younger age-groups was only substantial for 16–17-year-olds, around 40 per cent of whom had already had vaginal intercourse. The prevalence of oral sex was somewhat less common, though still reported by around 60 per cent or more of the sample in all age-groups except the youngest and oldest; it was noticeably lower among women aged 45–59 than among men of the same age. By contrast, the prevalence of anal sex—though comparatively low—declined very little with rising age-group and the sexes reported similar levels of this type of sex.

It is important to bear in mind that simple counts of sexual acts such as those in Figure 7.1 are not an indication of

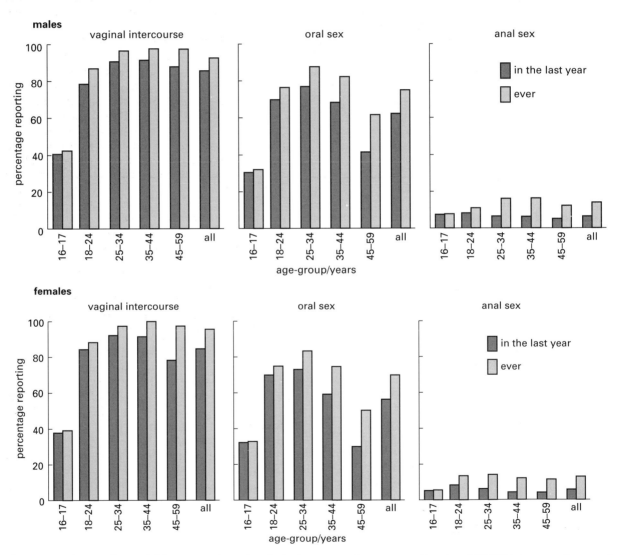

Figure 7.1   *The prevalence of different sexual practices in the last year, and ever, reported by almost 18 000 heterosexual men and women in different age-groups in Great Britain, surveyed between May 1990 and November 1991. (Data derived from Wellings, K., Field, J., Johnson, A. M. and Wadsworth, J., 1994,* Sexual Behaviour in Britain, *Penguin, Harmondsworth, Table 4.6, p. 155)*

sexual identification. Frequency of performance of sexual acts reveals little of people's ideas about their own sexuality or the choices they might like to make. This becomes obvious when we consider that for example, more than one-third of single people of all ages reported no vaginal intercourse in the last year (Wellings *et al.*, 1994, p. 163). Yet probably, if asked, most of these people would describe themselves as heterosexual and seeking a partner, rather than celibate out of choice.

Simple counts of 'disembodied' sex acts leave us in the dark about the larger social connections that shape sexuality; that is, the complex links between society, individual identity, choice, and the performance of individual sexual behaviours. This point is made powerfully by the American historian Ellen Ross and anthropologist Rayna Rapp, who warn against assuming that the sexual identities and experiences of black slave women and white plantation women, for example, were the same, although both may have had sexual intercourse with plantation owners (Ross and Rapp, 1984, p. 107). They argue that sexual feelings and activities express all the contradictions of power relations—of gender, class, and ethnic group. Looked at this way, it is not surprising that sex acts and sexual identity have the potential to provoke outrage and are regulated in every society. Many individuals campaigning for the right to express their sexuality in the way they choose see themselves as engaged in a political struggle for human rights.

Consenting to sexual relations

The principle of **consent** is one of the mechanisms through which the abstract 'right to choose' is translated into a concrete reality. It describes the right of an individual to make decisions that are respected, regardless of whether that decision is considered foolish or wise by others. In many respects, adulthood, citizenship and the capacity to consent are closely linked: our consent to be governed forms the basis of modern civil society. People deemed not to have the capacity to consent are often denied the right to vote; they may also be denied the right to make decisions in relation to sex, fertility and whether or not to undergo medical treatment and participate in medical research. Hence sex, which appears to be a deeply private and personal activity, cannot be talked about in isolation from medical, legal and political considerations.

Most adult heterosexual men have enjoyed fully the modern idea of rights, including the right to consent to sexual intercourse, for over 400 years; slaves, women and children who were seen as these men's property, and people with learning difficulties and severe mental health problems, have had to, or are still having to, fight for these rights. Acquisition of rights proceeds piecemeal; for example, in 1928, British women achieved the right to vote on an equal basis with men, but a woman's right to refuse sexual intercourse with her husband was only recognised in law in 1991 when rape within marriage was recognised as a criminal offence (*R v. R (rape: marital exemption)*, 1991, p. 481). Before then, a husband enjoyed conjugal rights over his wife's body and could demand sex irrespective of whether or not she agreed to it.

During the twentieth century there has been grudging recognition of children's rights. They now have the right to certain resources, such as education, and the right to protection from harm. Although pressure is being put on politicians to extend children's rights in other areas, few people support children's right to consent to sex. The denial of this right to children (and others deemed incapable of consenting, especially adults with learning disabilities) is justified on the grounds that it might expose them to risky situations which they may come to regret. Many people fear that such a legal right will lay them open to exploitation and abuse by more powerful people. Another worry is that foolish decisions might jeopardise the health and wellbeing of a child's adult self. As the sociologist Priscilla Alderson puts it:

> ... the future adult is implicitly seen as a butterfly imprisoned in a chrysalis (the child) and needing protection from any harm the careless child might do it before the date of magical release (the age of consent). (Alderson, 1993, p. 31)

The extent of the disagreement over the age at which the future adult is released from the chrysalis with sufficient maturity to consent to sex is evident in the variation in the legal age of consent specified by different industrialised countries (Figure 7.2, *overleaf*).

☐ Think back to Chapter 6 and the ages at which the biological changes of puberty take place in males and females. Compare these ages with those in Figure 7.2. What do you notice?

	heterosexuals	lesbians	gay men
Austria	14	14	18
Belgium	16	16	16
Bulgaria	14	14	14
Cyprus	16	16	illegal
Czech Republic	15	15	15
Denmark	15	15	15
Finland	16	18	18
France	15	15	15
Germany	14	14	18
Hungary	14	18	18
Iceland	14	14	14
Ireland	17	17	17
Italy	16	16	16
Liechtenstein	14	14	18
Luxembourg	16	16	16
Malta	18	18	18
Netherlands	16	16	16
Norway	16	16	16
Poland	15	15	15
Portugal	16	16	16
San Marino	14	14	14
Slovak Republic	15	15	15
Spain	12	12	12
Sweden	15	15	15
Switzerland	16	16	16
Turkey	18	18	18
United Kingdom	16	16	18

Figure 7.2 *Age of legal consent to sexual intercourse in Council of Europe countries, 1993 (1994 for United Kingdom). (Data compiled by the* Guardian, *published 8 February 1994)*

■ The development of secondary sexual characteristics does not coincide well with the legal age of consent, which is the same for heterosexual males and females in all these countries. Girls in industrialised countries become fertile about two years later than boys and take even longer to mature physically. In several countries different rules apply depending on whether the sex being consented to is heterosexual or same-sex; where a difference exists, the age of consent for homosexual males (though not, on the whole, for females) is higher than for heterosexuals, despite the fact that males reach physical maturity at an earlier age than females.

According to English law, it is unlawful for a boy or man to have sexual intercourse with a girl aged under 16, although she commits no offence in participating. Heterosexual sex between a woman over 16 and a boy under 16 is also criminal because it would constitute an indecent assault. Even consensual sexual activity between 15-year-old boys and girls is criminal in the eyes of the law because, according to the Sexual Offences Act 1956, the consent of people under 16 does not count.

Before The Criminal Justice and Public Order Act 1994 lowered the age of consent for same-sex sex between men from 21 to 18, Britain's age of consent for gay men was the highest in the developed world. The Sexual Offences Act 1967 had partially decriminalised male homosexual activity by introducing a number of provisos, including an age of consent set at 21 (the age of majority at that time, that is, the age at which voting was first allowed). Current British medical and psychiatric opinion is in favour of an equal age of consent for heterosexual and same-sex acts, albeit for health reasons: the British Royal College of Psychiatrists first said so in 1976, and in 1994 the British Medical Association publicly supported a reduction of the age of consent to gay sex at 16.

□ What might the 'health reasons' be?

■ Consent at 16 would allow young gay men to seek advice about 'safe sex' without fear of criminal prosecution. Those who are 'queerbashed' may fail to report the matter to the police for fear of being investigated themselves; they may also be open to blackmail.

Although the law is silent on the matter of sex between two women, lesbians in England effectively share the heterosexual age of consent of 16, because the Sexual Offences Act 1956 states that it is an offence for a person to sexually assault a girl under 16. Female homosexuality has never been criminalised in England; among the apocryphal explanations for the law's silence on lesbian sex are that Queen Victoria thought sex between women impossible or, alternatively, that she saw nothing wrong in it.

Without careful analysis, it is impossible to account for national differences in laws regulating sexual relations. Ireland provides a good example of the dangers of jumping to hasty conclusions. There is copious evidence to suggest that many Irish people are not prepared to flout Roman Catholic teaching on sex and fertility. In 1986, a majority rejected a proposal to vote in favour of making divorce legal. The notorious case of X, a 14-year-old victim of rape who, in 1992, was prevented from travelling to Britain for an abortion, provides another illustration of Ireland's laws in relation to matters of sex.[3] Yet in 1993, without any opposition, the Irish Dail agreed to the introduction of a common age of consent of 17 to heterosexual and same-sex relations. Furthermore, the Roman Catholic Church refrained from being obstructive when a change in law was made necessary by a ruling in 1988 of the Court of Human Rights in Strasbourg that the Irish ban on homosexual sex was a breach of human rights. The reason why many Irish people supported the new legislation was because the old laws, which banned homosexuality, had been introduced by a decision of an English court in 1855. As David Norris, a lecturer at Trinity College, Dublin, a Senator in the Dail and a leading campaigner for gay rights, put it, '[W]e want to move away from the British psyche which seems to need to discriminate' (quoted in Duval Smith, 1994, p. 16). It was his appeal against the banning of homosexual acts that led to the ruling by the European Court of Human Rights.

When compared to many other countries, English laws in relation to male homosexuality seem harsh. Most Western countries do not recognise the offence of 'gross indecency' under which men in England can be prosecuted for consenting to same-sex sex in public. Public opinion seems to favour a repressive attitude towards male homosexuality. A survey by Kaye Wellings and Jane Wadsworth (1990, p. 110) found that more than two-thirds of British men and more than half of women believed sex between two men to be always or almost always wrong (there was only marginally less condemnation of sex between two women).

British gay rights activists exploit the fact that accepted types of sexual behaviour vary widely between different cultures. As the celebrated British artist and film-maker Derek Jarman put it, in Britain, 'heterosexuality isn't normal, it's just common' (quoted in Robinson, 1994, pp. 4–5). Britain can claim to be marginally more tolerant of homosexuality than the USA, where homosexual acts are illegal in 14 States, and where three-quarters of respondents in the national 1989 General Social Survey judged them to be always or almost always wrong.

Paradoxically, opponents of gay rights portray male homosexuality as so attractive that, once experienced, a young man will be lost to it, and sacrifice his physical and

CHOOSE SAFER SEX.

Except in 'safe sex' campaigns (like this poster produced by the Health Education Authority), prejudice against gay men ensures that they are rarely portrayed as attractive, romantic and affectionate people—attributes commonly assigned to young heterosexual couples. (Photo: Health Education Authority)

mental health (similar fears are almost never expressed in relation to same-sex sex between women). Perhaps that is why the present law in Britain appears to support the claim that young gay men are in greater need of protection than young women. Indeed, there is evidence to suggest that the present law, far from offering protection to young gay men, is liable to have a number of damaging consequences, as outlined earlier.

[3]The European Court of Human Rights subsequently ruled that a member state could not restrict freedom of travel between European Union countries.

Consent and fertility

Some people hold that if it is a criminal offence for a man to have sexual intercourse with a young woman aged under 16, then it must be an offence for a doctor to prescribe her with contraception as that is tantamount to causing or encouraging her to agree to sexual intercourse. This was the official point of view until 1974, when the Department of Health and Social Security (DHSS) decided that contraceptive services should be made more readily available to girls under 16. The DHSS advised doctors that they might lawfully treat and prescribe contraception for a girl under 16 without contacting her parents; indeed, the doctor should *not* contact parents without the girl's agreement. Subsequently, the DHSS revised its advice to doctors, but it still held that if the girl was adamant her parents must not be told (a more detailed account of the events can be found in Margaret Brazier's book, *Medicine, Patients and the Law*, 1992, pp. 331–4).

The DHSS's advice undermined parents' rights to decide what is best for their children. It enraged Victoria Gillick, a mother of ten, who, in August 1982, went to court for the first of several hearings to seek a declaration that none of her five daughters should be given advice on contraception or abortion without her prior knowledge and consent. Mrs Gillick had been campaigning against the 1974 circular for several years before her first appearance in court. She believes that easy availability of contraception encourages young women to agree to sexual intercourse. By refusing them access to contraception without parental approval, her argument goes, young women will be deterred from starting to have intercourse for fear of pregnancy and parental disapproval; furthermore, it would provide them with a defence against pressure from their peers to have sex with someone. Opposing Mrs Gillick are those who claim that significant numbers of young women under 16 are going to continue having sexual intercourse, irrespective of whether they have lawful access to contraception. Hence, they argue, it is in their best interests to protect them from pregnancy by making contraception available.

Mrs Gillick's case was finally decided in 1985 by the House of Lords, the highest court in the land. It was a majority decision: not all the Law Lords agreed, which left the door open for dissenters. The decision held that if a doctor judged that a young woman had the capacity to understand the implications of contraception, then she could be offered advice on it. The decision ruled that it is a medical judgement whether or not a young woman is sufficiently intelligent and mature to understand the implications of sexual intercourse and her request for

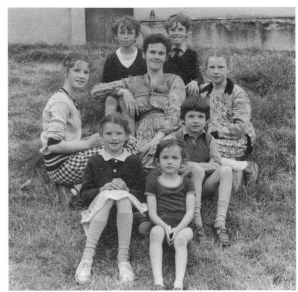

Victoria Gillick with seven of her ten children, photographed in 1983, when she sought a declaration that none of her five daughters would be given contraceptive advice or treatment by a doctor without her consent. (Photo: Gerry Free)

contraception. The *Gillick* ruling (*Gillick v. West Norfolk and Wisbech Area Health Authority*, 1985) suggests that young women can make legally recognised choices if they understand the decision. In effect, it extended medical power at the expense of that of parents. The ruling probably applies also for abortion to girls under 16.

Despite the *Gillick* ruling and the availability of contraception, under-age pregnancies rose steadily throughout the 1980s (see Figure 7.3): in 1989, the conception rate was 9.5 per 1 000 girls aged 13–15 years and by 1990 it had risen further, to 10.1 per 1 000.

□ Briefly describe the trends in the outcomes of under-age pregnancies, revealed by Figure 7.3. What do these data suggest?

■ The rates of both outcomes rose throughout the 1980s, but the increase was steepest for conceptions leading to maternities, so that by 1990 they had reached almost the same rate as conceptions leading to an abortion. Motherhood seems to have become more popular among very young women, perhaps because it became more acceptable during this period.

In its 1992 publication, *The Health of the Nation*, the Department of Health set the target of halving the

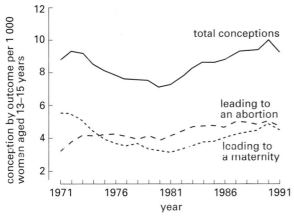

Figure 7.3 *Conception rates (per 1 000 girls in the age-group) and their outcomes for girls aged 13–15 years, 1971–91, England and Wales. (Source: Babb, P., 1993, Teenage conceptions and fertility in England and Wales, 1971–91, Population Trends, No. 74, Winter, OPCS, London, Figure 2, p. 13)*

pregnancy rate in under-16s to 4.8 per 1 000 girls by the year 2000. It proposed achieving this through the development of family planning services that are

> … appropriate, accessible and comprehensive, and which meet the needs of those who use or may wish to use them. (Department of Health, 1992b, p. 23)

This aim presumably includes services for young women under 16. The Department of Health's intention is to attract and satisfy individual 'customers' of family planning services, and not placate hostile public opinion. The ambiguity of the House of Lords' *Gillick* ruling threatened to undermine this ambition. In 1994, the Health Education Authority, the British Medical Association, the Royal College of General Practitioners, and other interested organisations, issued guidance which reminded general practitioners of the duty to confidentiality owed to patients irrespective of their age (BMA *et al.*, 1994). Doctors are only entitled to breach confidentiality where circumstances suggest that a vulnerable person is at risk of serious harm.

The 'management' of fertility

Social pressures and biological constraints

The Health of the Nation assumes that all conceptions in girls under 16 are 'unwanted' (Department of Health, 1992b, p. 22)—although it doesn't say by whom. Underlying this assumption is the idea that women acquire the capacity to 'manage' their fertility, and 'plan' their families during the course of their development as adults. A

mark of adulthood in women is that the babies they have are 'wanted'—having an 'unwanted' baby denotes immaturity.[4] It is important to note that discussions of 'wanted' and 'unwanted' babies have almost invariably focused on women; only rarely are men given any responsibility in managing fertility or asked whether or not their children were 'wanted'.

Preventing 'unwanted' pregnancies entails the expenditure of an enormous amount of energy by women.

> ☐ Make a rough estimate of the maximum number of menstrual cycles a present-day British woman could experience in her lifetime. How many of these cycles are likely to result in a birth?

> ■ On average, she will menstruate 13 times per year between the ages of approximately 13 and 50, so she could experience as many as 480 menstrual cycles in her lifetime; yet according to current social norms for most ethnic groups in the United Kingdom she should produce a baby only twice.

Social norms also dictate that on one of these occasions, her baby should be male, and on the other, female. It has also become increasingly the norm to 'delay' the first

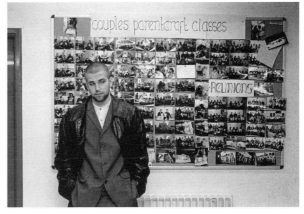

Discussions of whether babies are 'wanted', 'unwanted' or 'unplanned' rarely include prospective fathers. (Photo: Mike Levers)

[4] The terms 'wanted' and 'unwanted' are being used here in a social and personal sense, but demographers also make this distinction when analysing counts of conceptions and births, although they recognise that great difficulties surround any attempt to define or enumerate them, or to distinguish 'unplanned' from 'unwanted'. They sometimes refer to a continuum of 'wantedness', with an area in the middle where the mother 'doesn't mind'.

conception, which took place at an average age of 27 years in the United Kingdom in 1990 (as Chapter 2 described). Motherhood is increasingly popular in the 30s age-group, whereas it continues to decline in favour amongst women in their 20s, among whom it is at its lowest level of popularity since 1945.

Not every woman is capable of performing according to the exacting cultural standards set for reproduction, as Table 7.1 shows. On average, one in every five conceptions (20 per cent) was legally terminated in 1988.

Table 7.1 Number of conceptions and percentage ending in legal abortion in 1988, by age-group of mother, residents of England and Wales (excludes abortions to non-residents)

Age-group/years	Number of conceptions /thousands	Percentage ending in abortion
under 16	9	53
16–19	112	34
20–24	256	21
25–29	267	13
30–34	143	14
35–39	51	24
40 and over	11	45
total	**850**	**20**

Data from Botting, B. (1991) Trends in abortion, *Population Trends*, No. 64, Summer, OPCS, London, Table 4, p. 22.

☐ What does Table 7.1 tell us about the relationship between the woman's age and the likelihood of a conception ending in abortion?

■ Abortion is commonest among the youngest and oldest women: between a third and a half of conceptions to teenage girls and women aged 40 or over ended in abortion, the age-groups in which pregnancy is least acceptable or affordable. (An additional factor in older women is the increased possibility of conceiving a baby with Down's syndrome.)

The abortion rate also varies with the marital status of the pregnant woman: in England and Wales in 1985, outside marriage, 37 per cent of all known conceptions ended in a legal abortion; inside marriage, the proportion was 7 per cent. Not all 'unwanted' pregnancies are terminated: in 1981, it was estimated that about 42 per cent of 'un-

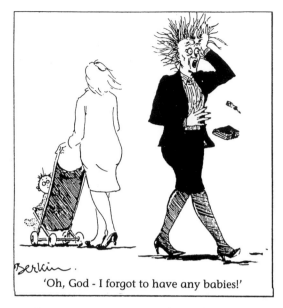

'Oh, God - I forgot to have any babies!'

Social pressure on women to produce children conflicts with the trend to enter full-time employment and delay reproduction until their 30s. (Source: Daily Express Syndication)

wanted' pregnancies resulted in live births. There were about 15 unwanted births that year per 1 000 married women who wanted no further births: this represents almost 10 per cent of the marital fertility rate (Coleman and Salt, 1992, p. 133).

Women who fail to meet the reproductive targets set by social convention risk being stigmatised and having opprobrium heaped upon them for having a child at the 'wrong' time, or for having too many or none at all. Men are rarely held to share responsibility for these 'failures'. The conception of an 'unwanted' pregnancy is taken as a sign of female immaturity and fecklessness; it is commonly stated that contraception is readily available and women have no excuse for not using it. Conversely, significant numbers of adults are unable to have a baby when they want one: estimates of the number of involuntarily childless women range from around one in six to one in twelve. Women who are unable to conceive are frequently characterised as emotionally unstable and desperate individuals, states that are rarely attributed to infertile men. The inability to conceive a wanted child often leads to episodes of emotional distress and for some individuals these can become chronic, but infertile women are portrayed in the media and by some of the doctors who specialise in treating infertility as desperate all the time. A short critique of this pervasive representation (by Naomi Pfeffer, the author of this chapter) appears in the *Reader* under the title 'The stigma of infertility'.[5] You should read it now; then answer the following questions.

☐ Why is it misleading to equate physical infertility with involuntary childlessness and what are the consequences of doing so?

■ Some infertile people never discover their infertility because they never attempt to have a child, either from choice or because of social impediments; others know about their infertility but do not want children. Some people who are physically capable of having a child are prevented from doing so by adverse personal circumstances. (You might have added that, after the menopause, all women become physically infertile regardless of whether they have previously had a child.) The equation of infertility with involuntary childlessness assists the portrayal of everyone who cannot have children as 'desperate' seekers of medical intervention.

☐ In contrast, infertility is described by Pfeffer as a 'self-imposed' rather than a 'medically-imposed' definition. Explain why.

■ There is no medical agreement about the length of time it 'normally' takes to get pregnant, nor about the number of different options a person with a fertility problem should try in attempting to have a child. Thus, whether or not to refer to oneself as 'infertile' is a personal decision.

This is summed up in these extracts from a poem by Chris Gothard, which also expresses her despair at the failure of medical science:

BARREN: INFERTILE: CHILDLESS
the names they wouldn't say
labels I gave myself
definitions of this lack.
I am less, reduced by this
unwomanly, abnormal. …
They had given up.
I was abandoned to the grey, flat, second-best
future of the childless.
(in Butler, C. (ed.), 1994, *If not a Mother*, p. 57)

[5] *Health and Disease: A Reader* (second edition, 1995).

In order to be successful managers of their fertility, adult women (and to a lesser extent men) have to negotiate more than the twin tyrannies of biology and social pressures. The government, the law, medicine, money, science, ethics and religion define the parameters within which women's endeavours to regulate their fertility take place. There is no equivalent attention to male fertility— indeed it is almost totally neglected.

Medical, scientific and legal controls

A number of significant developments in law and science have extended doctors' authority over women's fertility and also regulated women's *access* to the reproductive technologies they need if they are to manage their fertility successfully. Before 1967, except in exceptional circumstances, it was illegal for a doctor to terminate a British woman's pregnancy; those who did so committed a criminal offence and ran the risk of prosecution. The Abortion Act 1967 permitted the introduction of more liberal policies towards termination of pregnancy by removing the legal sanctions on doctors who carry out the procedure. The Act enlarged the circumstances under which a registered medical practitioner may legally terminate a pregnancy. As a result, most abortions are now carried out in safe conditions, unlike the so-called 'back street' abortions before 1967, in which many pregnancies were terminated, sometimes at great cost to women's health.

Until 1974, when the government agreed to pay GPs a fee for the service, many family doctors were loathe to offer advice on contraception to adult women. Some considered it immoral; others felt that it would be beneath their dignity after many years of training in medicine to be expected to dispense condoms, diaphragms and spermicides. Most people who could afford contraceptives bought them either by post, at chemist shops, barbers, or so-called rubber goods shops. In some parts of the country, contraceptive advice was dispensed by doctors at family planning clinics run by the local authority or the Family Planning Association.

The 'pill' and the intra-uterine contraceptive device (IUCD or 'coil'), developed by scientists and doctors in the 1960s, transformed contraceptives from 'rubber goods' into medicines whose safety and efficacy depended on women's supervision by a qualified medical practitioner. So-called 'scientific' contraception became widely available to women when, in 1974, the Department of Health and Social Security issued a circular outlining arrangements for a comprehensive family planning service within the NHS (Department of Health and Social Security, 1974). This circular represented a major change in government attitudes towards

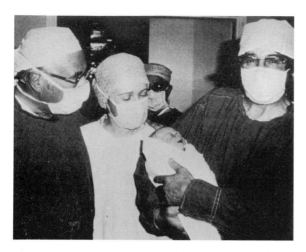

The research and medical team of (left to right) Patrick Steptoe, Jean Purdy and Robert Edwards presenting Louise Brown to the press immediately after her birth in 1978—the first baby ever to be conceived outside the womb. (Central Office of Information)

contraception by allowing contraceptives, for the first time ever, to be prescribed free of charge by doctors working within the NHS.

Although involuntarily childless women (and sometimes men) have always sought and received medical help, infertility treatment became regulated by law for the first time through the Human Fertilisation and Embryology Authority Act of 1990. The Act set up the Human Fertilisation and Embryology Authority (HFEA), which licenses the clinics that can legally offer **assisted conception techniques**, for example *in-vitro* fertilisation (IVF, described in Chapter 3), artificial insemination using donated semen (AID), and other techniques permitted by the HFEA. Before providing any woman with treatment, the HFEA's *Code of Practice* obliges clinics to take account of the welfare of any child who may be born or who may be affected as a result of the infertility treatment, by 'vetting' all would-be parents (HFEA, 1993a, p. 10).

☐ Can you identify an inconsistency in this practice?

■ The overwhelming majority of babies are conceived without medical assistance and no one judges whether these children's welfare is likely to be safeguarded by their parents. Extending vetting to all would-be parents would be considered a major intrusion into people's personal lives and would offend against our ideas about civil liberties. Only involuntarily childless couples receive this scrutiny ahead of infertility treatment (or adoption).

Note that with respect to abortion, scientific contraception and assisted conception techniques, the law licenses registered *medical practitioners* to undertake certain specified procedures. It does not confer on *women* the right of access to the means of managing their fertility. There may be a lot of talk about 'reproductive rights', and of 'a woman's right to choose' but, according to British law, it is medical judgement, and not a woman's personal decision, that determines whether she has legal access to abortion and to certain of the new reproductive technologies.

Financial constraints

Even where their circumstances pass muster in relation to medical and legal criteria, many British women have to pay for an abortion and couples have to pay for certain infertility treatments, or go without. This is because these procedures have been given a low priority within the NHS and they have failed to attract sufficient resources to meet demand. In 1991, for example, 47 per cent of the abortions carried out were within the NHS; the remaining 53 per cent were performed on a private fee-paying basis (*Hansard*, 1993). Relatively low-cost abortions are available because the voluntary sector has stepped in to fill the breach left by the NHS. However, the majority of involuntarily childless couples who seek assisted conception techniques are forced to turn to the private medical sector, where profit is the primary motivation. Some couples spend large sums on infertility treatments and it is not unknown for people to re-mortgage or sell their homes. The situation is summed up by Tim Gordon, from personal experience:

> … an attitude of 'you want it, you pay for it' has arisen in respect of childless parents who are now 'offered' DI (donor insemination) at £30–60 per cycle or IVF (*in-vitro* fertilisation) at £1 500–2 000 per cycle. At half a dozen cycles for any real hope of success, these prices clearly discriminate against those who are unable to pay. (Gordon, 1991, p. 4)

There is considerable regional variation in what treatments are available and at what cost. For example, in Scotland in 1992, IVF treatment was free in Glasgow, subsidised in Dundee (the cost to patients was £350–500 per cycle), but only available in Edinburgh and Aberdeen if the patient met the full cost of at least £1 500 per treatment.

☐ On what grounds could it be argued that abortion and infertility treatments should not be funded by the NHS?

■ Critics of NHS funding have argued that 'unwanted' pregnancies and infertility are not illnesses and so should not be 'treated' by the NHS.

Not every country accepts this point of view. For example, IVF is provided by the national health scheme of Denmark; in France the Social Security system reimburses the clinical costs of such treatment (Gunning, 1990, p. 5). In Italy, abortion is available on demand up to 90 days gestation, but only in state hospitals where no charge is levied.

Despite the high profile of assisted conception techniques, the majority of involuntarily childless women and men reject them either because they are too expensive or for personal reasons. According to the HFEA's *Second Annual Report*, in 1992 around 7 000 women underwent assisted conception techniques (HFEA, 1993b), out of at least 70 000 women who find themselves having difficulty in conceiving each year.[6] The decision to seek medical assistance to overcome infertility is simply one of many options available to women and men who have not been able to conceive a child.

Political, religious and ethical concerns

Like the age of consent for heterosexuals and homosexuals, access to reproductive technologies and the adequacy of resources made available for them are shaped by political, religious and ethical concerns. In the United Kingdom, some opponents of reproductive technologies have used them as the prime example to articulate their objections to the secular view of the world, which has come to dominate legal, medical and political thought. In general, the debate about abortion and certain assisted conception techniques generally focuses on whether or not the autonomy of the embryo or that of its mother should be paramount.

Those who oppose both abortion and the manipulation of embryos in the treatment of infertility do so on the grounds that at the moment of conception, a fertilised egg acquires the status of a human being. Deliberate death of the resulting embryo (or fetus, at later stages of development) is considered by them to be murder. However, according to British law, a fetus does not acquire the

rights attached to personhood, and hence cannot be murdered, until it has been born alive. As a compromise measure which probably satisfies none of the interested parties, the Human Fertilisation and Embryology Act 1990 forbids the development *in vitro* (in laboratory culture) of a human embryo beyond 14 days, when the neural tube emerges (recall Chapter 3). The neural tube is the earliest manifestation of a nervous system and brain, and hence putative consciousness.

Given the thorny nature of procedures to manipulate human eggs, sperm and embryos, it is probably in the best interest of any political party in a democracy not to become too closely identified with one or other extremes of point of view: to do so might cost votes. The 1967 Act which liberalised the law on abortion was piloted through Parliament not by the government of the day, but by David Steel, a member of the Liberal Party. It was not until twelve years after the birth of the first 'test-tube' baby in 1978, that the government introduced into Parliament the Human Fertilisation and Embryology Bill, which set up the HFEA. Nevertheless, governments clearly have an interest in the type of policies enacted in relation to fertility. As we pointed out above, the government's *Health of the Nation* targets in relation to fertility cannot be achieved by the year 2000 without women having easier access to contraception and abortion.

The political investment in fertility is more explicit and visible in countries governed by totalitarian regimes, which are often characterised by draconian laws with respect to abortion and contraception. The harshness of China's one child policy can be matched by the notorious anti-abortion and anti-contraception regulations introduced in the 1970s by Nicolai Ceausescu, President of Romania, in order to force Romanian women to bear as many babies as possible.

Choice and adequacy of contraception and infertility services

In Britain, around seven out of ten of the population of childbearing age use a contraceptive (Berer, 1994). Table 7.2 (*overleaf*) shows trends in use of different methods of contraception by British women between 1970 and 1989.

[6]The figure of 7 000 women receiving assisted conception techniques in 1992 includes some who came to Britain from overseas; the figure of 70 000 women experiencing difficulty with conception is arrived at by assuming that the 650 000 women per year who have a baby represent 90 per cent of the total who tried to conceive that year.

Table 7.2 Contraception: trends in use, 1970–89: percentage of ever-married women, aged 16–39/40 years, using each method

Form of contraception	% in 1970, England and Wales (1)	% in 1976, Great Britain (2)	% in 1983, Great Britain (3)	% in 1989, Great Britain (4)
pill	19	32	29	25
IUCD (coil)	4	8	9	6
condom	28	16	15	16
cap	4	2	2	1
withdrawal	14	5	4	4
safe period	5	1	1	2
abstinence	3	0	1	–
other	–	1	1	1
currently using at least one non-surgical method	71	61	58	50
female sterilisation	4	8	12	11
male sterilisation	4	8	12	12
total currently using at least one method	**75**	**77**	**81**	**72**
not using any method currently	25	23	19	28

Sample sizes surveyed in each column: (1) 2 520, Family Planning Services Survey; (2) 3 378, Family Formation Survey; (3) 2 850, General Household Survey; (4) 4 776, General Household Survey. 'Non-use' figure inflated by new 'no sexual relationship' option in questionnaire in 1983 and 1989. (Source: Coleman, D. and Salt, J., 1992, *The British Population: Patterns, Trends and Processes*, Oxford University Press, Oxford, p. 125; data derived from General Household Survey, 1983, Table 5.5; OPCS Monitor SS 90/3, Table 17)

☐ Look at Table 7.2. What do you notice about the trends in contraceptive use and how might you explain them?

■ In the 1970s, the 'pill' became the most widespread contraceptive, and use of previously popular methods such as condoms declined. Use of the 'pill' peaked in the late 1970s and then fell as fears about the health risks attached to it began to emerge (e.g. in 1977 attention was first drawn to the risks from thrombosis in older women). In the 1980s, the proportion of people being sterilised or not using any form of contraception increased.

Given the wide range of contraceptive techniques available in the United Kingdom, the impression conveyed is that with respect to their fertility, the needs of the adult population are being catered for. Indeed, the term 'cafeteria' is often used to describe family planning services, suggesting that women are free to pick and choose from the methods on offer (men have almost no choice). But just as cafeterias may not offer the type of food people prefer, or which meet their cultural requirements, so reproductive technologies may not suit or be appropriate to the needs of individuals.

Furthermore, it takes a great deal of knowledge, assertiveness and experience to make an appropriate choice in the contraception cafeteria; the risks and benefits attached to each method vary enormously. However, studies show wide differences in how much women know about all the methods of contraception; levels of knowledge vary with respect to age and social class (see the review by Marge Berer, 1994). Relatively few women, for example, know which factors might lessen the pill's effectiveness (Smith, 1992), and asking a doctor for advice is not always beneficial. Some surveys have found that many GPs lack knowledge about the various methods (Berer, 1994). In fact, GPs prescribe the pill to four out of five of their family planning clients and

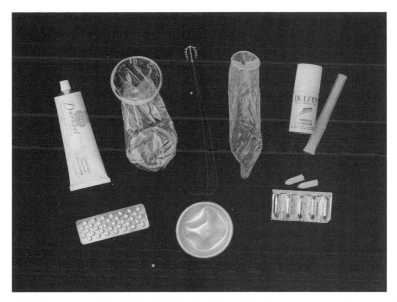

The wide range of devices in the contraceptive 'cafeteria' disguises the reality that most women have very little choice, once the drawbacks of each method have been considered; several methods require medical approval before they can be 'chosen'. Left to right (top row): spermicidal gel, female condom, intra-uterine contraceptive device (IUCD), male condom, spermicidal foam and applicator; (bottom row): the 'pill', diaphragm (Dutch cap) and spermicidal pessaries. (Devices from the Family Planning Association's contraceptive display kit. Photo: Mike Levers)

most neither fit IUCDs, nor offer post-coital contraception.

Many adults appear to be unhappy with the contraceptive technology developed in their name. For example, a survey carried out in 1993 found that 81 per cent of women aged 16–49 wanted new methods of contraception to be made available to them because established methods were unsuited to their needs (Editorial, *Journal of the National Association of Family Planning Nurses*, 1994). A survey of men attending a busy genito-urinary clinic in an area of south London revealed that condoms fit relatively few of them: one-quarter of respondents reported difficulties in putting condoms on and nearly one in five men found condoms too tight (Tovey and Bonell, 1993).

Similar criticisms have been levelled about the appropriateness of the technologies developed to overcome infertility. Some people argue that more resources should be devoted to finding ways of preventing women and men from becoming infertile, rather than on developing new, perhaps controversial, methods of treating infertility. Other critics are less concerned about the technology itself, but take issue with the poor standards of medical care meted out to infertile patients, who have

little 'choice' and scant knowledge of the methods on offer, nor of variations in the quality of the services available. More than a decade ago, Robert Winston, consultant gynaecologist at the Hammersmith Hospital, London, claimed that:

> … women are given drugs to induce ovulation when they ovulate already, much tubal surgery is performed with instruments more suitable for sharpening pencils, infertile men are fobbed off with drugs which have no proven effect on sperm quality and many women are advised to adopt bizarre coital positions or employ peculiar douches which add unwelcome variety to their sex lives but do little for fertility. (Winston, quoted in the *Observer*, 13 May 1982)

The appropriateness of medical treatment for infertility remains an issue in the 1990s not least because, as scientific knowledge advances, so the scope for medical intervention in reproduction increases. We return to this theme in Chapter 9, which refers to assisted conception after the menopause.

Conclusion

The right to consent to sex is one of the key social transitions in the human life course: almost every adult engages in sexual behaviour with a partner at some stage in their lives. In the United Kingdom in the 1990s, heterosexual identities and acts are socially accepted by a majority of the population, providing the participants are over the age of 16. Gay and lesbian identities are far less accepted and there are greater restrictions on homosexual behaviour between men than there are between women or between heterosexuals. For heterosexuals, consenting to sex also results in the use of methods to regulate their fertility. Discussions of fertility control tend to focus on the adequacy of women (rarely men) as individual 'managers' of their reproductive potential. The reproductive targets society sets as a mark of adulthood may not be physically or financially feasible or desirable for some people, and little attention is paid to the availability, appropriateness and adequacy of the techniques provided to help achieve them. Sex and fertility are matters of extreme concern, not just to adult women and men, but to doctors, politicians, religious leaders, legislators, ethicists and health-service providers—all of whom exert some power over the individual's ability to make and carry out decisions about their sexual and reproductive behaviour. In the next chapter, we turn to another major source of concern in adult life: paid work and domestic work, the stresses involved in having a job or in being unemployed.

OBJECTIVES FOR CHAPTER 7

When you have studied this chapter, you should be able to:

7.1 Comment on the limitations of survey data on reported sexual behaviour as indicators of sexual identity and sexual practices.

7.2 Give examples to support the assertion that the legal age of consent to sexual intercourse is determined more by social forces than by biological maturity.

7.3 Discuss the means by which doctors and medical scientists have assumed an unprecedented level of authority in the management of fertility in the United Kingdom in the 1990s.

7.4 Outline other (i.e. non-medical) external constraints on the ability of women and men to manage their own fertility.

QUESTIONS FOR CHAPTER 7

Question 7.1 (*Objective 7.1*)

In an interview study of homosexually-active men by Andrew Hunt and Peter Davies, published in 1991, respondents were asked the following question:

> Suppose someone asked you 'How many sexual partners have you had this month?', what must have happened sexually for someone to 'count' as your sexual partner? (Hunt and Davies, 1991, p. 46)

The responses are recorded in Table 7.3. What light do these data shed on the need for caution in interpreting surveys of sexual behaviour?

Table 7.3 Categories of answers given by respondents in a sample of 930 homosexually-active men when asked to define a sexual partner; interviews conducted in England and Wales in 1990

Counts as a sexual partner if following occurred:	Number responding	Percentage*
genital contact	449	48.2
orgasm	241	25.9
bed/naked/sleep with	208	22.3
physical contact	69	7.4
eroticism/arousal	25	2.7
aim for orgasm	15	1.6
must see more than once	14	1.5
privacy	4	0.5

*Percentages total more than 100 as some people mentioned more than one category. (Source: Hunt, A. and Davies, P., 1991, What is a sexual encounter? in Aggleton, P., Hart, G. and Davies, P. (eds) *AIDS: Responses, Interventions and Care*, The Falmer Press, London, Table 3.1, p. 47)

Question 7.2 (*Objective 7.2*)

Look again at Figure 7.2. What aspects of these data suggest that the legal age of consent to sexual intercourse is socially determined? Are there any features of the data to suggest that biological development is being taken into account? (You will have to think back to the discussion of puberty in Chapter 6 to answer this question fully.)

Question 7.3 (*Objective 7.3*)

Read the following extract from the book by Robert Edwards and Patrick Steptoe, *A Matter of Life: The Story of a Medical Breakthrough*, in which they describe their early attempts at *in-vitro* fertilisation.

> Once the eggs had started their indomitable ripening programme no hesitations were allowed. There was no turning back. Patrick had to be prepared to carry out the laparoscopy to obtain the eggs; Jean and I had to be at Kershaw's on the dot to obtain those same eggs prior to fertilisation. Alas, we discovered slowly that we were fertilising fewer eggs than had been the case at Oldham ... As a result Jean and I too often drove back to Cambridge silent and deflated, having achieved little or nothing though we had stayed several days up north. (Edwards and Steptoe, 1981, p. 121)

Who is missing from this account and what does it suggest about the role that doctors and medical scientists have assumed in the management of fertility in recent years?

Question 7.4 (*Objective 7.4*)

What policy issues would need to be addressed to enable adult women and men to have greater autonomy over the management of their own fertility?

ISLE COLLEGE
RESOURCES CENTRE

8

Work and stress in adult life

This chapter builds on the discussion of contemporary inequalities in health between people in different occupations in the United Kingdom, and between social classes when defined by occupational grouping, which occurred in another book in this series, World Health and Disease, *Chapters 9 and 10.[1] During your study of this chapter you will be asked to listen to an audiotape entitled 'Working lives: choices and conflicts'. You could also usefully study an article by Elizabeth Paterson, 'Food work: maids in a hospital kitchen', which appears in the Reader[2] and is optional reading.*

The principal authors of this chapter are: Howard Kahn, Lecturer in Organisational Behaviour in the Business School at Heriot-Watt University, Edinburgh, who has a background in business systems analysis and researches topics in organisational psychology such as job satisfaction, motivation and stress; and Cary L. Cooper, Professor of Organisational Psychology in the Manchester School of Management, University of Manchester Institute of Science and Technology, who is Editor of The International Journal of Organizational Behavior, and whose main research interest is in occupational stress. Basiro Davey, from the U205 Course Team, developed the distance-teaching aspects of this chapter and contributed some original material.

Introduction

One of the first questions most people ask of others is 'What do you do?' or 'Where do you work?'. A person's job appears to carry a great deal of information about who they are *as a person* and their occupation is a major determinant of their social status. Official statistics such as those presented in reports of the Registrar-General for England and Wales classify the whole population into six social classes, based on groups of occupations. This is just one example of the central importance of work to the way in which people see themselves and others in our culture. Work is a defining characteristic of adult status: there are fears that the rising numbers of school-leavers who cannot find a job may experience difficulty in making the psychological and social transition to adulthood (already discussed in Chapters 2 and 6 of this book). In the 1980s and 1990s, the million or so long-term unemployed have been described as an 'underclass', increasingly excluded from adult society. This chapter considers the psychological effects of working or not working, and of combining paid work with domestic labour. It also discusses the problems facing researchers in establishing whether 'stress' arising from work or the lack of it has measurable effects on health.

Abundant evidence exists that certain occupations expose their workforce to direct hazards to health such as chemical toxins, radiation, excessive noise or vibration, cold or heat, heavy lifting and danger of falls or falling objects. The indirect hazards are also well documented in terms of the additional health risk experienced by people in low-paid jobs, who can afford relatively poor standards of housing, heating and nutrition and who often live in districts with inadequate provision of, or access to, amenities such as sports facilities that might have a bearing on health status. Another important direction that research has taken in an attempt to explain the gradient of illness and disability between professional and manual occupations has been to evaluate the contribution of so-called 'lifestyle' factors, such as consumption of tobacco and alcohol, or obesity and lack of exercise, which tend to be greatest among blue-collar workers. These *social inequalities* in health have been extensively discussed elsewhere in this series (see footnote 1).

---

[1] *World Health and Disease* (1993) Open University Press.

[2] *Health and Disease: A Reader* (second edition, 1995).

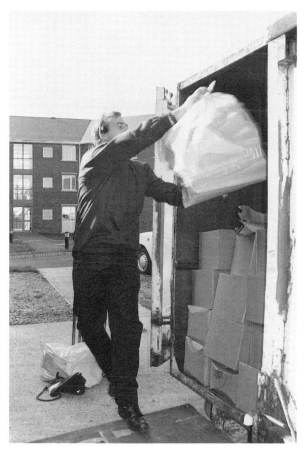

Occupational hazards, such as heavy lifting, which can have a direct effect on physical health, have been extensively researched among male manual workers; in the 1990s, work-related threats to psychological health are of increasing concern. (Photo: James McCarthy)

However, when all the measurable influences on health arising from direct hazards in the workplace, poor socio-economic circumstances and 'lifestyle' factors are taken into account, a gradient between the occupational classes still remains. For example, these factors taken together explain roughly 40 per cent of the health differences between employees in the highest and the lowest occupational grades in the civil service, a finding established by Michael Marmot and colleagues in two widely respected studies of Whitehall civil servants (Marmot, 1986, and Marmot *et al.*, 1991).[3]

[3] The findings of the Whitehall studies in relation to occupational gradients in coronary heart disease are discussed in *Dilemmas in Health Care*, Chapter 10.

In seeking an explanation for the remaining health gradient in these and other studies, attention has increasingly focused on the possible effects of the *organisation* of the work itself: factors such as its perceived stressfulness, the level of 'job satisfaction', the distribution and use of power in an organisation, job security and career progression. Could differences in factors such as these between different kinds of jobs, even within the same organisation such as the civil service, contribute to the very different health experience of workers at different levels in the organisational hierarchy? Moreover, these organisational factors are beginning to be investigated in the context of the *psycho-social environment* of a specific workplace and its 'culture'; this involves study of the psychology of the workers as individuals, their behaviour at work and the ways in which they interact.

The need to combine responsibilities at work with responsibilities at home has also come under scrutiny as a possible source of stress in adult life, particularly for working women who generally take the largest share of domestic labour and childcare.

Collaborative research into this complex arena by psychologists and sociologists, anthropologists and political scientists, has gradually coalesced into the discipline of **organisational psychology**. This chapter gives a view of the impact of work on health and wellbeing from this perspective.

Work and non-work

Attitudes to work

There are many ways in which individuals view the meaning of work, and these are affected by pay, hours of work, working conditions and also by how different occupations tend to be defined in terms of status. There is general agreement from a wide range of studies by organisational psychologists in different industrialised countries that the 'higher' the occupation in terms of an accepted hierarchy of jobs in that country (for example, the Registrar-General's classification of occupational social class in the United Kingdom), the more challenging and motivating workers find it, and the more stimulated and fulfilled they tend to feel. Jobs higher in 'status' in this sense also tend to be better paid, offer shorter hours and more paid holidays, and have greater time flexibility. In contrast, the 'lower' the job in terms of the occupational hierarchy, the more likely the job-holder is to see work as primarily a means to an end, that is, gaining a wage.

A group of management and social researchers, led by Alan Cowling of Middlesex University, has distinguished three different types of employee orientation to work: instrumental, bureaucratic and solidaristic, which they describe as follows:

> *Instrumental* [orientation], where the primary meaning of work is as a means to an end—a way of acquiring the wherewithal to support a way of life of which work itself is not a valued part. People with this orientation see their paid employment in calculative terms; effort and attachment to the occupation are balanced coolly against the rewards on offer. Emotional involvement in the job is low and 'work' is sharply separated from other segments of life. On the whole, manual workers are seen as the most likely group to have work orientations approximating to this type.
>
> *Bureaucratic* orientation, where the meaning of work is in terms of a commitment to the organisation in return for a steady rise in the status/income hierarchy, but material rewards are not primary—it is the intrinsic rewards and opportunities for personal achievement that are important. Other areas of social life are orchestrated to link with work life so that the separation of work from non-work is not sharp. On the whole, this orientation is strongest among non-manual workers.
>
> *Solidaristic* [orientation], where work is defined as a group activity involving an immediate set of workmates or even all those participating in, say, a small enterprise. Economic rewards are only maximised where this does not threaten group solidarity: loyalty to workmates or the firm might mean accepting lower material rewards. But involvement in work is high and, again, there is no sharp separation between work and other spheres of social life. (Cowling *et al.*, 1988, p. 22)

As an example of this last orientation, they suggest coal-miners, dockers and ship-building workers.

While this formulation greatly simplifies the meaning of work to individuals, it does indicate that different people have different views of and needs from their job. Another example occurs in Table 8.1, from the work of British management researcher, author and broadcaster, Charles Handy.

Table 8.1 Analysis of 2 000 replies to the question 'what is the most important aspect of your work?', when British workers (from across the social spectrum) were asked in 1988

Responses	Per cent answering
having control over what to do	50
using knowledge and experience to make decisions	50
having a variety of things to do	39
amount you earn	35
being with and making friends	21
doing a job that you know people respect	19

Note: The highest socio-economic group put money even lower at 25 per cent and variety higher at 62 per cent. (Source: Handy, C., 1990, *The Age of Unreason*, Arrow Books, London, p. 164)

A job provides money, which allows the individual to purchase the goods and services that indicate that he or she has an accepted status as a member of society. For many young people, money means independence, and the chance to move away from the parental home. Work also provides a social framework to life, a chance to make friends, and gives structure to the day. To most adults, work is a psychological necessity and without it the individual feels marginalised and excluded from the mainstream of society. For many people, *any* paid work is better than not working.

Women's work

The intrinsic satisfactions of certain jobs have often been used as an argument for keeping pay low. Interestingly, this is usually in occupations with a large proportion of women, e.g. teaching and nursing; this may be yet another example of the way in which women's work—in or out of the home—is devalued because it *is* performed by women. Studies of attitudes to work (and non-work) have concentrated on men rather than women, who have rarely been asked the question 'Why work?'. Comparatively little is known about the particular relationship in women of stress, work and health,

> ... nor do we understand the implications for women's health of their increased involvement in the labour force. In addition, research has often treated women as a homogeneous group,

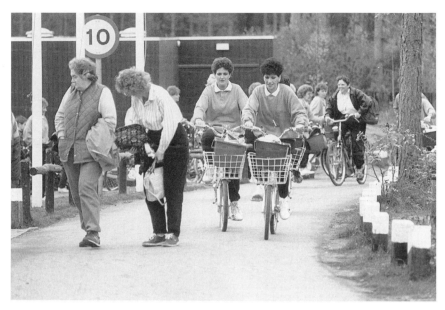

Compared with current knowledge about the effect of work on men's health, much less is known about the implications for women's health of their increased involvement in the labour force. (Photo: Mike Levers)

'averaging' across the effects of different types of occupation and jobs as well as across the different life stages of women ... clearly, the research to be conducted during the 1990s must move to a more complex understanding of the effects [of stress] on women and their greater participation in paid employment. (Ross and Altmaier, 1994, p. 24)

The relative neglect of workforce issues focused on women may be because women's work outside the home came to be regarded in the twentieth century as temporary work, as a means of supplementing family income to obtain items such as holidays or consumer goods, performed in addition to their 'real' work within the home and family. Women are not paid for the work they do in the home, although this supports the national as well as the household economy in various ways.

☐ What aspects of women's domestic labour support the national economy?

■ Childbearing, child rearing, education and socialisation of future workers; care and maintenance of economically active adults and (increasingly) older relatives, who would otherwise need state-funded health and social care; tension management, health promotion (e.g. through nutrition) and lay health care during sickness within the family.

Voluntary work, which also relies heavily on women's labour, has tended to be even more invisible than domestic work in most research studies. Retired and semi-employed people, the voluntarily and involuntarily unemployed, as well as those in full-time jobs, often also undertake voluntary work, which further indicates the importance of work to the individual.

Unemployment and uncertainty about the future

Unemployed people are often seen as having failed, or as somehow being outside society's norms. Not having a job not only excludes an individual from taking his or her place in the formal economy, but results in the loss of many social and communal activities. The adverse consequences of unemployment for mental and physical health have been convincingly demonstrated by epidemiologists and social researchers and are discussed elsewhere in this series.[4]

Even *before* finding their first job, young adults in the 1990s are confronted with problems and difficulties which their parents did not have to face. For instance, in some inner-city areas unemployment rates are over 50 per cent, and many young adults perceive that they have

[4]*World Health and Disease*, Chapter 10.

little chance of obtaining a job. As an extension of this problem, counselling services at many universities and colleges in Britain are in crisis, with more students (and staff) seeking help than ever before for severe psychological problems.

In a time of recession and redundancies, those in work face problems associated with an uncertain future. When an organisation has to lay off employees, it may well not re-employ them if the economy improves, but require existing staff to work harder. The remaining staff may also consider each other as potential threats. If there are to be more redundancies, people worry about who will be selected. This kind of anxiety about the future is more prevalent at a time of increasing and/or high unemployment, as in the United Kingdom throughout the 1980s and into the 1990s.

The changing work environment

Hazardous machinery in the workplace, noise, vibration, dust, exposure to toxic and carcinogenic chemicals, and so on, still have a serious impact on health in certain manual occupations, even though they are subject to legal controls. These direct occupational threats to physical health are discussed elsewhere in this series.[5] However, as the manual industries declined in the 1980s and white-collar jobs in businesses and the service sector increased, so the problem of stress-related illness arising from the organisation of the workplace came to the forefront of research.

The psychological stresses of the changing workplace include loss of control of the work environment, greater psychological demands, social isolation, lack of decision-making power and so on. We will look more closely at these stresses later in the chapter. New forms of work, such as the development of organisations which employ a relatively small number of permanent 'core' employees supported by temporary staff, staff working from home via telecommunications systems, an increase in part-time working, etc., may be attractive to organisations, and to a number of individual employees, but bring with them new stresses. Of course, the psycho-social problems associated with the 'older' forms of work such as night-work and shift-work continue. These changes have contributed to the widespread perception that the workplace is becoming ever more stressful. According to some commentators, simply being alive in modern society is so stressful it may present a threat to health and wellbeing:

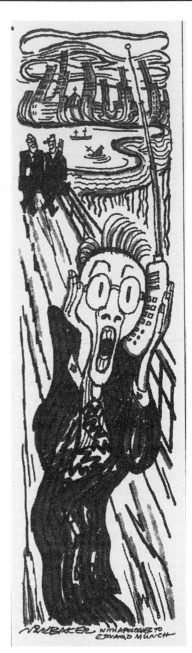

Simply being alive in modern society is stressful, according to this cartoon which appeared in the Financial Times *on 23 May 1994. (Drawn by Nick Baker)*

[5]*World Health and Disease,* Chapter 9.

... each individual not only is beset by the pressures of his or her own daily life but is privy to every disaster in the country and the world through modern news media and communication methods. Perhaps the gains of modern civilisation will be outweighed by the stress-created side effects if we do not come to understand, control, prevent or adapt to stress and anxiety. (Kutash *et al.*, 1980, preface, p. xii)

Defining and measuring stress at work

Each month sees the publication of dozens of new articles reporting research into stress and its effects upon a particular group in society. Rightly or wrongly, stress has become a major concern to individuals, to the organisations in which they may work, and to the national economy. The popular view is that technological change, recession and ever-increasing demands for higher productivity have produced an unprecedented level of stress. The premature deaths of MPs, the suicides of undergraduate students, and the high alcoholism rates of professionals such as doctors and airline pilots are seen as linked with increasing levels of stress. But is there indeed a relationship between stress and health? This question leads us to examine a persistent problem in stress research: the definition of **stress** itself.

Two American academics and stress researchers, Debra L. Nelson and James Campbell Quick, summarise the problem and offer their own definitions:

Stress is one of the most creatively ambiguous words in the English language, with as many interpretations as there are people who use the word. Even the stress experts do not agree on its definition. Stress carries a negative connotation for some people, as though it were something to be avoided. This is unfortunate, because stress is a great asset in managing legitimate emergencies and achieving peak performance. Stress, or the stress response, is the unconscious preparation to fight or flee a person experiences when faced with any demand. A stressor, or demand, is the person or event that triggers the stress response. Distress or strain refers to the adverse psychological, physical, behavioral, and organisational consequences that *may* occur as a result of stressful events. (Nelson and Quick, 1994, p. 202)

Researchers into occupational stress have variously used the term 'stress' to denote the environmental factors impinging upon the individual, or the individual's perceptions of them, or their immediate or long-term effects. This confusion makes it difficult to compare the results of different studies or to understand the causal relationships reported in research.

Nelson and Quick referred to a common definition of stress, derived from the well-established physiological responses known collectively as the **fight or flight reaction**. Coordinated physiological responses have evolved in humans and many other mammals which prepare the individual for a rapid reaction if he or she feels threatened by a possible attack. Perception of such a threat automatically evokes nervous and hormonal responses in preparation for 'fight or flight'. The rate of respiration, heart rate and cardiac output increases, blood pressure rises and the flow of blood to the tissues and organs shifts so that the muscles get more at the expense of the gut and skin. Hormones from the adrenal glands cause stored fuels to be released into the bloodstream in the form of glucose and fatty acids as sources of extra energy for the working muscles.[6] As soon as the attack and the effort associated with it are over, regulatory mechanisms bring the body back to its 'resting' state.

In modern humans, stressful situations occur numerous times each day, and may produce aspects of the physiological responses to stress, but there is rarely an opportunity for a physical outlet such as 'fight' or 'flight'. Persistent activation of the physiological responses involved in the fight or flight reaction has often been taken as proof that an individual is under **physiological stress**. There is sufficient evidence from animal experiments to justify the expectation that sustained physiological stress in humans could cause changes to the bodily organs over the medium and long term, and that these may result in physical and/or mental disorders.

Two American stress researchers, Brian Steffey and John Jones, have recommended that greater attention be given to research based on objective outcome measures, such as blood pressure and various biochemical indicators of stress obtained from blood or urine samples. However, physiological definitions of stress do not seem to correlate well with self-reports of how stressed an individual *feels* themselves to be. For example, their own research on clerical workers under stress

... did not uncover the expected relationships between perceived stress and a battery of blood

[6]The metabolism of fuels derived from the products of digestion is discussed in *Human Biology and Health: An Evolutionary Approach*, Chapter 7.

chemistry measures. The results ... resemble those of other studies that have also found weak relationships between self-reported stresses and biochemical measures. (Steffey and Jones, 1988, p. 695)

Partly as a consequence of difficulties such as these, but also as research tools in their own right, an ever-increasing array of questionnaires and rating scales has been developed to make systematic assessments of subjectively experienced **psycho-social stress**. These assessments have sometimes been criticised precisely because they *are* subjective and many studies are based on self-reports. Self-completed questionnaires and rating scales rely on the assumption that all respondents have interpreted the questions in the same way and have answered honestly; but questions about performance at work can elicit defensive answers which bias the outcome. However, it is essential to take full account of personal experience when evaluating the stresses associated with a particular job.

☐ Can you suggest why?

■ The experience of work situations differs from person to person: while one individual may work well under the pressure of deadlines, another may get 'uptight' and feel stressed; one person may find slow periods with little work boring and frustrating, while another finds the same situation desirable and relaxing.

A commonly used research tool, the Crown–Crisp Experiential Index, illustrates the ways in which organisational psychologists approach a definition of stress in psycho-social terms. The Index consists of 48 questions such as 'Do you often feel "strung up" inside?', 'Do you experience long periods of sadness?' and 'Can you think as quickly as you used to?'. The answers provide information about the person's mental health and the Index is widely used in clinical psychology. The mental states of most interest to many organisational psychologists are: *free-floating anxiety* (described by Crown and Crisp, 1977, as anxiety evident in an individual who is afraid but, unlike normal fear, cannot discern the cause; it consists of dread, indefinable terror, tension without a cause, or panic); *somatic anxiety* (indicated by physical symptoms such as breathlessness, headaches and other aches and pains); and *depression* (sadness of mood, combined with difficulty in thinking clearly and slowing of actions and activity).

The methodological problems in stress research do not end with determining an operational definition of stress for the purposes of a particular investigation and adapting it to take account of individual differences arising from the personality of the worker. The **stressor**, the source of the stress, must also be defined and a method devised for measuring it reliably. This is tricky, given the huge variety of circumstances or events that could fit the following definition:

... all stressors have one thing in common: they create stress or the potential for stress when an individual perceives them as representing a demand that may exceed his or her ability to respond. (Hellriegel, Slocum and Woodman, 1992, p. 280)

A similar process of definition and measurement must be set up to detect any effects of the chosen stressor on physical and/or mental health. Establishing that there is a link between stressor and health outcome is particularly difficult, for reasons that two of the pioneers of organisational psychology, Robert Karasek, an American academic, and Tores Theorell, a Swedish physician, point out.

Another common characteristic of stress theories is that the nature of the causal link between environment and effect on the individual is less easily determined than is usually true for the physical sciences or for conventional medical science. Instead of a single unambiguous cause-and-effect linkage, as in the hard sciences, in stress models many causes may accumulate to produce a single effect. On the other hand, a single cause (stressor) may manifest itself in many quite different effects. Furthermore, there is usually a significant time delay between the cause and the effect ... The ambiguity of stress theory need not be mistaken for non-science or sloppy science; it is merely another form of cause–effect rationality. This form of rationality is probably very well suited to complex systems of all sorts that involve multiple, interacting subsystems. (Karasek and Theorell, 1990, p. 87)

Difficulties in demonstrating causal links between stress and health have led to a stress literature awash with studies that purport to establish these relationships and which cite numerous stress-related outcomes, but the methodologies used are often extremely weak, suffering from 'poor control groups, low response rates, crude statistical analyses and weak designs' (Sloan and Cooper, 1987, p. 117). Longitudinal stress research is essential, since most stress/illness links occur over time: some outcomes can take weeks or months to develop, as in the case of *post-traumatic stress disorder*, which has become an accepted diagnostic category in the wake of accidental disasters and warfare. Studies looking for effects on the incidence of chronic illness such as coronary heart disease or cancers, may require many years to complete. The problem is that researchers are rarely able to commit the time and resources necessary to long-term studies, and are often unable to obtain all the data that might be implicated.

Despite these methodological difficulties, a considerable body of research has been conducted since the mid-1970s in several industrial countries, primarily the United Kingdom, Scandinavia, the USA and Canada, and this has informed the building of models of how stress at work may lead to adverse health outcomes. A widely used model was developed by Cary Cooper, one of the authors of this chapter, indicating how the sources of stress at work interact with various characteristics of the individual to produce symptoms of occupational ill-health and consequent disease (Figure 8.1). In the remaining sections of this chapter, we examine the aspects of this model in more detail and illustrate some of the outcomes of stress at work by reference to selected research studies.

Sources of stress at work

If you have ever had paid employment outside the home, you are likely to recognise from your own experience some of the six major categories of stressors in the workplace listed in Figure 8.1, which have been identified in numerous research studies. We review them briefly here.

Stressors intrinsic to the job

Every job is thought to have a set of unique factors which job-holders identify as sources of pressure, but four major recurring themes reported by many employees are highlighted here. These are (i) physical working conditions, (ii) information technology, (iii) work overload and underload, and (iv) working long hours.

Physical working conditions

There is clear evidence of a positive relationship between stress and negative physical working conditions such as noise, extreme temperatures, pollution and crowding.

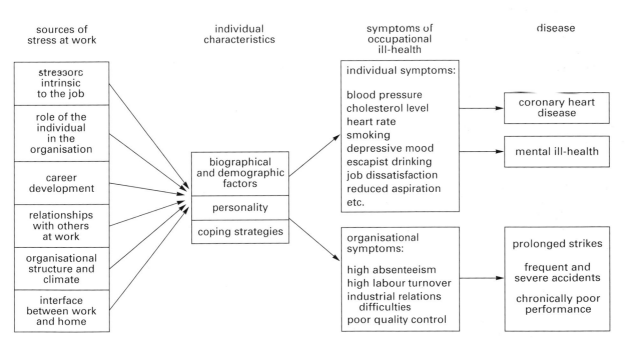

Figure 8.1 *A model of stress at work and its occupational and health outcomes. (Source: Cooper, C. L., 1986, Job distress: recent research and the emerging role of the clinical occupational psychologist,* Bulletin of the British Psychological Society, **39**, *Figure 1, p. 325)*

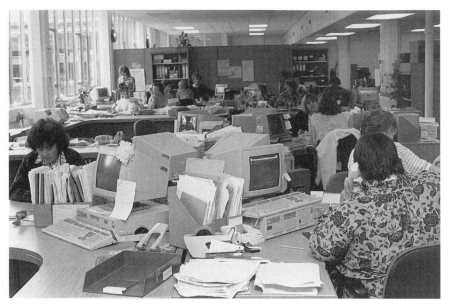

Open-plan offices can be stressful working environments for individuals who dislike being overlooked and overheard; lighting and ventilation cannot accommodate individual preferences and noise levels may be distracting; reliance on information technology can present stresses as well as support. (Photo: James McCarthy)

Within the office environment, stress has also been linked with badly designed offices and office furniture, automation, poor air conditioning and ventilation, artificial lighting, isolation or lack of privacy, and physical safety.

Information technology

More and more jobs are now being replaced or supported by information technology (IT) products such as computer terminals, communication systems including electronic mail (e-mail) and voice mail, and database management systems. Modern large organisations are almost totally dependent upon IT, but the overall stress effects on users are uncertain and are influenced by management attitudes to the proper selection, maintenance and operation of equipment, and the involvement of staff affected by new working methods.

There have been many reports of office workers who use a visual display unit (VDU) suffering negative psychological and physiological effects (Kahn and Cooper, 1986). VDU work is demanding on the eyes, and workplaces that provide little control over time spent at the screen and have poorly positioned or badly designed equipment can lead not only to eye-strain but also to backache and headaches. Depending on the context, using computer systems can result in worker alienation and dissatisfaction with the job, or make jobs more enriched and satisfying.

Work overload and work underload

Having too much or too little work can be stressful. *Quantitative overload* occurs when individuals are asked to do more work than can be completed in the time available. *Qualitative overload* occurs when individuals feel that they lack the skills and abilities needed to perform a given job. Work underload can also lead to stress.

> Quantitative underload refers to the boredom that results when employees have so little to do that they find themselves sitting around much of the time ... qualitative underload refers to the lack of mental stimulation that accompanies many routine, repetitive jobs. (Baron, 1986, p. 210)

Working long hours

Working long hours can lead to health problems. In one early study, it was observed that, for workers in light industry aged under 45 years, those who spent more than 48 hours per week at work had twice the risk of death from coronary heart disease than those working 40 or fewer hours per week (Breslow and Buell, 1960). A recent MORI poll, commissioned for a management training video, of 200 senior managers in a range of companies in the United Kingdom found that 1 in 6 started work before 7.30 a.m., 1 in 4 did not leave work until substantially after 6.30 p.m., and 1 in 4 often worked at weekends (Taylor Made Films, 1992).

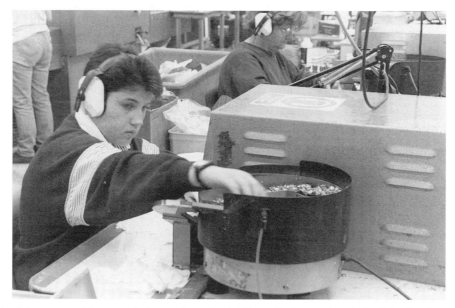

Routine, repetitive jobs may combine quantitative work overload with qualitative work underload, in that the worker experiences constant pressure to keep up with production targets while experiencing the tedium of repeating the same task. (Photo: Mike Levers)

The role of the individual in the organisation

Three important sources of stress arising from the role of the individual in the organisation have been identified by organisational psychologists: (i) role conflict, (ii) role ambiguity, and (iii) being responsible for the work of others.

Role conflict

Most people play several different roles simultaneously at any one point in their lives, for instance those of parent, partner, manager, subordinate, etc., and different behaviours are required from an individual in each of these roles. Often the needs and expectations of the significant others whom a person encounters in each of their roles are difficult, if not impossible, to reconcile. This can lead to 'role conflict' (also known as 'role strain') as a source of stress. If you have time, you could usefully read an article in the Reader which illustrates this concept: it is called 'Food work: maids in a hospital kitchen' by Elizabeth Paterson.[7] She describes how the hospital

kitchen maids she studied felt conflict between their role as 'bulk' food producers at work with little interest in the quality of the meals they prepared, and their role as caring producers of family meals at home. The maids found ways to signal to each other that their attitude to food preparation at work 'is not the real me'. We return to this subject later when we discuss sources of stress in the interface between work and home.

Role ambiguity

Role ambiguity occurs when an individual is uncertain about his or her job role, for instance about the latitude of their authority and responsibilities, or about the ways in which their work performance is evaluated. This may be due to the inadequacy of the training they have received to do the job, or to poor communication systems within the organisation, or to the deliberate withholding or distortion of information by a colleague. Many studies have indicated that role ambiguity is strongly related to the stress experienced by an individual.

Responsibility for others

Responsibility at work can refer to responsibility for 'things', e.g. buildings, machinery or money, but it is responsibility for 'people' which appears to carry the greater risk to health. Individuals who are responsible for others at work, and so must motivate, reward and admonish them, etc., generally experience higher levels of stress

[7]*Health and Disease: A Reader* (first and second editions, 1985 and 1995); this article is also set reading for *Dilemmas in Health Care*, Chapter 6, which discusses variations in autonomy and control in health service occupations.

than those who have no such responsibilities. The reasons for this are related to the interpersonal aspects of a manager's or supervisor's job: those in charge of other people at work have to face the human results of the decisions they make, which may cause an individual to be sacked, or not promoted, or not given a bonus, etc. Managers and supervisors often have to deal with personality conflicts between members of staff, and intervene in disputes, yet they must also promote cooperation and leadership.

Career development

This category of stressor includes the impact of over-promotion and under-promotion (when a person is given responsibilities that either exceed their capabilities, or are below their actual or self-perceived abilities); lack of job security or ambiguity about the future of the job; and thwarted ambition. A number of work stressors related to career development have emerged in recent years which reflect changes in national and international economies: these include *corporate takeovers, mergers and acquisitions*, in which career progression may be negatively affected and staff fear they may not fit into the new organisational structure; *retrenchment and budget cutbacks*, leading to job insecurity, role ambiguity and work overload; and occupational *'locking-in'* when an individual has minimal opportunity to move from his or her present job.

Relationships with others at work

It is clear that relationships at work can be both a stressor and a source of support. Heavy demand for cooperation with and from superiors and subordinates has been shown to be stressful for white-collar workers, and the largest proportion of stressful events occurring in paid work involves interactions with a colleague.

Organisational structure and climate

This source of occupational stress includes such factors as office politics, performance appraisal, little (or total absence of) effective consultation, no participation in decision-making processes, and restrictions on behaviour. The most important aspect of the 'culture' of an organisation seems to be **work control**: the extent to which the workers feel they have control over their working lives. If you look back at Table 8.1 you will see that half of all workers questioned rated 'having control over what to do' or 'using knowledge and experience to make decisions' as the most important aspect of their work.

Lack of participation in decision-making was found by one team of stress researchers to be the most consistent and significant predictor of job-related stress (Margolis *et al.*, 1974). They found that non-participation was significantly related to overall poor physical health, escapist drinking, depressed mood, low self-esteem, low satisfaction with life, low motivation to work, intention to leave

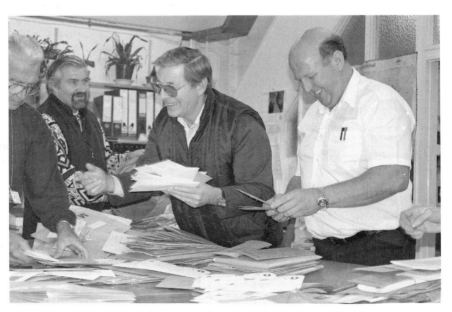

Relationships at work can be both a stressor and a source of support. (Photo: James McCarthy)

the job, and absenteeism from work. High demand coupled with low discretion produced the highest incidences of job dissatisfaction, pill-taking, absence from work, and reports of exhaustion.

Gender differences in the level of control in the workplace have been identified by Ellen Hall in a huge survey of over 13 000 workers in Sweden. She asked them whether they had never/sometimes/often had influence over a range of aspects of their working life, including setting the pace and varying the content of their work, planning of breaks, and learning new tasks. She concluded:

> Males, as a group, were found to have access to a larger and more diverse set of jobs than do females. Work control was found to be consistently higher among men than among women. The highest level of control was found among white-collar men in male-segregated jobs, while the lowest was found among blue-collar women in male-segregated jobs. It was notable that men had a higher level of control than women even in jobs that are traditionally considered to be 'women's work.' … White-collar workers of both sexes have more control than blue-collar workers. (Hall, 1989, pp. 725, 742)

Interface between work and home

This category of potential stressor consists of those events that occur outside the specific work environment but which affect the individual's behaviour at work. It includes *life events* such as 'births, deaths and marriages', a house move, traumatic incidents such as a burglary or accident, a financial windfall or sudden debt, etc. It also includes conflicts between personal and company beliefs and *role conflicts* (mentioned earlier) between workplace and family demands. The latter is the most extensively researched aspect of women's health in relation to work. Later in the chapter, we return briefly to this subject to summarise the findings of a large-scale study on the effect on women of working a 'double day', i.e. having a paid job outside the home as well as prime responsibility for domestic work and childcare. The increasing tendency in many countries for men as well as women to occupy multiple roles at work and at home has led to many areas of role conflict in the interface between the two domains.

☐ Can you suggest an example?

■ Pressures to spend long hours at work may conflict with demands or expectations from family members to spend more time at home.

Personal life events and family relationships may mitigate or exacerbate the effects of stressors from within the workplace. This is amply illustrated by the audiotape 'Working lives: choices and conflicts', which you should ideally listen to now.[8]

A revision exercise

The audiotape contains interviews with three Whitehall civil servants, at different levels in the organisational hierarchy, and a hospital porter. Two of the civil servants are in very senior positions: one is a married man with two grown-up children whose wife did part-time voluntary work for most of the years they were at home, and the other is a married woman with two school-age children whose husband also has a very demanding job which often takes him abroad. They reflect on differences in their experiences of conflicts between work and home life which emerge from the very different levels of support they can draw on from their partners. The other civil servant is a secretary in the same department, a young married woman who has a small child and a husband who would prefer her to give up work as soon as they can afford it. The hospital porter is a single man in his 40s who has a regular girlfriend and no dependents.

As you listen to the tape, try to identify the sources of stress the speakers describe as arising from the organisation of their jobs and the interface between work and home, and relate them to the six categories of stressors shown in Figure 8.1 and discussed above.

The four people interviewed on the audiotape display attitudes to their jobs that fit into the 'orientations to work' described earlier by Alan Cowling and his colleagues.

☐ Which of the worker(s) on the audiotape displays attitudes that most closely resemble the *instrumental* orientation to work, and who has the most *bureaucratic* orientation?

■ Amanda, the secretary, sums up the *instrumental* orientation when she says the best thing about her job is '… the money. I don't get any particular job satisfaction in what I do … I don't get home at the end of the day and think "Oh I did really well today" … I come to work because I have to have money.' Michael, the senior civil servant, shows the *bureaucratic* orientation when he says 'You don't work in the civil service for the money. The buzz that

[8]This audiotape has been specially recorded for Open University students, who should consult the Audiocassette Notes before listening to it.

we get, I think, out of our jobs relates to the feeling of being at the heart of government and playing a part in running the country.'

Work stress and health outcomes

Bearing in mind the need for caution in interpreting the results of stress research outlined earlier, there is now a great deal of evidence from organisational psychology to suggest that a high level of stress in a particular job, combined with the individual characteristics of the job-holder, can result in job dissatisfaction, mental and physical ill-health, accidents, high rates of sickness-absence, alcohol abuse and social or family problems. Note that, as the model in Figure 8.1 makes clear, work stress *alone* does not seem to be an adequate predictor of adverse health outcomes: the ways in which individual workers 'cope' with stress also have a strong influence, and this in turn is affected by their social circumstances as well as by aspects of their personal psychology. High stress levels combined with an ineffective coping style and inadequate personal and material support seem to pose the most potent threat to health. There must also be genetic and other biological factors contributing to an individual's vulnerability or resistance to the effects of stress, but these fall outside the realm of organisational psychology. Biological research on the effects of stress on human subjects has largely concentrated on specialised groups such as astronauts, fighter-pilots and deep-sea divers, and tells us little about everyday workplace situations.

Stress and physical health

Most of the basic research on stress as a cause of illness has been devoted to the impact it has on physical health. It appears to be the chronic diseases, that is, non-infectious diseases of long duration, which are particularly influenced by the experience of stress. A high level of stress may result—in some individuals—in high blood pressure and high levels of blood cholesterol and, as a consequence, an elevated risk of heart disease. Other common outcomes identified in stress research are ulcers and arthritis, headache, heartburn, backache and general fatigue.

☐ How might stress affect physical health *indirectly* through behavioural change?

■ Some people respond to stress by smoking more cigarettes, or drinking more alcohol, or abusing other drugs, all of which can have direct effects on health.

Not everyone responds to stress in the same way— individual personality, material circumstances and available support from friends and family all affect the experience of stress and whether or not it can be coped with. Of these mediating factors, personality characteristics have been of most interest to psychologists investigating the outcomes of stress; in particular they have focused on a possible link between the so-called **Type A personality** and physical illness. People with Type A personalities are described as competitive people, who drive themselves hard and have a strong desire to achieve, coupled with

> ... a strong sense of time urgency, hurried and explosive speech patterns, quick motor movements ... [they are] aggressive, hostile, restless and impatient. (Sutherland and Cooper, 1990, p. 74)

Research on Type A personalities has a long history, beginning in the late 1960s and continuing to the present day. People with Type A personality have been shown to be at greater risk of physical illness in a large number of studies, and the most consistent association has been with coronary heart disease (CHD). In the early 1980s, a Review Panel of 50 scientists assembled by the US National Heart, Lung and Blood Institute concluded that available evidence from American studies demonstrated that Type A personality was associated with an increased risk of CHD in employed, middle-aged people (cited in Rosenman and Friedman, 1983).

The earliest studies generally showed an association between this personality type and the incidence of CHD, regardless of whether or not the individual was under stress—but only for white-collar workers. More recent research has tended to view Type A as a *behaviour*— a 'coping style' for dealing with stress, rather than a fixed personality characteristic. In a review of earlier studies, Matthews and Glass (1984), two leading social researchers, concluded that people with Type A behaviour use more effort than other personality types in attempting to regain control over uncontrollable events.

Type A behaviour seems to interact with several other factors to produce ill-health. For example, a study by Cary Cooper and co-workers of 218 men and women who had been investigated for heart-valve disease at Wythenshaw Hospital, South Manchester, showed that the combination in a patient of work stress, Type A behaviour, adverse life events, and low social support from family and friends were significantly related to the patient's past history of high blood pressure and heart disease (Cooper *et al.*, 1985).

Another possible link between stress, personality and illness which has attracted considerable attention, but little agreement, relates to some forms of cancer, particularly breast cancer. Results have often been conflicting, perhaps because longitudinal studies of the relationship between stress and cancers (which take a long time to develop) have been relatively few to date. In a recent contribution to the debate, Cary Cooper and Brian Faragher (1993) surveyed perceived stress levels and stress-coping techniques in the preceding period reported by over 2 000 women in England who had been referred for specialist evaluation after complaining of breast lumpiness or tenderness. The researchers found that a high level of subjectively experienced stress, coupled with a tendency to 'deny' the problem and 'bottle-up' emotional reactions to it, was correlated with a greater probability that the breast problem would subsequently be diagnosed as cancer. However, there are as yet no satisfactory biological models of how such an interaction between stress, personality, coping styles and social support might affect the occurrence of cancer. A correlation does not prove causality.

Stress and mental health

While considerable attention has been given to the relationship between stress and physical health, especially within the medical community, less has been given to the impact of stress on mental health. Yet, at least indirectly if not directly, the psychological problems resulting from stress may be just as important to day-to-day job performance, absence from work and individual wellbeing. If we accept the broad definition of health adopted by the World Health Organisation as 'a state of complete physical, mental and social wellbeing' (WHO, 1958), then stress at work is a major cause of ill-health.

The psychological outcomes of stress include family problems, sleep disturbances, sexual difficulties, depression, anxiety, irritability and **job burnout**, a concept that has attracted increasing attention in recent years. Job burnout is said to be occurring when an individual feels that the stresses associated with the job are unavoidable and that sources of satisfaction and relief are unavailable. It results in physical, emotional and mental exhaustion; the person can no longer cope with the demands of the job and their willingness to 'try' drops dramatically. Burnout has been widely assessed in a number of occupations, forefront among them being nursing, using a specially designed questionnaire, the Maslach Burnout Inventory.

For example, a study of 95 nurse tutors in Northern Ireland by Hunter and Houghton (1993) assessed occupational stress using this inventory in combination with other rating scales of general health and the sources of stress at work. Significant levels of moderate and high burnout were detected, and this was more apparent among male tutors than among females. Respondents reported emotional exhaustion and depersonalisation, most commonly identified as arising from having too little time to perform their duties to their satisfaction.

As in the case of research cited earlier on the interaction of stress and physical health, the worker's personality and social support have an influence on mental-health outcomes. The results from studies in several countries identify certain personality characteristics among people most at risk of burnout in heavily stressed occupations: they tend to be perfectionists and/or self-motivating achievers who often seek unrealistic or unattainable goals.

☐ Can you suggest a way in which studies of individual personality might be used to reduce the adverse health effects of stress at work, and do you foresee any drawbacks in such an approach?

■ Workers whose coping style is likely to be ineffective in protecting their health could be counselled to avoid heavily stressed occupations; the drawback is that employers may seek to bar individuals from taking up certain jobs on the basis of a personality test which can be of dubious accuracy. Moreover, this approach focuses on changing the job-holder rather than changing the stressfulness of the job.

The health effects of combining paid work and domestic labour

As we said at the beginning of this chapter, studies of the health effects of work stress have largely been carried out on 'male' occupations—the notable exceptions being nursing (for example see Hunter and Houghton, 1993; Sullivan, 1993), and to a lesser extent school teaching. Very few studies have systematically compared the working lives of men and women or their health outcomes across a range of occupations. Conversely, although research into 'women's work' has increasingly taken account of paid as well as domestic labour, there has been little investigation of the health effects of managing conflicts between these two domains among men. One large-scale study that has attempted to address these shortcomings is in progress in Scotland.

Kate Hunt and Ellen Annandale are conducting a long-term study of the everyday life and health of a cohort of about 1 000 men and women, who were 35 years old in 1986 when they were recruited into the 'West of

Scotland Twenty-07 Study' (which runs until the year 2007). The influence of paid and domestic work on health was investigated in the 597 individuals in this cohort who were in any kind of paid work for 10 or more hours per week, and who also had a cohabiting spouse or partner of the opposite sex. These selection criteria ensured that the respondents had at least two roles: worker and spouse. The hours spent working (both domestic labour and in paid jobs), their domestic responsibilities and their conditions of employment, together with self-perceptions of stresses in their working lives, were obtained from interviews and questionnaires. Their health was assessed objectively by various measures of physical functioning and by subjective self-reports. Two dimensions of health status were recorded: the level of *malaise*, which includes difficulty in sleeping or concentrating, worrying, depression, poor appetite and feeling 'run down'; and common *physical symptoms*, which includes trouble with bowels, kidneys or bladder, colds and 'flu, painful joints, sore throat and haemorrhoids.

In common with other studies, women carried most of the responsibility for domestic labour: more than 75 per cent of the women contributed over 15 hours per week to domestic chores, compared with 14 per cent of the men. By contrast, men spent significantly more hours in their paid jobs than did women: 70 per cent of the women spent 36 hours or less per week in paid work, compared with the 80 per cent of men who worked longer weekly hours than this. The women in this sample had significantly higher malaise and physical symptom scores than the men. When the relative contribution of domestic labour and paid work to health outcome was assessed, Hunt and Annandale concluded:

> ... we have found that domestic work alone has some effect on women's health (and none on men, probably because too few of the men were engaged in any substantial amount of domestic work); that paid work alone has far more potent effects for both men and women; and that the combination of both (in conjunction with work-related stress indicators) has an enhanced effect over paid work alone, particularly for women. (Hunt and Annandale, 1993, p. 659)

They note that the overall level of self-reported conflict between work and domestic life was not significantly different for the two sexes, but suggest possible differences in the sources of that conflict: men may predominately experience conflict as a result of very long working hours keeping them away from home, whereas role conflict for women could arise from the 'greater underlying tension between the expectations or obligations of their roles' (p. 655).

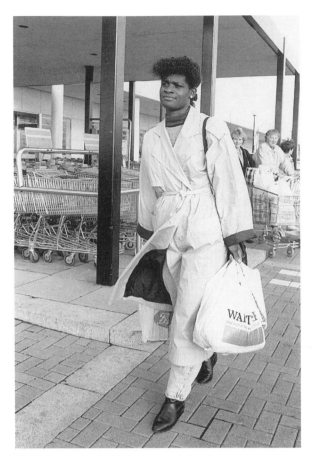

Shopping for the family in the lunch-break is a common experience for women who combine domestic responsibilities with paid work. But does working a 'double day' carry additional health risks or give some protection against depression and anxiety? (Photo: Mike Levers)

A key area of future research into work-related stress will be the health effects of women's increasing participation in the labour market and conflicts at the interface between work and home. The question of whether paid work is 'good or bad' for women's health is not easily answered, since there are wide variations between women in their experience of employment (e.g. the pay and status of the job), in the extent of their domestic responsibilities (e.g. the presence of young children in the household), and in their material and social support (e.g. adequate household income from another wage-earner). Several studies have shown that, in general, employed women report lower levels of anxiety and depression than non-employed women, including the study by Sara Arber published in 1991, based on an analysis of responses to the General Household Survey (GHS). However, Arber and her colleagues have been concerned about the effects of employment on women in poor material circumstances:

> … without a change in the domestic division of labour and with women constrained to low-status, low-paid, often part-time jobs, waged work may have little liberating effect for women. It may simply increase their burden and severely curtail or eliminate any 'unobligated time'. (Arber and Gilbert, 1992, p. 7)

The situation is also far from clear when higher-status jobs are considered. As more women enter the professions and managerial grades, they are increasingly becoming

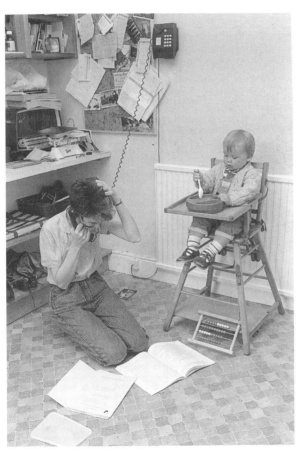

Stress for working women can arise from conflict between their roles at home and at work, but women in professional and managerial occupations may be allowed more flexibility to fulfil their dual obligations. (Photo: Mike Levers)

the subject of occupational stress research, but a review by Burke and McKeen (1995) concluded that there was not yet enough evidence to assess whether there are gender differences in the experience of work stress or its outcomes in these occupations. However, the general trend in these studies is in broad agreement with reports on the population as a whole: working women tend to report better mental and physical health than women who don't have jobs outside the home.

The economic costs of stress

Technological change, recession and ever-increasing demands for higher productivity have produced an upward trend in the level of stress-related **sickness absence** in recent years. In the 1980s, on average, over 37 million working days were lost annually in the United Kingdom through stress-related illness (Cox, 1985). In the early 1990s, the estimate has risen to 90 million working days per year lost through stress—30 times more than that lost through strikes (Confederation of British Industry/Department of Health, 1992). A survey of *Employment in Britain*, published by the Policy Studies Institute in 1993, revealed that 31 per cent of employees reported significant levels of stress as a result of their work and 54 per cent felt that the level of stress had increased over the last five years.

Stress may currently be costing medium-sized companies in the United Kingdom (those employing around 1 000 staff) an average of £200 000 per year each, or 10–20 per cent of profits (Landale, 1989). In 1993, the Confederation of British Industry estimated that absenteeism through illness in the United Kingdom (not all of which is stress-related) amounted to 171 million lost working days and cost employers £11 billion (CBI, 1994). A report commissioned by the United Kingdom Health and Safety Executive estimates that stress-related illness is the largest cause of sickness absence and costs British industry £7.5 billion per annum—around 10 per cent of GNP, the Gross National Product (Cox, 1993). Absenteeism was found to be highest in blue-collar workers and public sector employees; white-collar staff took roughly half the number of days off sick compared with other workers. Part of the explanation may lie in the organisation of the work itself, as in the Whitehall II Study of civil servants mentioned at the start of the chapter:

> Men and women who rated their jobs as low for control, variety and use of skills, pace, support at work or satisfaction had higher rates of short and long spells of sickness absence compared with those who rated their jobs high for these characteristics … For example, men who

reported low variety and use of skills had 72% and 82% higher rates of short and long spells of absence respectively, compared with those who reported high variety and use of skills. (North *et al.*, 1993, p. 363)

Stressful work organisation may cost employers in ways other than through lost productivity. The dividing line between an employer's and an employee's personal responsibilities for work-related stress was tested in 1994 by Britain's first-ever damages claim by a stressed employee: a social worker who suffered a second nervous breakdown successfully claimed damages from his employer for failing to protect him from excessive work-related stress after his health had failed the first time. United Kingdom businesses have generally not taken seriously the problem of noise at work (leading to deafness), nor the effects of passive smoking, both of which have cost organisations large amounts in employee compensation. As the evidence mounts, cumulative stress may eventually become classified as an industrial injury.

OBJECTIVES FOR CHAPTER 8

When you have studied this chapter, you should be able to:

8.1 Discuss the meaning of work in people's lives in the United Kingdom in the 1990s and distinguish between the instrumental, bureaucratic and solidaristic orientations to work.

8.2 Outline the main sources of difficulty in researching links between stressors in the workplace and health outcomes in the workforce.

8.3 Give examples of stressors in the workplace and discuss reasons for increases in the perceived stressfulness of work situations in recent years.

8.4 Illustrate the costs of stress at work by referring to examples of adverse effects on physical and mental health, and the costs to industry.

QUESTIONS FOR CHAPTER 8

Question 1 (*Objective 8.1*)

In the audiotape 'Working lives: choices and conflicts', which of the workers makes statements that seem consistent with the *solidaristic* orientation to work?

Question 2 (*Objective 8.2*)

Consider the following report of a study by Patrick Sullivan on 'burnout' among all of the 78 psychiatric nurses employed in acute in-patient facilities in two English Health Authorities. The nurses completed three self-administered questionnaires, one of which was the Maslach Burnout Inventory; the other two were devised by Sullivan specifically for this study. He also interviewed each nurse using a semi-structured interview design, followed by coding of responses for analysis. Correlations between the results of the questionnaires and interviews were generated by statistical methods. Sullivan concluded that these psychiatric nurses showed a high level of burnout and that

> … there was a correlation between burnout and problems relating to staffing levels, administrative duties and work overload. (Sullivan, 1993, p. 598)

What reasons arising from the research methods used in this study can you give for interpreting Sullivan's conclusions cautiously? (You should also think back to the discussion of qualitative research methods in an earlier book in this series.)[9]

Question 3 (*Objectives 8.3 and 8.4*)

The report commissioned by the United Kingdom Health and Safety Executive (Cox, 1993) found that sickness absence was highest in blue-collar workers and public sector employees; white-collar staff took roughly half the number of days off sick compared with other workers. What explanations can you suggest for this finding?

[9] *Studying Health and Disease* (revised edition, 1994), Chapter 3.

9 Change and crisis in mid-life

The principal author of this chapter, Mike Hepworth, is a Reader in Sociology at the University of Aberdeen, whose main research interest is the social construction of the life course and, in particular, mid-life. The distance-teaching aspects of this chapter have been developed by Julia Johnson and Bill Bytheway, and Basiro Davey contributed some original material.

Introduction

Conversations about 'middle age' or 'mid-life' are commonplace in Western culture in the late twentieth century. But how is mid-life defined, and what is normally expected to happen as one passes through it? In this chapter, we begin by considering the historical development of views about mid-life and the ways in which representations of this period in the life course have influenced our thinking about it in the present day. Then we focus on three 'events' associated with mid-life, which have received considerable attention during the last twenty years: the *menopause*, the *male menopause* and the *mid-life crisis*.

Although the labels 'menopause', 'male menopause' and 'mid-life crisis' are frequently used to mark out the boundaries of a certain period in the life course, there is considerable debate over their validity. This is because these events cannot be defined solely in terms of biology—they are also *social constructs*, that is to say, they are strongly shaped by the social beliefs and practices particular to a given culture or society at a given time.[1] These dominant beliefs and practices influence the ways in which 'stages' or 'phases' of the life course are

[1]Social constructionism is discussed in *Medical Knowledge: Doubt and Certainty* (revised edition, 1994), Chapter 7.

defined, and this in turn can have an impact on individual experience.

☐ Can you think of a group of people amongst whom the idea of a male menopause may not exist, or may be regarded as ridiculous?

■ You may not subscribe to the idea yourself and possibly you thought of many others who might not—Intercity train drivers, Cardiff dockers, or Chinese herbalists, for example. And if they do, they may characterise it differently. Indeed, in the United Kingdom, a hundred years ago, such ideas may not have existed, at least in their present form. You may even have thought that the idea of a male menopause was simply the invention of an imaginative journalist.

There is no dispute that most women experience the bodily changes known as the menopause at some time between the ages of 45 and 54 years. However, there is considerable diversity in personal experience of these changes, some of which may be due to the negative social meaning ascribed to this sign of 'middle age'. To this extent, the female menopause is a culturally as well as a biologically driven event. In contrast, there is little or no evidence of biological changes associated with mid-life in men, so if the male menopause exists, it does so entirely in the cultural realm. There is a similar uncertainty about whether middle age is indeed a period of 'crisis' in the life course. These uncertainties are significant: if such events exist, then people want to understand them and know how to manage them. A mentally and physically 'healthy' mid-life is often seen as an important ingredient of successful ageing.

In this chapter, evidence collected by social and biological researchers and other experts is compared with the personal experiences of individuals, to obtain the fullest possible picture of the diverse characteristics of mid-life and its positive and negative features. An important aspect of this analysis is the contribution of 'popular culture'—and in particular the news media—to the cultural construction of mid-life.

What is mid-life?

The term **mid-life** implies the mid-point in the human life course. This idea is not new, as social historians point out (see, for example, Cole, 1992; Sears, 1986). Consider Figure 9.1, an engraving by Jorge Breu the Younger, dated 1540. Breu depicted the life course as a series of steps rising to the mid-point of maturity before descending, through a number of fixed stages, towards physical decrepitude and ultimately death. Death itself is portrayed as a transitional stage to the everlasting life thereafter. This is a good example of the social construction of the life course, in this case in the sixteenth century.

One of the major differences between the time when Breu created his representation of mid-life and the present day is that many more people in industrialised countries such as the United Kingdom now live into and beyond middle age.

☐ What is the principal reason for this increase in longevity?

■ More people survive into middle age and beyond in the twentieth century largely because of the decline in perinatal and infant mortality rates; this decline is primarily a result of the decrease in infectious diseases as a cause of death due to the public health reforms of the late nineteenth and twentieth centuries, and improvements in nutrition and living standards,[2] coupled with better health care of babies and infants with congenital abnormalities (Chapters

[2]See *Caring for Health: History and Diversity*, Chapters 4–6, and *World Health and Disease*, Chapters 5 and 6.

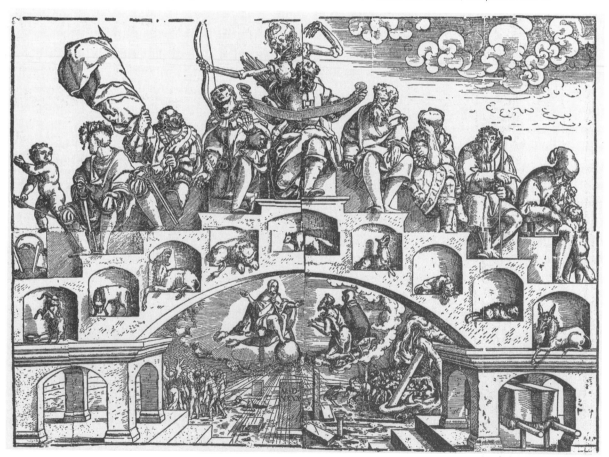

Figure 9.1 *An engraving entitled 'The Steps of Life' by Jorge Breu the Younger, dated 1540. (Source: The British Library)*

2–4 of this book). In addition, mortality from accidents in childhood and adolescence has also fallen in recent decades (Chapters 5 and 6).

Before the Industrial Revolution, although there was some appreciation that the life course had a maximum span, this was attained by few and the actual length of life averaged less than half this age.[3]

☐ Christians and Jews are led by the Bible to hope for 'three-score years and ten' (i.e. a lifespan of seventy years). How might those living in (e.g.) the sixteenth century have interpreted their thirty-fifth birthdays?

■ Given the much lower life expectancy in the sixteenth century, most people would have been acquainted with many deaths in childhood and in early adulthood. Even though they may have recognised that their thirty-fifth birthday was only halfway to the end of a 'full' life, most would also have recognised that death could come at any time and that existence in mid-life remained a continuing battle for survival.

As a result of huge improvements in life expectancy in the wake of industrialisation, mass education and health care, there has been a conspicuous increase in the number of men and women who are achieving a 'full' lifespan in the twentieth century. The expectation of life at birth for babies born in the United Kingdom in 1989 was 72 years for males and 78 years for females, according to United Nations estimates (1991). The present time is unique because mid-life has become a statistically 'normal' experience. Most people expect to live into old age and are able to interpret certain events as characteristic of their mid-life. For this reason alone, there is increasing interest in the quality of mid-life and, in particular, in its positive and negative features.

We are living in an increasingly age-conscious society, a society with a noticeable tendency to regard ageing and old age as a 'problem' (a tendency we return to in Chapter 10). This negative attitude towards the second half of life is resulting in more and more attention being paid to the 'ageing population'. There is a strongly held view in medicine that many of the illnesses of old age can be prevented by the adoption of healthy habits

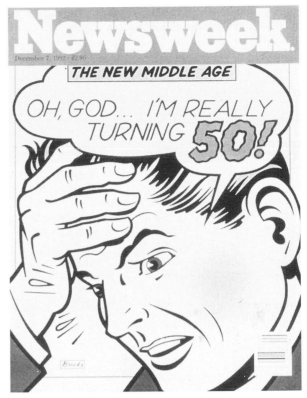

Western culture increasingly represents ageing as a problem and the realisation of middle age as a personal crisis, as this cover of the American magazine Newsweek, dated 7 December 1992, illustrates. (© 1992 Newsweek Inc. All rights reserved. Reprinted by permission.)

before mid-life. Against this background, it is hardly surprising that health and wellbeing in mid-life have become a focus of popular concern.

It has been argued that many of the popular cultural attitudes of the late twentieth century are based upon visual and verbal media images, such as those portrayed in television soap operas. Typically these are the stereotyped images of the mid-American lifestyle. Alex Kalache, for example, has argued that these images have had a significant impact on the lifestyles of even the very poorest people in countries such as Brazil (Kalache, 1993).

[3]There is a debate within biology about whether humans and other species have a maximum lifespan which is genetically 'programmed' regardless of the accumulation of wear and tear during life; this is discussed in *Human Biology and Health: An Evolutionary Approach*, Chapter 8.

□ The cartoon in Figure 9.2 is a popular image of the life course in the 1990s. What is the message it suggests to you about middle age?

■ The cartoon conveys an image of middle age as the peak of the life course: an ecstatic couple are linked in abandoned celebration. This reinforces the traditional idea (as in Figure 9.1) that mid-life is the peak experience of the life course, a brief time of exuberance, after which life is 'downhill all the way'.

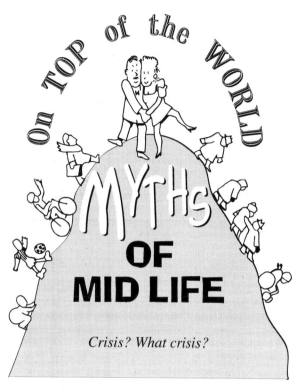

Figure 9.2 *A popular image of the life course in the 1990s. (Cartoon: Bill Bytheway)*

The traditional image of the life course as a journey up and down a hill, of mid-life as a brief, pleasurable period of maturity and of later life as a long, slow period of social, mental and physical decline, reinforces one of the 'myths' about middle age. The myth of mid-life, as the peak experience of the life course, derives its persuasive power from the deeply entrenched belief that the ageing process in later life is one of biological decline. The biological time-clock begins to run down in middle age, it is believed, and it is assumed that our mental and physical capabilities begin to deteriorate. In Western culture therefore, mid-life is highly ambiguous: it is simultaneously the peak of maturity and the 'beginning of the end' of physical life in this world.

However, if our quest for an accurate and comprehensive definition of mid-life is going to reflect the wide range of experiences of middle and later life, it is necessary to recognise all the myths and stereotypes that surround it. Myths have an important part to play in the cultural construction of mid-life.

Jenny Hockey and Allison James have studied popular images of the human life course. They have argued that the belief that life can be divided into an 'upward curve to adulthood' and a 'downward path to old age' (Hockey and James, 1993, p. 29) is dangerous—not because human beings do not grow older biologically, but because this belief imposes a mythical and misleadingly negative image of the complex reality of later life. Although there can be no doubt that our bodies do age and do ultimately lose certain capabilities, it does not follow that later life is—or should be—a time of disengagement from an active life. There is no evidence to support the view that later life has less potential for personal growth than earlier years.

□ Why is it dangerous to assume that decline is characteristic of the ageing process?

■ The word 'decline' implies a valuation: that one is moving from a desirable state to a less desirable one. What we judge to be desirable or undesirable, however, depends not upon our changing biological constitution but rather upon cultural norms. It is change, not decline, that is characteristic of ageing.

One change that is often represented negatively is the menopause.

The menopause

The association of the menopause with a negative stereotype of ageing and old age can have poignant implications for the sense of personal 'selfhood':

I searched for the truth about the menopause but what I found didn't help me. All the books I read and all the people I talked with told me it was nothing at all. Some said 'Think positively and don't gain weight'. Others said 'It's all in the culture'. I had to validate my own experience. No one would acknowledge or could explain why I had a hard time whenever my hormones shifted. I thought I was going mad. (Quoted in Doress, Siegal and Shapiro, 1989, p. 191)

The **menopause** is the name given to a period of several years in mid-life when natural, biological changes occur in a woman's body, which gradually reduce her fertility and ultimately bring to an end her capacity to conceive a child.[4] It is widely referred to as 'the change of life', and is often interpreted as a mid-life 'crisis' for women since it involves complex and sometimes difficult interactions between bodily changes and potentially far-reaching psychological and social responses. The medical term for the menopause—the *climacteric*—seems to encapsulate this: it comes from the Greek word 'klimacter' meaning 'critical period'.

How is the menopause defined and when does it occur? What are the boundaries that distinguish the pre-menopausal from the menopausal and the post-menopausal woman? These questions are difficult to answer, even when apparently objective biological measurements are made. The levels of two hormones secreted by the ovaries—oestrogen and progesterone—fall in the bloodstream to the point where they no longer promote ovulation—the release of a mature egg from the ovary in a regular monthly cycle (as described in Chapter 3). The woman may continue to menstruate (i.e. shed the lining of the womb) even if a cycle has not resulted in ovulation, but the regularity and duration of menstruation generally becomes increasingly erratic, before ceasing altogether, usually within two or three years either side of the fiftieth birthday.

However, this sequence of events varies widely between individuals: for example, some women simply stop menstruating 'overnight' without any preceding signs that the menopause is under way, while others experience irregular bleeding and other signs for several years before their last menstrual period and continue to feel menopausal symptoms for several years thereafter. For a minority of women, the menopause can start unusually early in their 30s, and for a very few even earlier. As a consequence of these variations in individual experience, the only sure way to define the menopause is retrospectively: it is over when it is over and it can only be said with certainty to have occurred when a year has elapsed after the last menstruation. It is for this reason that Germaine Greer has appropriately defined it as 'a non-event, the menstrual period that does not happen' (Greer, 1991, p. 25).

The incidence of physical and psychological signs commonly associated with the menopause (especially those that are regarded as 'problem symptoms') in the *general* population of women in mid-life has been a neglected area of research. A frequently-voiced criticism of research into the menopause is that, until recently, it has been marred by the use of non-representative samples of women with unusual symptoms. Most accounts have been based on those women who have sought medical help for symptoms which were having a negative effect on their lives: until recently, we knew rather little about the experience of the majority of women who passed through the 'change of life' without consulting a doctor. This has reinforced the belief that the menopause is universally negative in its consequences. Drug companies have reinforced this view in advertising the benefits of **hormone replacement therapy (HRT)**, which aims to alleviate problem symptoms by regular intake of small doses of oestrogen and progesterone until the menopause is over. Consider the following extract from a leaflet, *Mastering the Menopause*, written by two (male) doctors for the drug company Organon.

> The occurrence of symptoms and particularly the development of irregular vaginal bleeding are signs that a woman should consult her doctor to discuss the problem. Although some women do go through the menopause without experiencing any symptoms at all, we know that almost all women will experience the longer term problems of oestrogen deficiency unless they receive treatment.[5]

This medical view highlights a further cause of concern to an increasing number of feminist critics such as Germaine Greer and Emily Martin: most of the vast literature on the subject is written by men whose perspective on the menopause is derived from stereotypical assumptions about women's bodies and the nature of female reproductive organs.[6] Noticeably absent from their accounts are references to women's actual experiences of their own bodies. It is important to take into account the fact that male doctors, whom Germaine Greer

---

[4]Menopause is unique to humans; a discussion of the evolution of menopause as an adaptive strategy which may enhance the survival of the human species occurs in *Human Biology and Health: An Evolutionary Approach*, Chapter 8.

[5]See Daly *et al.* (1992) for an evaluation of the costs and benefits of HRT during the female menopause; this subject is also discussed in *Dilemmas in Health Care*, Chapter 9, which refers to the promotion of HRT by doctors and drug companies.

[6]A discussion of the work of Emily Martin in analysing negative imagery and language in descriptions of female reproductive biology in medical textbooks occurs in *Medical Knowledge: Doubt and Certainty* (revised edition, 1994), Chapter 7.

dismissively describes as the 'Masters of Menopause', will never undergo the experience themselves (Greer, 1991, p. 3).

Yet another subject of major public debate concerns the use of sex hormones to reverse the physiological changes of the menopause, enabling a post-menopausal woman to become pregnant and give birth to a baby in her 50s or 60s. The social outrage reported in the news media in response to these mothers demonstrates the extent to which the menopause is 'owned' by society as much as by the women themselves.

In a moment we will consider the findings of a large-scale study of experiences of the menopause in Scottish

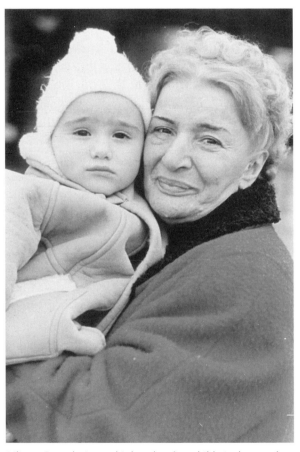

Liliana Cantadori gave birth to her first child, Andrea, at the age of 61 in July 1992, after hormone treatment to reverse the menopause and in-vitro fertilisation using an egg donated by another woman. (Photo: Mirror Syndication International)

women, conducted by Maureen Porter and her colleagues from the Department of Obstetrics and Gynaecology at the University of Aberdeen (Porter *et al.*, 1994). They divided the problem symptoms of the menopause commonly reported by women who seek medical help into three categories: classic, somatic and psychological. The *classic* physical symptoms are: hot flushes, night sweats, sleep problems, dry or sore vagina. The *somatic* symptoms are aching or painful joints, headaches, sore breasts, nocturia (passing water often at night), palpitations and dizziness. The *psychological* symptoms are irritability, concentration or memory problems, anxiety, depression and feelings of inability to cope.

The main difficulty with lists of **menopausal symptoms** such as these is that they do not in themselves tell us whether the symptoms are normal or abnormal characteristics of the menopause: it is necessary to discover whether they are widely experienced by women, and if so, whether or not they are experienced as a 'problem'; and for those women who do find them problematic, how intense the negative experiences may be. Furthermore, there is uncertainty over whether or not the hormonal changes related to the gradual cessation of ovulation are the *cause* of any of these problem symptoms, and if so which, or whether other factors (such as social and personal circumstances) are also involved.

These uncertainties were addressed in a study of women's perceptions, expectations and actual experiences of the menopause by Maureen Porter and her colleagues, mentioned earlier. One objective of the research was to assess the degree of distress caused by the symptoms commonly believed to be associated with the menopause; another was to relate the occurrence of individual symptoms, and whether or not they were experienced as problematic, to a woman's *menopausal status* (defined in terms of an irregular pattern of menstrual bleeding, or time since last menstrual period). Between February and April 1993, over 6 000 women aged between 45 and 54 years completed a lengthy questionnaire concerning their health and wellbeing, and aspects of their lifestyle, including the occurrence of major 'life events'. These women were a random sample of the population in the Grampian region. They were asked whether, during the last six months, they had experienced any of fifteen symptoms frequently associated with the menopause, and if these had caused them problems. The results are shown in Table 9.1.

Table 9.1 Responses of 6 084 Scottish women aged 45–54 years to questions about menopausal symptoms in 1993

Symptoms	Per cent experiencing symptom	Per cent experiencing symptom as a problem
Classic symptoms		
hot flushes	57	22
night sweats	55	24
sleep problems	66	33
dry/sore vagina	34	14
Somatic symptoms		
aching/painful joints	67	29
headaches	60	23
sore breasts	51	14
nocturia	48	16
palpitations	37	13
dizziness	35	11
Psychological symptoms		
irritability	72	25
concentration/memory problems	64	30
anxiety	58	26
depression	51	22
feeling unable to cope	43	19

Source: Porter *et al.* (1994) *A Population-based Study of Women's Perceptions of the Menopause*, Table IV. Final report submitted to the Scottish Home and Health Dept, Edinburgh. Copies obtainable from the Department of Obstetrics and Gynaecology, Aberdeen University.

☐ What do the responses in Table 9.1 suggest about the experience of the menopause as 'a problem'?

■ Most of the individual symptoms investigated were experienced by between a half and two-thirds of the 6 000 women. However, a far lower proportion—a third or less—reported that they perceived individual symptoms as a problem.

The researchers noted that when problems do arise they tend to be as a result of clusters of symptoms occurring in the same person. The 25 per cent of women who reported problematic symptoms tended to be taking HRT or to

have had the menopause medically induced (usually when their ovaries were removed during a hysterectomy). When each woman's menopausal status was defined and related to their experiences, it was found that

… components of menopausal status were good predictors of classic symptoms but not somatic or psychological. Having a history of depression or anxiety, poor health status, and experience of recent life events were the best predictors of somatic and psychological symptoms … health and lifestyle problems women experience at this time are as likely to be due to pre-existing poor mental and physical health. (Porter *et al.*, 1994, pp. 6, 7)

The researchers concluded:

Women have realistic expectations of the menopause and accurately anticipate the types of symptoms they are likely to experience. These symptoms are not as problematic as studies of clinic populations have suggested. (Porter *et al.*, 1994, p. 7)

This conclusion is borne out by the Massachusetts Women's Health Study—the largest study in the USA—which found that the overwhelming majority of women reported positive or neutral feelings about the cessation of their menstrual cycles (Avis and McKinlay, 1991).

Until relatively recently, the menopause was described as a 'silent crisis'—women who were experiencing a difficult menopause were not supposed to speak about it openly. A glance at a selection of women's magazines shows that this is no longer the case, but the images of the menopause presented to women in the media are rarely as positive as the personal account (below) from an American book, *Ourselves Growing Older*. (In the USA, a hot flush is known as a 'hot flash'.)

I never felt that I should suffer hot flashes in silence, so my husband and kids called me 'Flash'. When I told my husband it was the first anniversary of my last period he said, 'Congratulations, Flash. You've done it.' So we went out to dinner and celebrated that night. (Quoted in Doress, Siegal and Shapiro, 1989, p. 202)

The growing openness about the body and about physical changes in mid-life in recent decades has increased the opportunities for women whose menopause is distressing to seek personal and medical help, but it has also tended to reinforce negative myths about the menopause as a prolonged 'crisis' that all women must endure.

The male menopause

Men do not menstruate and so they cannot experience any cessation of the menses, nor is there any significant reduction in male fertility during mid-life. There is no evidence of a sharp reduction in male hormone levels in the majority of the male population; testosterone declines by about 1 per cent per year from middle age onwards but remains high enough to ensure that most men produce fertile sperm throughout life. So, in a biological sense, the term **male menopause** (or 'andropause' as it is sometimes called, meaning a pause in the output of male hormones) is a misnomer. But this has not prevented the idea of a male climacteric being given serious academic consideration since the 1970s (see, for example, van Keep *et al.*, 1979), and from being actively promoted in the popular media.

How menopausal men go mad

Don't blame it on hormones—it's just the triumph of frustration over embarrassment …. There are happily married men who have never looked twice at another woman who wake up one morning with the burning conviction that they will never rise higher than Assistant Deputy Sales Manager, and suddenly these men will start looking twice, or three times. (John Diamond, *She* magazine, March 1992, p. 89)

Why men don't act their age! When the hot flushes start you know it's the Maleopause

10 signs to watch out for:
1   He takes up jogging and All Bran.
2   He begins buying his own underwear.
3   He starts putting 40 watt bulbs in the bathroom.
4   He cuts out ads for male cosmetics.
5   He thinks Joanna Lumley is much too old for him.
6   He wears tinted contact lenses at all times.
7   He asks the kids to call him by his first name.
8   He buys pastel coloured trousers and matching jacket.
9   He starts watching *Top of the Pops* on the telly.
10   He thinks he's a ringer for Brando 1965 instead of 1994.
(Joan Burnie, *Daily Record*, 4 May 1994, p. 21)

There are many supporters of the concept of a male menopause who tend to adopt a much broader definition of the indicative symptoms. A term gaining currency in the USA in the 1990s for this experience is *viropause*, meaning a pause in a man's virility. Aubrey Hill, an American medical practitioner, published a book in 1993 called *Viropause/Andropause*, which contained a series of case histories drawn from his medical practice. Although he accepts the current scientific view that there is no conclusive biological evidence to support the existence of a male menopause, he argues that there can be no doubt that 'most men undergo what could be called a male menopause' and it is 'a significant problem among men in societies of the industrial nations' (Hill, 1993, pp. xiv and 49).

Hill's evidence for this conclusion is typical of the way in which the male menopause generally has been described and analysed. He bases his assertions on selected cases that are not representative of the population at large, and divides the symptoms into two categories: physical and emotional. The physical symptoms are 'reduced sexuality' and 'cardiovascular disease'. These are different from the physical symptoms associated with the menopause in women, and relate to problems that are only very loosely associated with middle age. The emotional category includes depression, anxiety, fear, a sense of inadequacy, reduced self-esteem, and a fear of death.

☐ How do these emotional symptoms compare with the psychological symptoms ascribed to the female menopause?

■ Some of the symptoms are commonly associated with mid-life in both sexes: depression, anxiety, and a feeling of being inadequate or unable to cope. But there are differences: men are said to experience fear of death and reduced self-esteem, whereas women are said to be irritable and to have problems with concentration and memory. What might amount to very similar psychological symptoms, appear to be described differently—to be given different cultural ascriptions.

Hill estimates that 15 out of every 100 men will experience symptoms which are sufficiently severe to warrant them being considered ill. The viropause/andropause syndrome is, according to Hill,

… a naturally occurring psychological state that occurs in men's middle years, producing feelings of unhappiness and undermining men's sense of self-worth, identity and competence. (Hill, 1993, p. 197)

The conclusion of this and other recent books on the subject is that, although the biological causes of the male menopause have not been identified with any precision, it is nonetheless a real phenomenon, and popular and professional belief in it has increased substantially since the 1970s (for example, see Bowskill and Linacre, 1976; Aquilina Ross, 1984; Sheehy, 1993). An extension of this belief has been the growth in interest in hormone replacement therapy for men—using testosterone—as a 'treatment' for the symptoms of the male menopause, particularly sexual impotence.

This is a highly controversial intervention for two reasons, which have been highlighted by the largest study of health in middle-aged men—the Massachusetts Male Aging Study, part of which has focused on impotence (Feldman *et al.*, 1994). First, there is only a weak association between testosterone levels and sexual potency, except in the small minority of men whose testosterone output has fallen extremely low; the great majority of cases of impotence in mid-life are not affected by testosterone treatment. Second, like hormone replacement therapy for women, there are health risks associated with giving testosterone to men; in particular, it may increase the risk of heart disease. Despite these reservations, private medical clinics have begun to appear in the USA and the United Kingdom, offering testosterone therapy to middle-aged men. The medical director—Malcolm Carruthers—of one in Harley Street in London, describes his patients and the future of HRT for men thus:

> Suddenly, their libido goes and their virility goes, and from being the high fliers in their professional field, from being the tigers of industry, they've become the sheep ... Just as I think women will be looking to estrogen replacement therapy to maintain their health and happiness, so I think men can look with confidence to testosterone replacement therapy. (Quoted by Chen, 1994, p. 22)

A different view of the same future is taken by John McKinley, the director of the Massachusetts Male Aging Study:

> The pharmaceutical companies are already capturing half of the population through the medicalization of menopause, which is a normal physiological event for women. Now they are moving on to capture the other half of the population through the medicalization of normally aging men. (Quoted by Foreman, 1993, p. 55)

The emphasis on treatments for loss of vigour and confidence in mid-life seems all the more strange in the context of the relative neglect of treatment for the physical ailments that do increase in middle-aged men. The commonest causes of impotence (which the Massachusetts Male Aging Study revealed increases in prevalence steadily from 40 years onwards; Feldman *et al.*, 1994) are cardiovascular disease and diabetes. The screening of men for early signs of prostate cancer (which is the second-largest cause of cancer deaths in men, after lung cancer), or prostate enlargement which interferes with urination, has not been given the same funding or publicity as the screening of breast and cervical cancer among middle-aged women (Pfeffer, 1985), although doubts remain about the effectiveness of prostate screening programmes (Schröder, 1993).

The neglect of physical illness and its prevention may be related to the promotion of mid-life itself as the 'disorder' requiring 'treatment'. In the final section of this chapter, we examine the pervasive belief that mid-life *is* a time of personal crisis.

The mid-life crisis

A crisis is a 'turning point' or a decisive change. There is an element of threat: in a crisis one is at risk. So, as in the course of a disease, the outcome of a crisis can be for better or for worse.

The term **mid-life crisis** was first used by the psychologist Elliot Jaques in 1965 in an article with the rather awesome title 'Death and the Mid-Life Crisis'. Jaques suggested that the mid-life crisis occurs between the ages of 35 and 39 and was caused by the awareness of the ageing individual that time is running out and that death is becoming an increasingly inescapable reality. He argued that the mid-life crisis was a turning point in the life course because the awareness of one's biological limitations must lead to either a positive or a negative outcome. The basis of this conclusion was his analysis of the lives of 310 painters, poets, composers, writers and sculptors. He found evidence that some creative artists ran out of steam in mid-life but others, such as Goethe, Shakespeare and Beethoven, went on to produce great works in later life. Although his conclusion was based upon a sample that was by no means representative of the wider population, Jaques' work was an important antidote to the belief that mid-life was necessarily the beginning of the end.

Jaques' theory of the mid-life crisis supports the more general view (derived from sociological and psychological research into later life) that all human beings have the

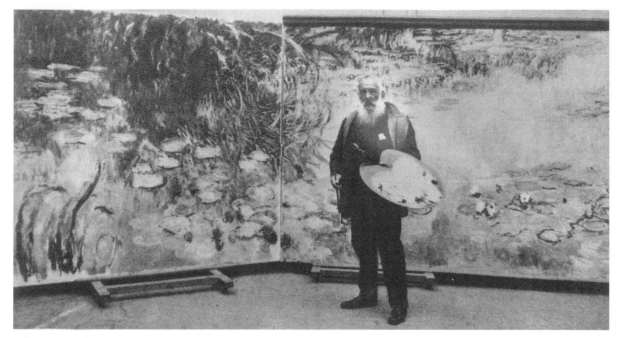

Claude Monet, like many others who remain creative into old age, continued to produce major works of art until his death at the age of 86, three years after this photograph was taken in 1923. (Source: Mary Evans Picture Library)

capacity for personal development throughout the life course. Personal growth does not necessarily cease as one grows older, although, as you will find out in the next chapter, social factors such as income, class and gender may have an important part to play in realising or constraining one's potential. However, there is a dearth of information about the experience of mid-life among contrasting groups in society.

Jaques' view—that the mid-life crisis results from an awareness that time is running out and that death is closer than before—is a **psychological model** of mid-life change. For other influential psychologists, such as Daniel Levinson and his colleagues (1978), mid-life is the testing time of a dream: the hopes one had for one's life and the state of one's plans for realising these hopes. Levinson's work was based on intensive interviews with a small number of men. Following a long historical tradition (as you saw in the work of Breu, Figure 9.1), he argued that life is divided into a number of stages and, in order for a man to make a successful mid-life transition, it is necessary for him to examine his dream and to resolve his disillusionment about those aspects of the dream that must remain unfulfilled. The alternative is stagnation.

> I'm 38 and I sort of look back and think 'What have I really done? What have I really been?' I think there is a big pressure that I feel, and that is one of time. I don't know how long I'm going to live but I've lived for 38 years and I've seen so little of the world for example … And to have been ten years in the one company, at one stretch, yeah, I feel I suppose that time seems to be running out. (Stewart, interviewed in 1994 for an Open University radio programme, 'The mid-life crisis')

Both these psychological models of the mid-life crisis are based upon very small samples, largely of men. Yet, despite the fact that our knowledge of the everyday experience of mid-life is so scanty and unrepresentative, these models continue to be extremely influential. There is considerable evidence of the existence of a strong popular belief that mid-life *is* a time of crisis.

Allin Coleman and Tony Chiva (1991) have developed a more open-ended approach to change in mid-life. Their 'coping with change' model (see Figure 9.3) is designed for use on mid-life planning courses and on courses to prepare people for retirement. In this psychological model, they put a strong emphasis on 'gaining insight' as distinct from 'accumulating information'.

Coleman and Chiva argue that there are no 'experts' in mid-life and retirement: the experience of mid-life is rapidly changing and is so diverse that each person needs

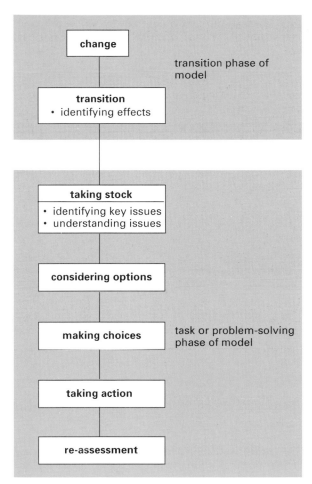

Figure 9.3 *Coping with change model (from Coleman, A. and Chiva, A., 1991,* Coping with Change: Focus on Retirement, *Health Education Authority, London, Figure 1, p. 7)*

to explore—with others—his or her resources and potential and on this basis make personal decisions for the future. In this model, mid-life is seen not simply as a phase in the biological process of physical ageing, but as a creative social process which involves taking stock of one's past life and considering options for the future. It is a reflective process of self-assessment and adjustment through which individuals actively create their future lives. This is very different to the traditional images of middle and later life, as exemplified by the 'steps of life' model.

> I like getting older, I quite enjoy getting older, because I think the sort of traumas and anxieties you have as a teenager, as well as when you are in your twenties, and your worry about your image and what you look like, has *gone*. I don't feel I need to—you know—make any false pretensions about what I am and what I want to do, etcetera .... Now it is 'So what!'. It doesn't really matter what people think about you as long as *you* know what you are, and that is a single woman, living very happily and very comfortably on my own. (Meena, interviewed in 1994 for an Open University radio programme, 'The mid-life crisis')

Coleman and Chiva's approach recognises the diverse range of situations people may find themselves in during mid-life towards the end of the twentieth century, and the impossibility of generalisation.

☐ Think back to earlier chapters of this book. What changes to the nature of work and family structure this century might make generalisation difficult about mid-life today?

■ In the twentieth century there have been major demographic changes, most notably in the divorce rate and in re-marriage, in lone parenthood, in the proportion of people living alone, and in completed family size; there have also been major changes in patterns of working between men and women, in unemployment, redundancy and early retirement. All this makes for enormous possible diversity in individual circumstances for people who are middle-aged. For example, a woman in her early 40s may be a new mother and, at the same time, a grandmother; she may never have had a paid job or she might be taking maternity leave from a demanding career.

The experience of mid-life and of the mid-life crisis can best be understood by considering the interaction between biological and social factors: as a dynamic on-going process of interaction between one's view of changes in one's body and one's position in society.

> I think for a significant number of people it's about being able to let go of earlier expectations. Like so many things to do with all these changes in mid-life, they go on, they're not something that happened and then, like, it's tomorrow and it's different. It's a continual sort of process. It's not 'Well here I am and I'm different now'. It's going on every day. (Peter, interviewed in 1994 for an Open University radio programme, 'The mid-life crisis')

Conclusion

Over the last 150 years, Western society has been transformed and people can now expect to survive to enjoy a long lifespan. In consequence, age has become an increasingly important factor both for society and the individual. In contrast with the sixteenth-century image of the 'Steps of Life', the model of the life course in the late twentieth century is much more complex. As Coleman and Chiva's work suggests, the establishment of mid-life as a contemporary social institution is an unfinished project—it is still being actively created. Contemporary norms, based on the expectation of good health, place an emphasis upon positive self-development and growth throughout the life course. Success in this is seen as a vital part of preserving health and wellbeing in later life. This helps to explain popular interest in the mid-life events we have considered in this chapter.

A comparative study of the symptomatology of the menopause, both female and male, is instructive because it provides further evidence that ageing cannot be understood simply as a biological process divorced from social and cultural circumstances. For those who adopt a purely medical model, the problems associated with mid-life are seen essentially as the result of specific processes of biological ageing, which may be remedied with such interventions as HRT. Critics of this model argue that the contribution of negative and discriminatory social attitudes towards ageing cannot be ignored in accounting for problems in mid-life. Reducing everything in mid-life to a biological explanation can lead to middle-aged women, for example, finding that many of their health complaints are being ascribed by doctors to the menopause, even though there may be evidence to suggest other causes.

Current controversies surrounding the existence, definition and appropriate responses to mid-life events can perhaps be regarded as symptomatic of a society (which means all of us, of course) coming to terms with massive historical changes in the structuring of the life course. In these circumstances, most of us continue to follow our cultural traditions in defining life as a series of stages, and mid-life as the highpoint of maturity, a stage which is also the first step 'down' towards old age. The main struggle for those who believe the reality is or could be otherwise, is to create more positive attitudes towards the later life that so many of us will come to experience.

OBJECTIVES FOR CHAPTER 9

When you have studied this chapter, you should be able to:

9.1 Discuss the contribution of popular beliefs about the life course to the experience of middle age in Western culture in the 1990s.

9.2 Distinguish between those aspects of the menopause, the male menopause and the mid-life crisis that can be construed as social and cultural constructs and those that have a biological basis.

9.3 Illustrate the diverse range of situations people may find themselves in during mid-life towards the end of the twentieth century, and relate this to psychological models of mid-life change.

QUESTIONS FOR CHAPTER 9

Question 9.1 (*Objective 9.1*)

How might popular beliefs about mid-life have an effect on personal experiences of mid-life changes?

Question 9.2 (*Objective 9.2*)

Which aspects of mid-life change in women and in men appear to be associated with alterations in the hormonal state of the body, and which do not?

Question 9.3 (*Objective 9.3*)

Summarise the main features of the three psychological models of mid-life change described in this chapter.

10 *Experiencing later life*

This chapter builds on the discussion of the biological changes associated with ageing, and scientific explanations for those changes, which occurs in another book in this series, Human Biology and Health: An Evolutionary Approach, *Chapter 8. The television programme for Open University students, 'Accumulating years and wisdom', is relevant to the present chapter and to the next one. The author of this chapter, Robert Slater, is a Lecturer in the School of Psychology at the University of Wales, Cardiff. He has conducted research in various age-associated areas, from tinnitus (ringing in the ears, experienced more often by older people) to aspects of the external physical environment that handicap vulnerable groups. His principal research interest is in the quality of life of residents living in old people's homes. The distance-teaching aspects of this chapter were developed by Julia Johnson, a member of the Open University Course Team.*

Old age is the most unexpected of all the things that happen to a man. (Trotsky, *Diary in Exile*, 8 May 1935)

Introduction

I do not like writing about being old. This is no doubt partly vanity—we all tend to think of ourselves as perennially young, but partly because society too has such a negative image of what it is like to be old. But it is also that the subject bores me. I am never conscious of being old, merely of not being able to see very well or take my dogs for as long walks as I used to, or do as much gardening. Otherwise, my life style remains broadly unchanged because it is domi-

nated by the same interests I have had all my life. There are also certain positive advantages. With the ending of the pressures to bring up a family, hold down a job or follow a career one can relax and take time to enjoy the little sensual delights of life like a lovely summer's day. I have learned to live in the moment and worry much less than I used to. (Castle, in Bernard and Meade, 1993, p. v)

The above passage was written by Barbara Castle, Baroness Castle of Blackburn, in her foreword to a book called *Women Come of Age*. Barbara Castle was born in 1910, and served in various Ministerial capacities in the Labour governments of the 1960s and 1970s. The book is one of several recently published books which attempt to give the reader some understanding of what it means to be old, especially an older woman, in the 1990s. Many are based on in-depth biographically-orientated interviews with selected samples—random or otherwise—of older people.

In her foreword, Baroness Castle continues by noting that she is one of the lucky ones, and clearly her perspective on later life might have been very different had she been powerless, poor, and prone to ill-health and depression in her earlier years or on the receiving end of 'do-gooders' in her later years, as is Mrs Williams, about whom you will read in Chapter 11. In the television programme associated with this chapter (and Chapter 11) you will also meet individuals whose histories illuminate their present perceptions.[1] What Barbara Castle says nicely encapsulates some of the points we make later: that older people don't tend to feel 'old'; that society has negative attitudes to ageing; that while there are physical and mental changes there is also continuity; and that there can actually be advantages to later life—grandparenting, for example, which may in many, but by no means all instances, bring a lot of pleasure without much responsibility.

[1] The television programme 'Accumulating years and wisdom' was made for Open University students studying this book as part of an undergraduate course.

Expectations and attitudes: past, present and future

In Chapter 2, and its associated Reader article by Peter Laslett,[2] and in Chapter 9, the tradition of dividing life into stages was noted. The last 'stage' often consists of caricatures of old age as decline and decay. Western European societies in the 1990s have inherited and tend to perpetuate this sort of negative imagery about, and attitudes towards, later life—fostering a view that what we witness as 'health' in old age is all to do with intrinsic internal and unmodifiable processes, and little to do with extrinsic factors.

When consulting a GP over some health concern, older people might well be asked 'what do you expect at your age?', and many might accept the implied answer—'ill-health'. This attitude is considered again in the next chapter, in the context of daily activities. Such an expectation is bound to be unhelpful in the management of later life, especially if it leads to a belief that nothing can, nor indeed should, be done because later life is all about 'natural', 'normal', ubiquitous and inevitable decline. (The problematic notion of 'normality' was considered in Chapter 1 and also in other books in this series.) Although there may be an increase in age-associated disabilities, their cause may not necessarily be 'intrinsic ageing',[3] nor are such disabilities an inevitable accompaniment of age. Age is a *cause* of nothing, it is an elastic index—a crude proxy—for other processes, the nature of which are currently being unravelled. It is these biological and social mechanisms that contribute to what we describe as ageing, and to the age-associated diseases and disabilities that arise over time. By understanding such processes we may be in a better position to influence them.

Moyra Sidell, a research fellow at the Open University who is investigating the health of older women, suggests that for many individuals in the current generations of older people, health in old age is bound up with a complex combination of psychological, spiritual and functional factors: 'feeling fit enough to carry on with the daily routine as it comes along without worry', 'being free in body to do what you want to do, not to be cramped with rheumatic pains', or 'when you can get about and get your own shopping and not depend on people to run and get your errands' (Sidell, 1995).[4]

Chapter 2 pointed to the success story of increasing life expectancy at birth. Largely as an outcome of public health policies in the late nineteenth and early twentieth centuries which reduced infant mortality, more and more people will have a chance to experience old age.[5] Even life expectancy for people in their 80s has been lengthening. However, a quick flick through a dictionary of quotations looking for 'wise sayings' about youth and old age would reveal the obvious: youth, by and large, is seen as being a more positive state than old age.

☐ Suggest possible reasons for being more optimistic about old age nowadays than our ancestors were.

■ You may have suggested that people in the 1990s have a better understanding that what is witnessed as 'old age' is not simply an unmodifiable production of genetics and physiology. Indeed, you may have considered that researchers are increasingly in a better position to understand the biological 'causes' of age-associated changes and, therefore, to offer ways to ameliorate some of their unwanted effects. You may have noted that the way people age is likely to be influenced by such things as diet, income, education, housing, and access to health and social services resources—commodities over which at least some older people can exert more control than in the past, as active citizens with a vested interest in their own futures. You may think that nowadays there are positive but realistic role models for older people who are increasingly visible, counteracting traditional negative expectations—perhaps on the front cover of *Active Life: the magazine for the years ahead.* You may have considered that information technology and consumer electronics are reducing the physical effort required by those older people who are frail or disabled to control their environment.

[2]The article 'A new division of the life course' can be found in *Health and Disease: A Reader* (Open University Press, second edition 1995).

[3]The biological nature of ageing processes is described in *Human Biology and Health: An Evolutionary Approach,* Chapter 8.

[4]Definitions of health and ill-health have many dimensions, as Chapter 1 of this book and the Reader article by Mildred Blaxter 'What is health?' made clear. See also the discussion of lay health beliefs in *Medical Knowledge: Doubt and Certainty,* Chapter 2, and its associated television programme for Open University students, 'Why me? Why now?'.

[5]See also the discussion of the world-wide increase in longevity in *World Health and Disease,* Chapter 3, and the underlying reasons for the increase in the United Kingdom since the Industrial Revolution, in Chapter 6.

There are healthy retired couples, where each partner has a good occupational pension, who live from October to April on the Costa Brava and who can genuinely say they are having 'the time of their lives'. There are, however, problems with re-packaging old age into an 'all-singing, all-dancing' version. Perhaps optimism should be tempered with caution lest unrealistic expectations about both genetic and social change may be generated; or lest people are made to feel guilty that somehow it is their own fault that they are not ageing quite as well as they should be and we 'blame the victim'. Notions of 'successful ageing' inevitably raise yardsticks by which many will fail. And failure is not good for anyone's self-esteem—something of particular importance in later life. Images of 99-year-old marathon runners may not help in this respect.

Are the expectations set up by cosmetics industries about keeping looking younger—and implicitly healthier—shaping negative attitudes to old age? A brief glance at the rack of women's magazines (and, increasingly, men's) at the local newsagent's would provide some evidence. Is it 'normal' to want to keep looking younger; to have plastic surgery to achieve it; to attempt to deny that one is, in fact, growing old? Why is it that wrinkles can (for the time being) be perceived as a sign of character in men? What strength and fortitude does it take for a woman to wear her wrinkles with pride, as evidence of life's experiences, as something not to be smoothed away and hidden?

Another feature of later life to be smoothed over and hidden has been sexuality.

☐ What is your reaction to the drawing in Figure 10.1, which featured in an article on sexuality in later life in a professional journal for nurses? (You might think back to the discussion in Chapter 7 of the contentious nature of sexual behaviour.)

■ We cannot guess your reaction, but it may have resonated with the comments of nurses who wrote to the *Nursing Times* about the illustrations. One wrote to say how pleased, touched and impressed she was by the article, which she was sure would help to open up minds and attitudes. Another wrote in to protest at the repulsive sketch of a 'leery old man copulating with an old crone' and suggested that such images were enough to put one off sex for the rest of one's life!

It is clear from various surveys that sexual activity can and does go on among people in later life, although—interestingly—the survey of *Sexual Behaviour in Britain* (Well-

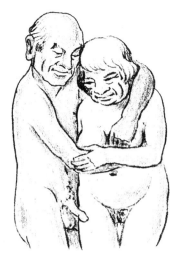

Figure 10.1 *This illustration appeared in 1989 in an article on 'Sexuality in later life' by Anne Roberts, which appeared in the professional journal* Nursing Times, **85**(24).

ings *et al.*, 1994; already discussed in Chapter 7 of this book) was based on interviews with a random sample of 18 876 British residents, all of whom were under the age of 59. One reason for excluding older people was that the main purpose of the study was to provide data for modelling the epidemiology of AIDS, and it was thought that there were few HIV-positive people over the age of 60 in Britain. However, the authors note that 'many of the topics for which data were collected are known not to affect older people greatly' (p. 23). Yet, of the 4 246 Americans aged between 50 and 93 who supplied the *Consumers' Union* with information about their sex lives, some 79 per cent of men and some 65 per cent of women aged 70 and over reported that they were sexually active (Brecher, 1984). Like the British survey, the *Consumers' Union* report ran to over 400 pages, suggesting that there *are* topics concerning the sexual behaviour of older people that merit attention.

Some argue that it is healthy to be sexually active in old age. Books like *Living, Loving and Ageing* (1989) by the Director of Age Concern, Sally Greengross, and the media doctor, Wendy Greengross, suggest how older people can avoid letting physical and medical complaints constrain sexual and personal relationships. Conversely, many older people may be relieved that they are no longer under pressure to 'perform' sexually. Prescriptions or proscriptions about the healthiness of sexual behaviour in later life seem to have more of a basis in value judgements than they do in scientific knowledge.

Terminology, stereotypes and discrimination

If there is at least some truth in the notion that the pen is mightier than the sword, then questions can be raised as to how the use of language might shape prevalent social attitudes to older people.

☐ Think of some terms—like 'old folk'—that are used as collective phrases for older people.

■ You may have thought of 'the elderly', or 'the aged', or perhaps 'the retired', or 'senior citizens'. More disparagingly or patronisingly: 'old ducks', 'old dears', 'old crones', 'old codgers', and now 'wrinklies', 'nearly-deads', and 'coffin-dodgers'.

Such terminology suggests that all people over a certain age are the same, despite the fact that they might span over thirty years in age-range, and be experiencing marked differences in, for example, health and income. It also suggests differences from other groups—that 'the elderly' for example, are categorically different from the 'non-elderly'. One reason why we write of *older people* in this book is that the term suggests relativity rather than some categorical state. And while many older people may prefer to be called 'senior citizens', many others might find it strange to be called anything of the sort. The correspondent to the *Nursing Times* who liked the line

drawing shown in Figure 10.1 also wanted to know how someone who feels like a 22-year-old can have adult children, wrinkles and grey hair. Certainly the 55 grandparents aged 55 and over, interviewed by Paul Thompson (1990), a historian at the University of Essex, and his colleagues, could say with sincerity that they didn't feel old, but young, albeit within an ageing body. It is less the passing of time that brings an 'old' identity, and more an event like a stroke, heart attack, or bereavement. (The five older people interviewed in the television programme 'Accumulating years and wisdom' express such feelings too.)

But when others perceive you as one of the category 'the elderly', you become a clearer target of prejudice, as the American feminist Barbara Macdonald found to her annoyance on a women's march to 'Take Back the Night':

I don't know exactly when I sensed that something was wrong and noticed that Cynthia was no longer beside me but a few feet away where the monitor was talking to her. I joined them. At first the conversation was not clear to me and I glanced at Cynthia's face for some clue. There was none. The monitor was at first evasive and then chose her words with care: 'If you think you can't keep up, you should go to the head of the march'. Gradually, I took in, like a series of blows, what the situation was, that the monitor

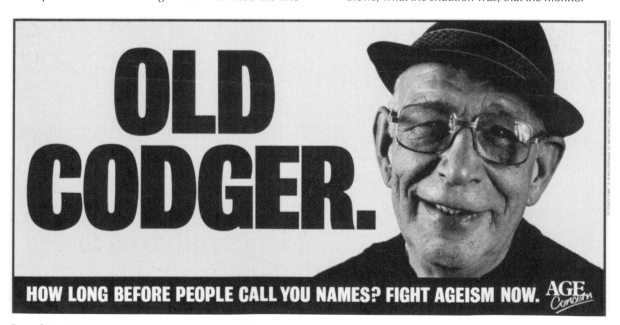

Part of Age Concern's campaign against age prejudice. (Poster courtesy of Age Concern)

thought that, because my hair is grey, because I am sixty-five and because I look sixty-five, I might be unable to keep up … I faced the monitor with rage. 'You have got to be kidding; I don't believe this.' My fists were clenched at the injustice as I felt the all too familiar wave of helplessness and fury engulf me … She wanted to apologize. I said it was all right but it wasn't all right. Sometimes I wonder if it will ever be all right. (Macdonald and Rich, 1984, pp. 28–9)

Age prejudice (sometimes referred to as ageism) is not quite like sex and race prejudice: individuals do not turn into persons of the opposite sex or of another race. Hence age prejudice is against our future selves—which is hardly self-serving. Age prejudice against older people is, then, potentially even-handed: if *you* believe people should be discriminated against on the grounds of age, rather than need—as newspaper headlines in the early 1990s claimed was happening in the health service—then you cannot complain when you are on the receiving end of age prejudice as you grow older.

But is age prejudice in attitudes being translated into **age discrimination** in the distribution of services? Are older people actually denied treatment on account of their age? This is difficult to research systematically, but anecdotal accounts from older people seem to be borne out by the personal experiences of at least some doctors. In 1994, David Jolley, Chairman of the Old-Age Section of the Royal College of Psychiatrists, wrote a letter to the Prime Minister, which was published in the *Guardian*. It began:

> Dear Mr Major,
> I was surprised to see you were taken aback when informed that elderly people were being denied treatment by the NHS. It is part of my everyday experience that old people are less likely to be offered admission to hospital because of acute illness than younger patients with less or similar problems. If they gain admission to hospital they are immediately exposed to pressure concerning arrangements which can be made to ensure early discharge. (Jolley, 1994, p. 25)

Life in retirement

Retirement is something that is largely taken for granted, but its often compulsory nature makes it a form of age discrimination. Dulcie Groves (1993), herself retired but

---

From The Guardian, 8 July 1994

NHS care for old to be limited

Long-term sick and elderly face charge

From The Times, 13 August 1994

AGE CONCERN

Care of the elderly should not be a lottery

From The Times, 22 April 1994

Pensioner wins fight for therapy

FORMER band leader who was told he was too old for physiotherapy treatment at his local hospital has forced health chiefs into a U-turn.

From The Times, 13 August 1994

Cradle-to-grave care undermined

Elderly patients lose right to hospital bed

In the early 1990s, the accusation that health services were being rationed on the basis of chronological age began to be hotly debated.

still actively engaged in research, points out that for those without an occupational pension, many of whom will be women, income is drastically reduced by retirement—literally overnight. This contributes to **structured dependency**, that is dependence on others and on the state as a consequence of older people being forced to retire from work and live on an inadequate pension (this is considered in more detail in the next chapter). Age discrimination in employment often occurs earlier than retirement age, in terms of hiring and firing, and it is clearly visible in many job advertisements. Justifying age discrimination is often impossible, which is why it is illegal in some countries—the USA, for example.

As you have seen in earlier chapters, the state of not being in paid work in recent years is less of a categorical or novel condition than at any time since the 1930s, as more individuals (mainly men) experience lengthening spells of unemployment before they reach 65. As sociologist Graham Fennell and his colleagues point out (1988), increasing numbers take early retirement for reasons other than ill-health. In the United Kingdom in 1971, for example, just over 86 per cent of men aged 60–4 were economically active, together with 30 per cent of men aged 65–9. Fennell estimated that in the 1990s the comparable figures is likely to be closer to 50 per cent and 9 per cent. This prediction is in broad agreement with estimates by Chris Phillipson, Professor of Applied Social Studies at the University of Keele (Phillipson, 1993).

Whatever the reason, significant numbers of older men and women in the United Kingdom still go from a full-time job one day to no job the next. In Finland, however, a flexible form of retirement has been introduced which enables employees to tailor their exit from work more to their particular needs. Having such control over their working lives contributes to positive self-esteem and may protect some individuals from the effects of stress (as discussed in Chapter 8); this in turn may be beneficial to health. But, as Chris Phillipson suggests, we should perhaps be wary of seeing retirement as a dislocation that affects everyone alike. During the last twenty years research has focused on

> ... variations in the experience of retirement, here reflecting lifelong inequalities and differences produced by class, gender and ethnicity. (Phillipson, 1993, p. 193)

In 1991, Michael Young and Tom Schuller (whose work was discussed in Chapter 2) interviewed 149 individuals living in Greenwich, London, all of whom were aged between 50 and the then statutory retirement ages (60 for women, 65 for men). All their respondents had left full-time employment, for a variety of reasons, within the two years prior to the interview. Their evidence led Young and Schuller to suggest that women often seem more able to cope with such life transitions as retirement, and that many women may still have less of a commitment to paid work as central to their identity when compared with men.

☐ Can you think of any challenges inherent in 'being retired' apart from perhaps having to adjust to a much reduced income?

■ You might have suggested some of the following: how will retired people fill those extra 40 hours a week and will they miss the company of their co-workers? How will domestic partners cope with each other when they have so much more potential time together? Will others think less of the retired person just because she or he *is* retired? 'Retirees' may be worried they have joined a club of which they didn't want to become a member.

Many retired people put their skills to use in working for voluntary organisations or in other forms of active citizenship which give them a real sense of purpose. For the first time in years some older people may be able to fill their time in just the way *they* want to fill it. They can attend those interesting-looking day-classes run by the extramural department of the local college of higher education or join the local branch of the University of the Third Age, or even start a course of study with the Open University. With a good pension, perhaps they will visit some of those National Trust sites they've always been meaning to, or join the local golf club, or go on a few of those cheaper winter package holidays. But for many of the 40 per cent of pensioners without an occupational pension, retirement means a reduction rather than an increase in choice and opportunity. In 1992, the state pension for a single person was worth 15.9 per cent of gross average male earnings, and this is likely to decrease in future years (Walker, 1993).

Health, finance and gender

Social Trends for 1994 (an annual survey by the Central Statistical Office) reveals that, of the poorest fifth of the population, 27 per cent are people over 65; if you compare this with the proportion of over-65-year-olds in the population as a whole—13 per cent—you can see that a disproportionate number of older people are living in poverty. Those in this poorest sector spend a higher proportion of their expenditure on necessities—fuel, food and housing—and less on 'non-essentials' such as leisure activities. They are less likely to own such consumer durables as a car, telephone or central heating. Older people, who are most at risk of **hypothermia**, may be less able to prevent this condition, which occurs when the body's temperature falls to below 35 °C (or 95 °F): conscious control over the muscles begins to ebb and mental processes start to slow down, which may load to further reduction in body temperature and ultimately death. And while the older rich may be getting richer, the older poor are not. The nation's increasing wealth is far from evenly distributed.[6]

Look at Table 10.1, which contains some of the data from a survey published in 1991 by British Gas.

[6]Inequalities in the distribution of wealth in the United Kingdom and the consequences for health are discussed in *World Health and Disease,* Chapter 10, and *Dilemmas in Health Care,* Chapter 11.

☐ What are considered to be the main problems facing older people in Britain? Where do the main age, sex and ethnic differences in perceptions lie?

■ Most striking is the identification of financial difficulties as one of the main problems facing older people: 45 per cent of retired people over 55 identified this as a problem, and 48 per cent of younger people agreed. However, when responses were analysed by ethnic group, older Asians were less concerned (25 per cent) about financial difficulties than other groups. Declining health and mobility was identified as a problem on average by 36 per cent of the over-55 age-group, rising to 40 per cent of white respondents over 75; rather more women than men saw this as a major problem, and there were no obvious differences between ethnic groups. Loneliness and isolation and lack of family was the next most problematic category for all groups except the older Asians (who, you may recall from Chapter 2, are the least likely to be living alone); women were

Table 10.1 Answers to the question 'What do you think are the main problems facing older people in Britain today?' from a survey in 1991; responses from the 'retired/over 55' age-group are presented according to sex and ethnic group: responses from the '16–24 age-group' are simple totals

Problem categories	Retired/over 55 age-group							16–24 age-group
	responses by sex (%)		responses by ethnic group (%)				total (%)	total (%)
	male	female	white 55–74 years	white 75+	black	Asian		
financial difficulties	47	44	45	45	45	25	45	48
problems with pensions	12	12	13	9	8	2	12	12
declining health/mobility	33	38	35	40	30	34	36	25
crime/fear of crime	9	13	12	10	13	7	11	15
loneliness/isolation/no family	15	23	20	18	25	9	20	12
transport/hard to travel around	9	11	10	11	7	6	10	5
lack of respect from society	8	7	8	5	13	5	7	12
no problems	6	4	5	3	7	27	5	1
total number responding	**333**	**429**	**401**	**113**	**122**	**128**	**764**	**475**

Other 'problems' which few respondents agreed affected older people have been omitted. Responses sum to more than 100 per cent because respondents could select any number of categories of problem. (Data derived from British Gas, 1991, *The British Gas Report on Attitudes to Ageing,* British Gas, London, Tables 24 and 25)

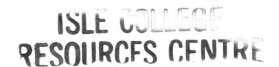
ISLE COLLEGE
RESOURCES CENTRE

more likely to see loneliness as a problem than men, and blacks more than any other ethnic group. No problems were reported by 27 per cent of the older Asian sample, compared with the average for the total sample of 5 per cent. The 16–24 age-group seemed to underestimate health and mobility problems as well as loneliness and isolation, but only 1 per cent thought that older people would not experience any major problems.

Perhaps to some extent these data reflect a wish on the part of respondents to present a favourable impression of their circumstances. For example, just 16 per cent of those aged over 55 described their health as poor or very poor. The survey also revealed that 30 per cent of those aged over 55 who rated their own health as good said they enjoyed life less as they got older, but this rose to 63 per cent of those who rated their health as poor.

Reviewing studies of social class differences in health in their book *Gender in Later Life* (1991), sociologists Sara Arber and Jay Ginn conclude that women are disadvantaged compared with men in terms of disability and health in later life, even though women have a longer life expectancy—a subject we return to in the next chapter. For older women, health disadvantages are compounded by worse financial resources. Women, who often have a discontinuous employment history, have fared badly in both state and occupational pension schemes. In particular, the older a woman is, the more likely she is to be poor and hence less able to afford, for example, repairs to her accommodation. Substantial numbers of older people, particularly women, live in some of the least satisfactory housing conditions and have less access to basic amenities than do younger people. Older people are, of course, more likely to be coping with disabling and chronic conditions associated with later life, including poorer vision and hearing.

□ Look at Figure 10.2, which is based on data from a survey of 9 000 adults in Britain in 1984–5, undertaken for the Health Promotion Research Trust by a multi-disciplinary team headed by Brian Cox.[7] Describe how the prevalence of symptoms reported during the last month varies with age and sex.

[7]Brian Cox and other members of the team, including Mildred Blaxter, talk about this survey in the television programme for Open University students 'Why me? Why now?', which is associated with *Medical Knowledge: Doubt and Certainty.*

■ Clearly, the prevalence of painful joints, trouble with eyes and palpitations or breathlessness increases noticeably with age (Figure 10.2a), but colds and 'flu, and headaches, decline as people get older (Figure 10.2b). Women, by and large, report a higher prevalence of symptoms than men, particularly at older ages; the exception is colds and 'flu for which the gap between the sexes declines with age.

Seven years later, Brian Cox, Felicia Huppert and Margaret Whichelow updated the earlier survey and published the results in 1993. They noted that men aged over 60 in non-manual occupations were twice as likely to report their health as having improved over the seven years, compared with men in the manual occupational class. For the oldest groups of women, more of those in the non-manual group reported better health than seven years earlier, whereas more women within the manual class reported a decline in health over the seven years. These results are a reflection of the fact that, as shown clearly in all large-scale surveys of morbidity as well as in mortality data, class inequalities in the prevalence of chronic diseases widen in middle age. This may be due to differences in the nature of the work done in different occupational classes, with unhealthy work taking a long-term toll; or it may be the cumulative effect over the life course of less healthy living environments, or poorer diets, or more smoking; it has also been suggested that a degree of 'programming' of chronic diseases in later life results from adverse perinatal experiences (mentioned in Chapters 4 and 14). Whatever the reasons, 'ageing' is an unequal process.

Multi-pathology—that is, having several disease conditions at once—increases with age. This was borne out by a major study conducted by the Centre for Disease Control in the USA in 1984 (published in 1990), of a representative sample of nearly 14 000 people aged 60 and over. It was estimated that 50 per cent of men and 58 per cent of women aged 80 and over had more than five chronic conditions; the older women tended to have conditions that limited their activities more than the conditions experienced by the older men. Around 49 per cent of the sample as a whole (i.e. all ages) were estimated to have some degree of arthritis; 42 per cent had hypertension; 20 per cent had cataracts; 14 per cent had heart disease, and 14 per cent had varicose veins. Between 5 and 10 per cent were having to cope with one or more complaints related to either diabetes, cancer, osteoporosis (thinning of the bones) and hip fractures, or the aftermath of a stroke. In the United Kingdom, more people aged over 65 die each year of 'heart disease' than

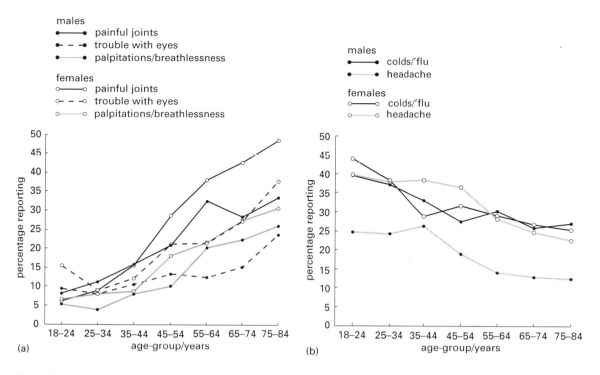

Figure 10.2 *Prevalence reported 'during the last month' of selected symptoms among adults in Britain surveyed in 1984/5, by age and sex. (Data derived from Cox, B. D. et al., 1987,* The Health and Lifestyle Survey, *The Health Promotion Research Trust, London, Table 2.6)*

any other cause, and many will have to cope with its main symptoms—breathlessness or extreme tiredness.[8]

The extent of health problems in later life means that older people are more in need of homes that are easy to run and maintain, but they are relatively less likely to be in possession of them, particularly if they are older women. The conditions under which many older people have no choice but to live clearly exacerbate health problems and diminish quality of life. Yet, as J. Grimley Evans, Professor of Geriatric Medicine at Oxford University, points out (1991), reducing such extrinsic causes of disease would actually prevent some older people from getting a disease, rather than merely postponing the age at which they get it—which makes this kind of intervention doubly worthwhile.

[8]Heart disease is the subject of a case study in *Dilemmas in Health Care,* Chapter 10.

Activity and passivity

'A woman's work is never done'—well, not quite. According to Eric Midwinter, the former director of the Centre for Policy on Ageing (1992), of an average 105 waking hours each week, the available leisure time for a British female in full-time employment is about 31 hours—compared with 48 hours for a male. (The health implications of this discrepancy can be deduced from the discussion in Chapter 8.) For a retired male, it is around 92 hours and for a retired female, 75 hours. Such figures are derived, in the main, from interviews undertaken annually with 3 000–4 000 individuals aged over 60, who are part of the national random sample selected for the *General Household Survey.* Somewhat paradoxically, active pastimes seem to be indulged in less among older generations: a 'typical' person over 65 may spend a lot of time watching television or listening to the radio, though many read, go to the library and visit friends and relatives. For many, retirement is a fairly sedentary existence (but, of course, work can be so, too), which hardly promotes health.

□ Can you suggest some reasons why older people may be relatively inactive in retirement?

■ Older people may be unused to the idea of making the most of leisure. Some may feel that jogging or aerobics is not what older people do. For many there may be financial barriers: certain activities need access to a car, which many older people have not got—especially older women who live alone. Older people may be worried about going out at night for fear of slipping on dark, wet pavements, or for fear of being mugged (even if in statistical terms the latter is very unlikely). Older individuals who have mobility difficulties may be handicapped by barriers in their physical environment, and those who have problems with continence may want to make sure there is always a toilet nearby.

The 'free time' that life in retirement can bring often requires structuring to replace that given by work; it requires activity that is goal-directed, not done just to 'kill' time. According to Michael Young and Tom Schuller, whose research we mentioned earlier, the

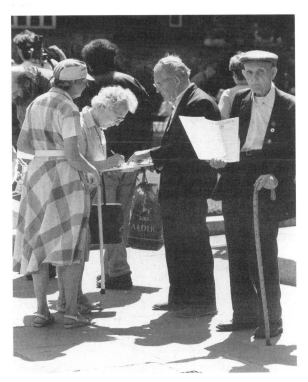

Pensioners at a mass protest against the imposition of VAT (Value Added Tax) on domestic fuel, 29 June 1993. (Photo: E. Hamilton West)

people in their sample of over-50-year-olds whom they labelled 'positive' third-agers, were those who enjoyed their hobbies, sometimes did things on the spur of the moment, and yet also planned for future events. Young and Schuller suggest that a life full of *contrasts* is needed, from a baseline of routine. But many cannot afford contrasts which require expenditure over and above that which is taken up by 'the basics'.

Many older people are far from inactive on political issues, as headlines like these reveal: 'Elderly residents take on local authority in High Court battle' (*Community Care*, 4 June 1992, p. 3); 'Greys protest over threat to activity scheme in Ely' (*Cardiff Independent*, 20 May 1992, p.4) and 'Armed pensioners plan to lobby parliament' (*Guardian*, 25 June 1993, p. 11). This kind of action is nothing new historically, but the difference is perhaps that pensioners are increasingly seen as members of a 'mass movement'. This could influence how individuals experience later life, for example in regard to their health or use of health services. The subtitle of the health manual written by the Boston Women's Health Book Collective—*Ourselves Growing Older: Women Ageing with Knowledge and Power* (British edition; Doress *et al.*, 1989)—succinctly suggests how some of the new psychological perspectives on health in later life, both mental and physical, are developing. We are moving from a view of older people as passive objects to one of active citizens.

Age-associated psychological change

The changes older people most commonly notice in themselves, and which are often noticed in them by others, and are confirmed by experimental evidence, concern slowing of behaviour and an increase in forgetfulness—particularly for names. These capacities are both major components of mental life that contribute to intelligence. Most psychologists agree that 'intelligence' has two qualitatively different components, often labelled as the *fluid* and *crystallised* forms. Tests of **fluid intelligence** assess the ability to solve problems quickly for which there are no solutions derivable from cultural practices or from formal training: this ability might commonly be called 'quick-wittedness'. **Crystallised intelligence**, however, is often assessed through vocabulary or other tests which attempt to measure the amount of knowledge a person has accumulated: it might be thought of as a form of 'wisdom'. Measurements of the intelligence of samples of individuals from different age-groups show that scores on the 'fluid' tests generally decline markedly with age, but scores on 'crystallised' ones decline much less, if at all.

☐ Why do you think caution should be exercised in attributing to 'ageing' the measured decline 'with age' in fluid abilities that such tests might reveal?

■ You might have suggested that, as people get older, the more likely they are to have one or more forms of illness, and it could be this, rather than their age *per se*, that is influencing their fluid intelligence scores; or that they are relatively unfamiliar with that sort of test material compared to younger people, or are less well motivated to perform optimally on it.

☐ The association between age and intelligence-test scores is usually determined by testing *cross-sectional* samples of people of different ages, and comparing the results of (say) people aged 41–50 with another group of people aged 71–80 who were tested at the same time. What is the major difficulty in interpreting the results of a study with this design and how might this be overcome?

■ The major difficulty with a cross-sectional study is that the tests are performed *simultaneously* by people of different ages, so the apparent decline in ability with age may in fact simply be due to *generational* differences between individuals—for example, the level of education when young may have been lower for the oldest people tested. To be sure of detecting a genuine decline with age, a large-scale *longitudinal* study of the *same* individuals over time would be required.[9]

However, even when such factors are taken into account, test scores for fluid abilities still show a decline with age, albeit a less marked one. Test scores also reveal more *variability* between individuals as they age, often because some individuals maintain pretty optimal functioning, while others decline at a variety of rates. Abilities are not set once-and-for-all: learning a new language in later life, for example, might require more effort, but that may be just what the older language learner is prepared to give it. Even performance on a test of digit span memory—how many numbers you can repeat back immediately after they have been read out to you—can be dramatically improved with sufficient training. Of course people with a dementing illness like Alzheimer's

---

[9]The advantages and disadvantages of using cross-sectional and longitudinal research methodologies are discussed in another book in this series, *Studying Health and Disease*, Chapter 6, and in Chapter 14 of the present book.

disease would find such new learning a daunting task, but that should not be a worry to the vast majority of older people. According to Elaine Murphy, Professor of Psychogeriatric Medicine at Guys Hospital in London, about 1 in 10 people over the age of 65 have a form of dementia, but it does not necessarily progress rapidly and many individuals 'appear to remain the same for many years without any further deterioration' (Murphy, 1993, p. 14).

Apart from the idea that *speed* of processing information is reduced with age, various psychological experiments suggest that there may also be a reduced *capacity* for processing. As task demands are increased, older individuals may be disproportionately disadvantaged. In particular, there may be a reduction in *working memory* capacity, that is the ability to hold onto information while, for example, you work out 16×18 in your head. There may also be differences in the strategies adopted to solve a problem, with older people adopting less optimal strategies under certain circumstances: for example, paying too much attention to irrelevant detail rather than the 'main point' when trying to remember a passage of text. These tendencies are known as *production deficiencies*.

Psychological changes such as these are often interlinked, so deficiencies are more likely to be apparent in complex situations. Consider car driving, for example. The driver has to concentrate on the road ahead, but look out of the side windows from time to time, and look in the rear view and side mirrors now and then. Sometimes the driver will be paying attention to the radio or to a passenger; some might even be steering with one hand while holding in the other a cellular phone into which they are conversing! Drivers make judgements about the speed of the car in front, about the likely actions of its driver, and about the articulated lorry bearing down from behind. They notice the traffic lights ahead, and the people who might be about to cross the road. They allow for the effects of weather conditions on the road surface. Sometimes many of these factors have to be considered simultaneously if an accident is to be avoided. It is not surprising, then, to find that older drivers' accidents occur disproportionately at complex junctions, as the researchers Carol Holland of the University of Leeds, and Pat Rabbitt, Director of the Age and Cognitive Performance Research Centre at the University of Manchester, have noted (1992).

Older individuals are more vulnerable to injury once a crash occurs and, as a group, experience a higher fatality rate than younger adults. Similarly, older pedestrians are more at risk and their vulnerability may be exacerbated by reduced visual ability and hearing. But unlike some younger drivers, older drivers *do* modify their driving in response to their own perceptions of how to put themselves and others at less risk, and to information fed back to them about their performance characteristics. They are less likely to speed, to drive in bad weather conditions and at night, and more likely to avoid routes they know to be problematic. And, if they are shown that their eyesight is not as good as they thought it was, they are likely to wear prescribed spectacles more appropriately (Holland and Rabbitt, 1992). This may partly explain the results of a MORI poll commissioned by the Direct Line insurance company, which showed that motorists aged over 50 have far fewer accidents and commit fewer driving offences than younger drivers, even though they use their car more often (reported in *Age Concern Information Circular*, October 1994, p. 12). However, American data suggest that this finding may not be quite as clear-cut as it appears.

Being able to drive may be important to an older person's sense of identity—reinforcing 'not feeling old', as well as being a practical necessity for those who are unable to walk far or use public transport, or for those living in rural communities.

It is not just with respect to driving that older people may modify their behaviour to bring continuity out of change. As you will see in the next chapter, older people make a variety of adjustments in order to achieve satisfactory lives for themselves, despite the many daily hassles and difficulties they have to face in a world that is often not designed to accommodate their needs, nor to be sympathetic to them. For example, consider the 'green-man crossing' that does not give older people enough time to cross a road; or the difficulty in hearing what is being said on the telephone, which might be ameliorated if the person could afford a phone with a volume boost and acoustic coupler; or the GP who tells older patients that 'it's your age' and therefore nothing can be done about their health problems. Perhaps, with the political will and individual initiative, future generations of older people may be even less prepared to 'put up and shut up' in order to experience more of the advantages that later life could bring.

OBJECTIVES FOR CHAPTER 10

When you have studied this chapter, you should be able to:

10.1 Give examples of age prejudice and age discrimination, and show how the experience of ageing—including health experience—contrasts with these negative attitudes and behaviours.

10.2 Describe how variations in material circumstances affect the health and quality of life of different groups (e.g. distinguished by age, sex, social class and ethnicity) within the population of older people, particularly after retirement age.

10.3 Use the example of driving to illustrate how older people may modify their behaviour to compensate for certain psychological changes in later life.

QUESTIONS FOR CHAPTER 10

Question 10.1 (*Objective 10.1*)

Stereotypes of 'the elderly' characterise older people as a homogeneous group in society. How would you criticise this view of the experience of later life?

Question 10.2 (*Objective 10.2*)

What reasons are there for suggesting that the experience of old age in the future might gradually improve, and what changes in society would promote this?

Question 10.3 (*Objective 10.3*)

Are older drivers better drivers?

11 Living with disability in later life

During your study of this chapter you will be asked to read an extract entitled 'Some bloody do-gooding cow' which comes from Tony Parker's book The People of Providence; *you can find it in the Reader.[1] The television programme for Open University students, 'Accumulating years and wisdom', is relevant to this chapter and to Chapter 10. The author of this chapter is Julia Johnson, a Lecturer in the School of Health and Social Welfare at the Open University; she is a social gerontologist whose principal research interests are social work and older people, residential care, and self-neglect in later life.*

Introduction

In writing about Parkinson's disease, Ruth Pinder comments:

> The way people deal with the daily contingencies and demands of living with the illness has been virtually ignored. Yet to understand this is an essential precondition to the many prescriptive statements of need which often characterize health care delivery writing. (Pinder, 1988, p. 68)

In this chapter, we are going to focus on how people experience and cope with physical limitations in later life. We also want to consider what it is like to receive help within a personal relationship. But before we do this we are going to look at what is known about the extent of disability in later life.

[1]Health and Disease: A Reader (second edition, Open University Press, 1995).

The prevalence of disability in later life

I went down the street and I got some things for Mrs Glyn and I came back and I went in her house and said, 'Dunno what's the matter with my bloomin' knees today' I said. 'they just won't go'. 'Ah', she said, 'you're getting old'. (Barbara Williamson, aged 76, quoted in Thompson *et al.*, 1990, p. 109)

□ Is disability an inevitable consequence of growing older? To answer this question, look at Figure 11.1,

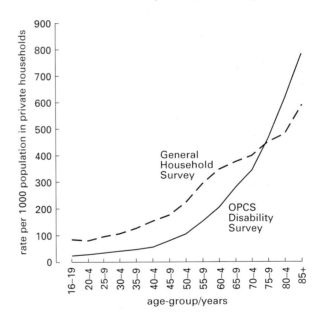

Figure 11.1 *Estimates from the General Household Survey (GHS) of the prevalence of limiting long-standing disability in different age-groups in Great Britain in 1985, compared with estimates from the Office of Population Censuses and Surveys (OPCS) Disability Surveys of adults in private households, 1985–8. (Source: Martin, J., Meltzer, H. and Elliot, D., 1988, The Prevalence of Disability among Adults, OPCS, HMSO, London, Figure 3.4, p. 20)*

which shows how disability, as measured in two different surveys, changes with age.

■ Figure 11.1 shows an association between age and disability: older people are more likely to experience disability than younger people. The rate per 1 000 adults living in private households rises slowly until the 50s and more steeply thereafter, particularly over the age of 70, when about 45 per cent of people reported a limiting long-standing disability. However, disability is not an *inevitable* consequence of growing older: 20–40 per cent of people aged 85 and over (depending on which survey you focus on) did not report a disability.

The General Household Survey (GHS) is a survey of a national sample of the population resident in private (that is non-institutional) households in Great Britain. It has been conducted annually since 1971. The sample includes about 10 000 households in which all members over the age of 16 are interviewed about employment, income, health, leisure and so on. The OPCS Disability Surveys were specially commissioned by the then Department of Health and Social Security, and were carried out between 1985 and 1988. Their aim was to provide up-to-date information about the number of disabled people in Great Britain, the level of severity of their disability and the circumstances in which they were living, in order to plan for benefits and services.

You may have noticed that, in age-groups under 75, the GHS estimates are higher than those of the OPCS Disability Survey. This probably reflects the different questions asked in each survey. The GHS asked about long-standing illness or disability which limited *any* activities, whereas the Disability Survey asked about limitations only on *specific* activities. Surprisingly, however, for those over the age of 75, the GHS rates are lower. The authors of the OPCS Disability Survey, Martin *et al.*, suggest that this may be because many older people regard limitations on their daily activities simply as part of growing old and do not see themselves as disabled or in ill-health. Thus, for many older people, it was only when they were asked about specific activities that their disability came to their notice. This indicates how important the form of questioning is in determining levels of disability in different groups.

☐ Study Table 11.1. For people aged 75 and over, what are the most common forms of disability and which of these increases most in later life? How do the rates for specific forms of disability in this age-group compare with the rates for people aged 60–74?

Table 11.1 Estimates of prevalence of disability among adults in Great Britain by type of disability and age (rate per 1 000), in 1985–6

Type of disability (problems with...)	Age-group/years		
	16–59	60–74	75+
locomotion	1	198	496
reaching and stretching	9	54	149
dexterity	13	78	199
seeing	9	56	262
hearing	17	110	328
personal care	18	99	313
continence	9	42	147
communication	12	42	40
behaviour	19	40	152
intellectual functioning	20	40	109
consciousness	5	10	9
eating, drinking, digesting	2	12	30

Source: Martin, J., Meltzer, H. and Elliot, D. (1988) *The Prevalence of Disability among Adults*, OPCS, HMSO, London, Table 3.14, p. 26.

■ Problems with mobility (locomotion) are the most common, followed by hearing difficulties, problems with personal care such as bathing and dressing, with eyesight, and with dexterity such as opening jars or turning on taps. The rate of disability in seeing is over four times greater in the 75+ group compared with the 60–74 age-group. For most of the other types of disability the equivalent ratio is less than three.

Forms of arthritis and rheumatism are the most common complaints causing disability in older people, followed by ear complaints (mainly deafness) and eye complaints, particularly cataract and glaucoma.

Michael Bury and Anthea Holme found high rates of sensory impairment (that is, of eyesight and hearing) in their survey of a representative sample of people aged 90 or over. Unlike the highly complex measure of severity used in the OPCS Disability Survey, Bury and Holme used self-reported chronic conditions to estimate the prevalence of disability in their sample. 46 per cent of the total sample reported 'relatively severe' or 'severe' trouble with their eyes, and 49 per cent with their hearing. Furthermore, of all the physical conditions mentioned by respondents, only deficient eyesight and hearing

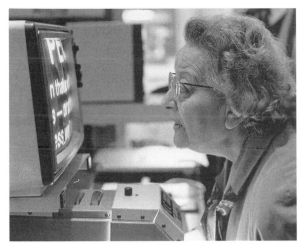

A large-print computer screen can assist someone with impaired vision. (Photo: Format Photographers Ltd/Pam Isherwood)

were reported as causing 'total incapacity' (Bury and Holme, 1991).

In 1986/7, the Royal National Institute for the Blind (RNIB) carried out the first ever nationwide survey of blind and partially-sighted people in Great Britain. It found that out of an estimated 500 000 people aged 75 and over who were eligible for registration as blind or partially sighted, only 97 000 were actually registered (Bruce *et al.*, 1991). The implication of this finding is that thousands of blind and partially-sighted older people may not be receiving enabling forms of support and services.

One feature of disability in later life is the presence of multiple conditions, or *multi-pathology* as we called it in Chapter 10. The RNIB found that 68 per cent of visually-impaired people aged 75 or more mentioned some other disability or illness: for example, 28 per cent had a hearing aid. Bury and Holme found that, with one exception, all the people in their study with five or more chronic conditions had a severe hearing problem. The exception, Mrs Storace, aged 91, reported a heart condition, arthritis, a chest condition, high blood pressure and 'agitation'.

Patterns of disability within the older population

The prevalence of disability does not simply rise with age: it is unevenly distributed within the population of older people along dimensions of social class, geography and ethnicity, which are similar to the patterns of health experience in younger age-groups.[2]

[2]Age, gender, ethnic and social class inequalities in health status in the United Kingdom, and possible explanations for these patterns, are extensively discussed in *World Health and Disease*, Chapters 9 and 10.

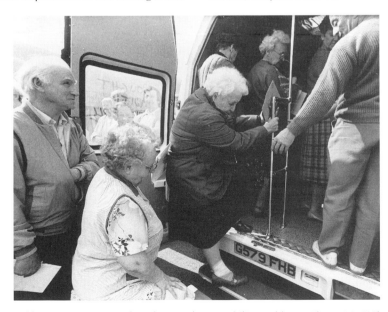

It is older women in particular who may have mobility problems. (Photo: Mo Wilson)

Although there is little difference in levels of disability between men and women aged 60–74, in people aged 75 or over, there is a substantial gender difference. The OPCS Disability Survey showed that 63 per cent of women aged 75 or over are disabled; the corresponding figure for men is 53 per cent. Men are likely to die earlier than women: between the ages of 65 and 74, the death rate for men in 1990 was 77 per cent higher than that for women, but the corresponding figure for men aged 85 or more was only 20 per cent higher. What all this means is that, generally speaking, there is a tendency for men to die at younger ages from illnesses such as heart disease and cancer, and for women to survive longer but to become disabled. It is women in particular who may face mobility problems, for example, in later life.

Christina Victor (1991), using data from the GHS for 1985, reports substantial social-class differences in the prevalence of disability in older people (see Table 11.2).

Table 11.2 Prevalence of limiting long-standing illness by social class for people aged 65 years and over, Great Britain, 1985

| Age/years | Percentage reporting limiting long-standing illness | |
| | Social classes* | |
	I and II (non-manual)	IV and V (manual)
65–9	35	44
70–4	34	45
75–9	42	52
80+	46	59

*Social classes defined by the Registrar-General's classification of occupations. (Source: Victor, C., 1991, Continuity or change: inequalities in health in later life, *Ageing and Society*, **11**(1), Table 11, p. 34, based on GHS reports of limiting long-standing illness)

□ Look at Table 11.2. What social-class differences in the prevalence of long-standing illness do you notice?

■ At all ages, there is a higher rate among people from manual working classes IV and V than among those from non-manual middle classes I and II. The

Table 11.3 Estimates of prevalence of disability (all degrees of severity) by region, per thousand population (all ages); Great Britain in 1985–6

Region	Disability rate per 1 000
Wales	170
North of England	166
Yorks and Humberside	156
Scotland	151
South West	145
West Midlands	139
North West	139
East Midlands	138
South East	132
East Anglia	130
Greater London	125

Source: Martin, J., Meltzer, H. and Elliot, D. (1988) *The Prevalence of Disability among Adults*, OPCS, HMSO, London, Table 3.9, p. 23.

prevalence of chronic illness among working-class people aged 75–9 is higher than that among middle-class people aged 80 and over.

Table 11.3 indicates that there are also extreme regional contrasts in the prevalence of disability. Although this table is standardised for age and covers all people with a disability, you should remember that 69 per cent of disabled people are aged 60 or over, so these data are largely about later life.

Statistical information on differences in disability in relation to race and ethnicity is harder to come by. It has been suggested that the major health problems of black and Asian older people in the United Kingdom are similar to those of the overall population, and that the distinctive problems for these minority groups are in obtaining the services they need (Bennett and Ebrahim, 1992). Ken Blakemore and Margaret Boneham, two sociologists with extensive research experience into questions arising from the ageing of Britain's post-war generation of black and Asian migrants, reviewed the evidence on the use of health services and on self-reported illness amongst minority ethnic groups. They suggest a complex pattern of differences between ethnic groups, and between men and women in these groups, and signs of rising ethnic inequalities in health in the poorer and industrial communities. Most of the problems, they argue:

> … centre around difficulties in communication and the slowness of the health services to adapt to the realities of a multilingual, multicultural society. (Blakemore and Boneham, 1993, p. 108)

Overall the evidence suggests that there are important differences in the prevalence of disability amongst different groups of older people. However, what lies behind the statistics is not just inequalities in health, but also cultural differences in the way different groups perceive and interpret their physical state and the need for help. As Bury (1988) points out, chronic illness and disability have different meanings independent of their functional consequences such as pain or restrictions on movement. For example, diabetes, stroke or arthritis present different issues for people in terms of how visible the condition is and the stigma attached to it.[3] And, what a disability means to someone is in part shaped by who they are—whether man or woman, older or younger, Irish or Bangladeshi, taxi driver or lawyer.

Definitions of disability and dependence

A commonly-used definition of disability is based on the distinction drawn by the World Health Organisation (WHO) between impairment, disability and handicap: poor eyesight (an **impairment**) may lead to an inability to read fine print (a **disability**) which may result in the failure to gain employment (a **handicap**). This definition of disability as resulting from impairment has been used in the statistics we have quoted above. It is an example of an **individual model of disability**, in the sense that it locates the disability in the person who has the physical impairment. Individual models of disability have been strongly challenged by some disabled people, for example, members of the Union of the Physically Impaired Against Segregation (UPIAS, 1976).

Michael Oliver, Professor of Disability Studies at the University of Greenwich, a disabled person himself, has argued that conceptualising disability as something that

stems solely from individual impairments is oppressive for disabled people. For example, the OPCS Disability Survey asked the question 'What complaint causes your difficulty in holding, gripping or turning things?'. Such a question, Oliver suggests, should be reframed as 'What defects in the design of everyday equipment like jars, bottles and tins cause you difficulty in holding, gripping or turning them?' (Oliver, 1990, pp. 7–8). This approach shifts responsibility for disability away from the individual: it is society, not the individual impairment, that is disabling. You may remember that in the first chapter of this book we made reference to these contrasting approaches to conceptualising disability.

Whereas the WHO and OPCS definitions of disability are aimed at determining the level of *need* for services, the **social model of disability** put forward by UPIAS is based on achieving equal *rights* for disabled people. In Chapter 1, we quoted the UPIAS definition of disability; we repeat it here, together with their definition of impairment.

> *Impairment* lacking part of or all of a limb, or having a defective limb, organ or mechanism of the body;
>
> *Disability* the disadvantage or restriction of activity caused by a contemporary social organisation which takes no or little account of people who have physical impairments and thus excludes them from the mainstream of social activities (UPIAS, 1976, pp. 3–4)

☐ Can you think of some ways in which society restricts the activities of older people with physical impairments?

■ The failure to make pavements safe places for walking, or to provide aids for daily living, or make adaptations to property, may restrict the activities of some older people who have physical impairments. An inadequate pension is also restricting: not having the money to keep the house warm or pay for a taxi. You may remember from the previous chapter that people over the age of 65 are disproportionately represented in the poorest fifth of the overall population.

Just as UPIAS has argued that disability is socially constructed, so Peter Townsend, author of *Poverty in the United Kingdom* (1979) and of *The Last Refuge* (1962) in

---

[3]The relative stigmatisation of certain disease conditions and the effects of stigma on the lives of people coping with such an illness is a major theme of *Experiencing and Explaining Disease* (first and second editions, Open University Press, 1985 and 1996).

which he mounted a devastating critique of Britain's old people's homes in the new post-war welfare state, has argued that dependency is 'socially structured' (1981). His theory of **structured dependency** (which we previewed briefly in Chapter 10) suggests that older people are made dependent on others and on the state when they are forced to retire from work and to manage on an inadequate pension, and when they are placed in residential care homes or made the passive recipients of community care services.[4]

Dependency, like disability, is not an attribute of individuals but of a relationship. Consider Mrs Smith, who is made disabled and forced to give up valued activities simply because the act of boarding a bus is too difficult and painful. The same problem has forced her to be dependent upon her husband to do her shopping. She may also depend on her husband for assistance with dressing, bathing and getting to the toilet. To describe her as 'a dependent older person' or more simply as 'a dependant' tells you little about the nature of the dependency relationships she is involved in: what she gives to Mr Smith, for example. What these descriptions do, however, is to reinforce stereotyped thinking about the characteristics of 'dependent older people' such as helplessness and incapacity. We considered these kinds of stereotypes in Chapter 10.

We also noted in Chapter 10 that women, particularly those over the age of 75 from social classes IV and V, are the most likely to be made dependent through poverty, ill-health and poor housing. Older disabled women are more likely to enter residential care. Older disabled men by contrast are more likely to be looked after at home by a spouse or other female relative (Arber and Ginn, 1991). These men may, therefore, interpret the care they receive as part of normal family life, whereas the women are more likely to experience it as unwanted and burdensome dependence (Qureshi and Walker, 1989).

But could, or should, everyone be *independent*? The reality is that within personal relationships most people depend on others in some way or another—financially, physically or emotionally. Everyone depends on the water companies for water, on shopkeepers to stock food for purchase, etc. so no one is really independent—rather, people are *inter*dependent. Despite this, a sense of independence is highly prized in our society.

☐ What do you think older people might say if asked what the term 'independence' meant?

■ Andrew Sixsmith, a gerontologist from Liverpool University, asked a sample of older people this very question. He found that the term independence has a variety of meanings for older people: not being physically dependent on anybody; being self-directing or in control; and the absence of feelings of obligation (Sixsmith, 1990).

Independence then is as much about autonomy and control as not needing assistance. So the challenge in sustaining a sense of independence in caring relationships is to provide **personal assistance** without undermining autonomy and control. Jenny Morris, a disabled person and a freelance researcher, suggests that the problem is that, once personal assistance is construed as 'care', the 'carer', whether professional or relative, becomes the person in charge and the disabled person is seen as being dependent—incapable even of taking charge of the personal assistance they require (Morris, 1993).[5]

For those older people who have been disabled for most of their lives, the challenges of ageing and the possible threats to independence may be even more acute. Gerry Zarb has been involved in a large study of people who have been disabled for most of their lives, some of whom are now well beyond retirement age. Interestingly, he found that for many of these people, ageing represented a threat to their independence, not just in the physical sense of being unable to do some things for themselves which they had previously been able to do, but in terms of 'losing control over how they wished to live their lives' (Zarb, 1993, p. 40). These people had been used to struggling to retain

[4]The conditions in residential care homes for older people in the 1960s, and Peter Townsend's attack on them, are discussed in more detail in *Caring for Health: History and Diversity* (second edition, Open University Press, 1993), Chapter 6. Townsend appears in the television programme for Open University students, 'A tale of four cities', associated with *World Health and Disease*, in the context of his research on material deprivation and ill-health.

[5]An extract from Jenny Morris's book *Pride Against Prejudice*, entitled 'Pride against prejudice: lives not worth living', appears in *Health and Disease: A Reader* (second edition, 1995). It discusses attitudes in the courts and media to severely disabled people who have campaigned for legal euthanasia.

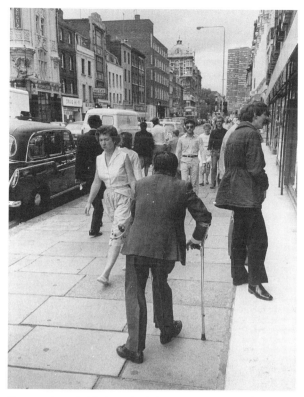

For people with life-long disability, the challenge of ageing may be particularly acute. (Photo: Sally and Richard Greenhill)

independence all their lives. Now, the effects of ageing were perceived as representing the onset of a 'second disability'.

Managing physical limitations in later life

But the picture that those we interviewed painted of themselves was very different from that implied by the surveys. For the most part, they did not perceive themselves as old, ill and disabled, in spite of being aged between sixty and 86 and having the whole range of chronic illnesses and disabilities that enabled them to be so labelled by others. None of them was helpless and incapable; and their diseases and disabilities appeared neither as major characteristics of themselves and their lives nor as how they characterized themselves. They gave a very different impression of themselves and

their world. The majority were still active and able to continue most of the activities they had participated in earlier in their lives, although on a smaller scale, in more limited ways. Essentially they perceived getting older—old age—simply as 'slowing down'. (Thompson *et al.*, 1990, p. 118)

These comments relate to the 55 grandparents aged from around 60 to over 80 interviewed in the study of later life which was referred to in Chapter 10.

☐ Think back to Chapter 10. Why do you think the respondents in this study did not perceive themselves as old, ill or disabled, despite their age and physical limitations?

■ Terms such as 'old', 'elderly' or 'disabled' label people as being different from others not so designated, and there is a stigma attached to this difference. These respondents (like those who feature in the television programme 'Accumulating years and wisdom', associated with Chapters 10 and 11) may be older and perhaps slower, but they are still the *same* people they have always been and are actively responding to the situation in which they now find themselves.

Rory Williams (1990) also interviewed a sample of people aged 60 and over living in two contrasting districts of Aberdeen. His enquiries focused on how they explained and coped with illness, old age and death. His interest in illness tended to focus upon chronic conditions entailing a degree of disability. Perhaps his crucial finding was that the way these Aberdonians explained and coped with the restrictions imposed by illness revolved around their notions of their *normal selves*. Most believed that their normal way of life generated health, and that normal living increased their reserves of strength in resisting and coping with a wide range of diseases and handicaps. It was very seldom the case that a person claimed to be categorically *unable* to do something because of a physical condition. Rather, they might think of the condition as making an activity 'not worth' the effort, pain, time or risk. Hence restrictions on activity could be construed as a choice and, therefore, remain a part of normal living.

The people whom Williams interviewed used a number of different tactics in their struggle to continue as normal. One was to shut out of their mind the threatening illness or condition. Such a response was generally considered admirable even if, at times, it made a treatable condition worse. More often, however, the condition was not denied but squarely faced. It was overcome by refusing to surrender to it. Thompson *et al.* describe how Mrs King, a widow of 80, faces up to her arthritis. Her day starts with the struggle to get out of bed and to get her breakfast, if possible in time for the ten o'clock news.

It takes me about twenty minutes or so to get dressed, and I crawl down the stairs … I come down backwards, because I feel safer that way … I crawl up the stairs when I'm going up although I've had a handrail up … But I feel a lot safer going up with me hand on until I get next to the top, and grab the side of the bannister, and pull meself up the last two steps. It's getting up the last two steps is worst. (Thompson *et al.*, 1990, pp. 165–6)

Despite these severe physical limitations, Mrs King leads an ordered, busy and normal way of life. She cooks and bakes and does knitting for sales. On Monday she does the washing and on Tuesday she irons. On Wednesday the home help comes and she goes to the church Ladies' Class. On Thursday she visits a neighbour to have her hair done and on Friday her elder daughter calls and takes her for a run in the car. On Saturday she prepares for her sister-in-law who comes for the night, and on Sundays one of her sons and his family sometimes visit. Another son, who lives close by, collects her pension and shops for her every week.

The struggle to maintain normality in the face of severe disability, however, is not always as successful as this. Williams cites a woman who, having been in bed for a year, had forced herself to walk again, despite many falls. In her view she had succeeded through 'determination' in controlling her condition, but she had had to acknowledge that she was no longer able to do nearly as much as she used to.

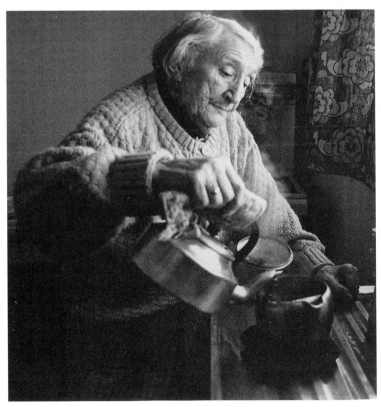

Being able to carry on as normal helps to generate health. (Photo: Mo Wilson)

A more positive reaction to restrictions, adopted by a minority of Williams' sample, was to search for new activities or revive old interests and to see these as a positive result of the disability: listening to 'talking books', knitting, painting and reading, for example. These were things that they would not have done *but* for the disability. On occasions this was linked to a welcome release from other disliked activities, such as cleaning.

Finally, by far the most common response was to cope by 'carrying on' with what was left, by stoically bearing an immutable sense of loss, and by contenting themselves by putting away frustrated wishes. A typical activity for these people was attendance at clubs associated with particular disabling conditions.

In summary, Williams identifies five broad responses to illness and disability:

- as controlled by normal living;

- as a continuous struggle;

- as an alternative way of life;

- as a release from effort;

- as a loss to be endured.

He draws out the conflict between disability as a continuous struggle on the one hand and as a loss to be endured on the other. The disappointment and frustration that arises from this conflict is eloquently expressed by May Sarton, an American novelist who published a journal of her own seventy-ninth year. She describes her struggle with constant pain and increasing frailty. During the year she lost fifty pounds in weight, could not tend her beloved garden and could no longer type. In describing to her doctor the anguish she sometimes experienced, she wrote:

> So I said, 'It's not grief that makes me cry, but frailty'. This is true, because it's when I can't do something that I very much want to do that I find myself in tears. Sometimes it's kind of shame for having so little strength, having to measure if I cross the room whether I have the strength to do it. (Sarton, 1992, p. 313)

In asking herself what value this journal has, she suggests that it shows:

> … how one old lady has dealt over a year with chronic pain; what the rewards are here of living by the sea, even old and ill; how I have had to learn to be dependent. (Sarton, 1992, p. 10)

Receiving help

Receiving help does not always create feelings of obligation. It can be experienced as an act of love and companionship, as it may have been for this man's dying wife:

> There's only me knows what it was like, the way the illness developed, the way she felt about it. I was having to prepare myself to lose her, and she was having to prepare herself to die. It was the hardest year's work either of us ever did in our lives, poor old girl. (Seabrook, 1980, p. 40)

There is, however, a dearth of research material on the experience of being cared for, compared to that on the experience of caring. Jenny Morris (1993) explored the experiences of younger disabled people who depended on someone they lived with for physical assistance. Her findings, summarised below, seem no less valid for older people who depend on a relative or friend living in the same household for assistance.

- Giving and receiving personal assistance can enhance a relationship.

- It can also stifle independence and lead to a dangerous, even abusive situation.

- Some people struggle to achieve a balance between maintaining some independence and recognising that personal assistance is a positive part of a relationship.

- Some people may want help from the statutory services to avoid being constantly dependent on relatives.

- A lack of services can exacerbate dependence and create additional stresses for both parties.

- Overprotection can be stifling and can create dependency.

- Some people may be neglected by family, causing physical and/or emotional damage.

- Retaining your own home is a way of preserving independence and sometimes safety.

- Reciprocity is an issue for many people who want to give as well as receive.

Remaining in one's own home can be important in retaining a sense of independence and normality. But when assistance is required because of restrictions imposed by chronic illness or disability, independence can be threatened.

Now turn to the Reader and read the interview by Tony Parker with Mrs Williams, entitled 'Some bloody do-gooding cow'.

☐ When you have done so, try to identify ways in which Mrs Williams' sense of independence is being undermined and ways in which it is being enhanced.

■ Clearly, Mrs Williams has had a hard life, struggling to feed and clothe her children when they were young. But she managed, without help. Now, through failing eyesight and arthritis, she finds that she needs help and is being offered it from a variety of sources, but she resents accepting it because it undermines her autonomy and control. It may be easier for her to accept help from her family because she has helped them in the past. But the others, for her, are 'do-gooders', who interfere and patronise and who have created a sense of obligation which she resents. (Not feeling obliged towards others, you may remember, was identified in Sixsmith's study as an important component of independence.) The neighbour who collects and delivers Mrs Williams' pension does not patronise or interfere and

manages, therefore, to assist Mrs Williams to retain a sense of independence. The well-meaning attempts to give Mrs Williams additional help and reassurance through the installation of a telephone, and subsequently the provision of a 'help' card, went badly wrong. Far from increasing her sense of security, they undermined it and created considerable anxiety.

These incidents demonstrate how easy it is to upset carefully-managed, familiar, daily routines through which people like Mrs Williams know how to get by.

The need for help and assistance which is associated with disability may, in time, contribute to a decision to enter a residential care home. At this point, the pattern of dependence might change radically. For example, Mrs Williams might find that someone else has taken control of her pension—deducting the home's charges from it and giving her what remains as 'pocket money'. She might also find that any prescribed medication she is used to taking for herself has been removed to a locked store, to be administered to her as and when she is meant to have it.

Not all residential care homes deprive their residents of autonomy and control, although there is a well-documented tendency for this to happen. In this chapter,

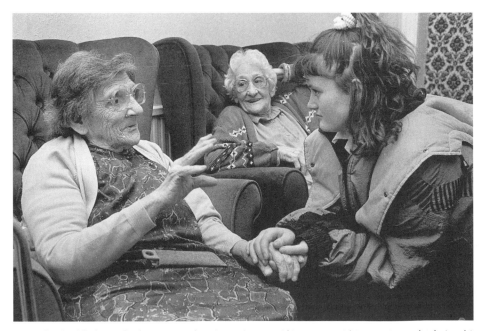

Personal assistance for disabled people does not undermine autonomy if it occurs within a reciprocal relationship: most people want to give as well as receive. (Photo: Sam Tanner)

we have described two older people—Mrs King and Mrs Smith—who, due to arthritis, take a long time to get moving in the morning. Both struggle to get up and dress, but they manage—in their own time. One of the problems in institutions is that the morning routine of getting a sizeable group of residents or patients up in time for breakfast, possibly before a staff shift-change, militates against people like Mrs King and Mrs Smith managing for themselves: they take too long to get ready. It is much quicker if a care assistant or nurse does it for them: indeed, staff may *have* to do it for them in order to meet deadlines. Although it is well established in theory that institutional routines should not take precedence over individual needs, in practice, they often do.

For some, like some of the older people Bury and Holme interviewed, residential care may be a welcome release from effort and worry. It can also alleviate the feeling of being a burden to relatives. Furthermore, it may be a refuge for those who have been neglected or abused by the people they lived with formerly. There are tried and tested ways of organising collective care so that it does not undermine people's autonomy and control, or their right to make choices and participate in decisions about their lives. Studies of older people living in small groups within residential care homes have demonstrated this (see, for example, the work of Lipman and Slater, 1977; Johnson, 1993). Stella Dixon, however, who as an action researcher tried, with the staff, to develop more resident-oriented practices in a residential care home, concluded that the stumbling block was staff attitudes. The staff seemed to see the residents as 'less than whole people' who were, therefore, regarded as not capable of making decisions about their own lives (Dixon, 1991). Dependency relationships are as much about power and presumptions of competence as they are about physical impairment.

Conclusion

We started this chapter by looking at the prevalence of disability in later life. But *how* disability is defined and measured will affect the findings of research into the levels of disability in society. Some of the evidence that we have reviewed here suggests that older people neither want to be classified as 'old' nor as 'disabled'. Their concern is to continue to lead what is for them a normal life, even in the face of physical limitation. If more attention were to be given to reducing ways in which society disables older people, then the physical limitations of later life could be regarded as more normal, less stigmatising and more manageable than is currently the case. We should be wary, however, that normalising disability is not used to justify the withdrawal of those health and welfare services which provide essential support to older people, and which help to sustain independence in later life.

OBJECTIVES FOR CHAPTER 11

When you have studied this chapter, you should be able to:

11.1 List the main physical impairments that older people are more likely to face than younger people and describe variations in levels of disability within the older population.

11.2 Explain the difference between an individual and a social model of disability and discuss the suggestion that social and economic factors create or contribute to dependency in later life.

11.3 Identify different ways in which people manage disability and dependence in later life and suggest ways of providing personal assistance that do not undermine a sense of independence.

QUESTIONS FOR CHAPTER 11

Question 1 *(Objective 11.1)*

What are the most common physical impairments and disabilities experienced by older people?

Question 2 *(Objective 11.2)*

Briefly explain the argument that it is society and not individual impairments that disables older people.

Question 3 *(Objective 11.3)*

It is not the provision of assistance but the way in which assistance is provided that has the potential to undermine independence and autonomy in later life.

Why is this so?

12 Dying

During your study of this chapter you will be asked to read an article by David Field, ' "We didn't want him to die on his own"—nurses' accounts of nursing dying patients', which appears in the Reader.[1] The author of this chapter, Clive Seale, is a Lecturer in Medical Sociology at Goldmiths' College, University of London; his principal research interests concern the experience of terminal illness, hospice care, euthanasia and old age.

Introduction

Most people in the United Kingdom are old when they die, yet this has not always been so. The prevailing age at death in a society has profound consequences both for the way in which death is managed and thought about, and for the personal experiences of those who die and those who are bereaved.

For the majority of people, the experience of dying is the final episode in a longer experience of old age, so the concerns of people who die are frequently those that are of relevance to older people in general. Just as the experience of old age can raise issues of bodily distress, dependency, material deprivation and social withdrawal, so the experience of people who die can—in the main—be understood as an intensification of these experiences, with death as the end point.

This is not to say that everyone is old when they die, or that illness and dependency always precede dying. There may be no warning of death in accidents, or of catastrophic physical events such as heart 'attacks' or 'strokes' (although these are usually preceded by some illness). The death of a child is a matter of great anguish, perhaps particularly in a society where people have become unused to seeing death in the young.

[1] *Health and Disease: A Reader* (second edition, Open University Press, 1995).

This chapter will describe a variety of experiences of dying, distinguishing between the deaths of older and younger people, and between different causes of death. It will also consider the different degrees to which death may be expected. We all know in a general sense that we are going to die, but not everyone who dies believes beforehand that they are 'dying', even when others may have felt that they were.

The chapter begins with a description of the various settings in which people die in the United Kingdom, indicating how this has changed over the years, and the implications of this for the care of those who die. The middle section of the chapter concerns varied experiences of dying, and the chapter ends with consideration of death in institutions—nowadays the main places where people die.

Where people die

Table 12.1 shows how the place in which death occurs has changed between 1960 and 1991.

☐ What does Table 12.1 show about trends over time in place of death?

■ Death in hospitals has increased from a half of all deaths in 1960, to about two-thirds in 1991. Deaths in other institutions have more than doubled to 7.7 per cent of all deaths. During the same period, deaths at home have nearly halved.

☐ What does the table show about gender differences in place of death?

■ Gender differences are greater in 1991 than in 1960. Women are considerably more likely to die in 'other institutions', which include residential homes, than are men.

☐ What could explain this gender difference? (Think back to Chapter 2).

Table 12.1 Place of death by gender, 1960 and 1991, England and Wales

	Hospital	Other institution*	Deceased's own home	Other private home and other places	Number of deaths (100%)
1960	%	%	%	%	
males	50.0	2.4	42.1	5.6	269 172
females	50.0	3.7	41.9	4.3	257 096
all	50.0	3.0	42.0	5.0	526 268
1991					
males	64.7	4.1	25.7	5.5	279 305
females	66.5	11.0	19.4	3.0	293 791
all	65.7	7.7	22.5	4.2	573 096

* Includes residential homes for older people. (Data calculated from General Register Office, 1962, *The Registrar-General's Statistical Review of England and Wales for the Year 1960: Part III, Commentary*, HMSO, London, Table CXIII, pp. 223–6; Office of Population Censuses and Surveys, 1993e, *Mortality Statistics: General. Review of the Registrar-General on Deaths in England and Wales, 1991*, Series DH1, No. 26, HMSO, London, Table 7, pp. 16–21)

■ Women live longer than men, and also tend to marry men who are older than themselves. They are therefore more likely to be widowed and enter long-term institutional care if they become unable to look after themselves.

The fact that more deaths occur in institutions, particularly hospitals, can be explained in a variety of ways. The growing elderly population, with increasing numbers living alone or with their spouse only, may be an underlying cause of the rise in hospital deaths. Hospital admission for older people has increasingly become a matter of acute care in times of crisis; admission may be precipitated by a marked episode of physical decline, or an intensification of symptoms, often causing problems for those looking after a dependent or very ill person at home. Hospitals are less likely than they once were to be treated as places for long-term care. This shift can be detected in the results of a study by Clive Seale, the author of this chapter, and Ann Cartwright (1994), which compared a nationally representative sample of 639 adults dying in 1987 with a similar group dying in 1969. They found that hospital admissions in the year before death had increased by 50 per cent between the two points in time, although the proportion dying in hospital had only risen by 4 per cent.

☐ What does this finding suggest about the number of discharges from hospital in the year before death?

■ These must have risen. People were going in and out of hospital more frequently at the later date.

Longer-term institutional care has increasingly become the province of residential and nursing homes, as is suggested by the statistics on place of death shown in Table 12.1. Seale and Cartwright's study reflected this, with 23 per cent of the people who died in 1987 spending some part of their time in such homes during their last year of life. Provision of places in such homes had risen between 1969 and 1987, official statistics showing an increase from 20.7 to 28.3 places per 1 000 people aged 65 or more in the population. The rise has been particularly dramatic in the case of residential homes run as private businesses, from 13 per cent of homes in 1969 to 40 per cent in 1987 (Department of Health and Social Security, 1982; Department of Health, 1990).

Although private households are not where most people die, most people spend most of their time living in their own homes in the months before death. Seale and Cartwright's study estimated that 81 per cent of people who died in 1987 spent most of the last year of their lives at home. Care in private households, either from family and friends, or from formal domiciliary services, remains very important. Yet here again, there have been shifts in recent years, as demographic changes have led to changes in the family and household composition of people who die, and health and social services have adapted to reflect changing patterns of need.

☐ From your reading of Chapters 2, 10 and 11, how might demographic change have influenced the care of older people at home by family members in their last months of life?

■ Increases in life expectancy have led to more people living alone or just with their spouse, who may find it difficult to look after a dependent person. There are likely to be fewer family members available to care for people at this time of life.[2]

Caring for people who are chronically or terminally ill at home can be very demanding, yet it is a task that many people take on. One study found that, in 1985, 15 per cent of the adult female population and 12 per cent of adult males were acting as informal carers for a mentally or physically disabled or elderly person (Green, 1988). As well as being experienced as burdensome, caring can also be experienced as deeply rewarding, particularly if the carer feels his or her efforts have contributed to a 'good' death. Here is the experience of a daughter who looked after her mother, not asking for the support of health services until shortly before the death.[3]

Three days before she died, we decided we must get the doctor; my cousin and myself. She couldn't eat or drink anything, it just ran out of her mouth ... The doctor came, he said she had Parkinson's Disease .... They said I should see the district nurse who came just the once, the day before she died ... She thought mother had been well looked after. She said I was doing very well. On the Friday she couldn't take the tablets. She was really bad. It was tea time. I cleaned up. She was such a mess. She was so distressed. It made me cry to see her. I went to wash the draw sheets. When I came in she was laid out stiff and making a noise. I sent for the doctor and my

[2]The experience of spouses caring for people in their final illnesses is described in an article by Ann Bowling and Ann Cartwright: 'Caring for the spouse who died' in *Health and Disease: A Reader* (first and second editions, Open University Press, 1985 and 1995). It is set reading for *Caring for Health: History and Diversity*, but you could usefully read it now if you have time.

[3]This account was given by one of the respondents in the survey by Seale and Cartwright (1994); at other points in this chapter and Chapter 13, examples of individual experiences are given which, unless indicated otherwise, come from the same source.

cousin ... She was dead when he came ... It was a labour of love. What else do you do? You look after old people when they are at the end of their life ... [I am pleased] that I was able to look after her, and that she had her wish and didn't go into hospital.

Dying at home, and caring for someone who dies at home, can be difficult, but is desired by many people who feel that institutional care is impersonal. Care in institutional settings will be described later in this chapter, but first something of the experience of dying will be conveyed.

The experience of dying

Predicted death

The moment at which a person is told of a life-threatening illness can be particularly dramatic and terrifying. The mother of a man who eventually died of AIDS described this:

They were very matter of fact. They told him to do whatever he wanted to do now and to make a will ... He became hysterical. He had a counsellor and a hospital doctor and several nurses there and they had to hold him down.

Elisabeth Kübler-Ross, a psychiatrist working with terminally-ill people with cancer, has written with great insight about the experience of dying under conditions such as these (Kübler-Ross, 1970). She has summarised the process of reacting to news of a terminal illness as a sequence of five stages:

Denial: is the first response. 'No, not me, it can't be true!' is the typical statement or feeling that is communicated. This stage can be expressed in many ways. Kübler-Ross cites, for example, a woman who insisted that her X-ray had been mixed up with some other patient's and who subsequently shopped around among doctors hoping to find one with a better prognosis for her.
Anger: wells up after the initial shock and denial has passed. 'Why me?' is the characteristic feeling at this time. Rage may be expressed against other people including doctors or family members and even against God. It is as though someone must be blamed for this overwhelming disaster.

Bargaining: is the middle stage. The dying person attempts to make some kind of deal with fate asking for an extension of life until a particular event has happened, which might be anything from making a world tour to awaiting the birth of a particular baby.

Depression: eventually follows as the person experiences increasing weakness, discomfort, and physical deterioration. It becomes clear that there will not be a recovery. The psychological picture of depression may include feelings of guilt and unworthiness. There may also be explicit fear of dying and a loosening of relationships with other people as the dying person withdraws and becomes less responsive. Thoughts and feelings are filled with a sense of loss.

Acceptance: the final stage, represents the end of the struggle. The person is letting go and this shows in a lifting of the depression. But acceptance is not necessarily a happy state: it may be almost void of feelings. One dying person described it as the 'final rest before the long journey'. (Adapted from Open University, 1992, p. 16)

The stages are devices which may help in making sense of experiences that are otherwise difficult to understand. Take, for example, the following account of a man who died of AIDS:

[The person] with AIDS never forgets for long the imminent approach of mortality. But what to do with this awareness? When my best friend died of AIDS I watched him in his last days juggle with two different senses of time, as though he were keeping two different sets of books on future accounts. He was intermittently lucid, knowing that all his efforts would soon be cut short; he wrote his will, saw friends, eliminated fools and finished his last book. At other times, however, he'd forget about his imminent death and would talk about projects five, 10 or 15 years hence. He was performing a delicate balancing act, fooling himself just enough to remain cheerfully engaged with the future, while being honest enough not to miss a second of the present. (White, 1993, p. 3)

☐ How might Kübler-Ross's stages be used to understand this man's behaviour?

■ He seems to be fluctuating between denial and acceptance.

Doctors in the USA and the United Kingdom have become more willing than they once were to tell people with life-threatening illnesses that they are likely to die from their disease. In the USA this change has partly been motivated by the more general onus felt by the medical profession to give patients full information about their condition, and about options for treatment. This is because of a heightened sensitivity to patients' rights in the USA, backed up by a fear of lawsuits from patients (or relatives) who feel they were given inadequate information at the time of major decisions.

In the United Kingdom, however, the shift in medical attitudes to truth telling has been more informed by psychological considerations, as it is commonly felt that open acknowledgement of dying gives people the opportunity to set their affairs, both of the internal and the external world, in order.

Death from old age

Another form of predicted death, and one that is more common than death from either cancers or AIDS, is death from extreme old age. It may seem odd to see 'old age' cited here as a cause of death. It is only very rarely written by doctors on death certificates as the cause of death, as the medical view of disease[4] usually involves the identification of a localised cause of death, such as stroke, pneumonia or 'respiratory failure'. However, in truth, many people die after a lengthy and gradual process of physical decline, where an accumulation of bodily events contribute to an eventual death. The task of the certifying doctor, in selecting a cause, or several underlying causes, of death is then somewhat unrealistic. Consider the following description, given by her sister, of the death of a woman of 84:

[She had] arthritis; hadn't been out for four years, had an infection of the bladder and arthritis in her hands and feet. The doctor said [she died of] old age [but wrote on the death certificate] bronchopneumonia … She was just fading away; she just faded out. She hardly ate anything—she was such a little thing … [When she came home from hospital] she was just

---

[4]This is discussed fully in *Medical Knowledge: Doubt and Certainty* (second edition, Open University Press, 1994).

waiting to die ... she gave up—she stopped eating. [When she died] she was so peaceful; she just waited for it, just lay there.

People who die in old age like this are often in situations rather different from those who die from AIDS or many kinds of cancer. In the survey reported by Seale and Cartwright (1994), the circumstances of adults who had died were described by their relatives and others some six months after each death. When compared with younger people with cancer, different patterns of symptoms were found in those over the age of 75 who did not die of cancer. In the older people, difficulties in seeing and hearing were more common, and troubles with pain and nausea were less commonly reported. Long-term restrictions (that is, experienced for more than a year before death) were also more common in the older age-group, concerning such things as mobility, dressing, washing and other aspects of self-care. At the same time, the older people in the survey were less likely to be living in households with family members who cared for them in their final illness; they were more likely to live alone, or to be in institutional care.

Deciding to die

You saw that in the death of the woman certified as dying of bronchopneumonia her sister said that at a certain stage she 'gave up' and stopped eating. In such a case there is a sense of the person actively anticipating, perhaps even seeking, his or her own death. Yet this would not be categorised as suicide, which is another form of predicted death in which the person who dies plays an active, if tragic, role in seeking death.

Suicide contrasts with other forms of self-willed death in being perceived by most onlookers as caused by an inability to cope with the pressures of life. Suicide may be committed by people with a history of psychiatric disturbance, as in the case of this man of 47, whose life and death is described by his wife:

He'd been ill for 15 years. He had a nervous breakdown and then became mentally ill—schizophrenic ... He had very dirty habits. He didn't flush the toilet and he wet the bed and dirtied his underclothes ... I daren't leave him to cut his nails; he would have stabbed himself ... [On buses] he would shout or stare at people and they didn't understand ... They took him into [psychiatric hospital]. He wasn't improving at all, and then while he was there he hung himself. They took him to [the general hospital] and put him in intensive care, but he was in a

coma. He never regained consciousness and died there.

Yet there is a point at which the category of death commonly called suicide can overlap with other forms of self-willed death. Consider the following case of a 50-year-old Dutch woman who had experienced one failed attempt at suicide through an overdose after her two sons had died. Her psychiatrist, Boudewijn Chabot, a member of the Dutch voluntary euthanasia society, eventually gave her pills which she used to end her life:

Chabot describes in his book ... how his patient remained adamant in her desire to die. He had to make a choice. She was, he believed, truly through with existence—not ill, but hurt by life. She had had enough ... [she wrote:] 'I long for the day that I do not have to stand at their graves any more, but will be allowed to lie there forever, between my darlings ... Why couldn't my boys live any longer? Why do I have to keep on living when I am already 50? I am not religious, but everything is so senseless. The grief, the despair, it is all so terrible.' ... [Chabot said:] 'I am not convinced that there is no other way out ...' It was the beginning of a long and melancholy dance, according to Chabot, with the psychiatrist trying to push her towards life. But she thought and talked only about death ... And thus ended [her] life. (Tromp, 1993, p. 16)

Euthanasia, the active ending of a life with medical assistance, is discussed in more detail in Chapter 13. In the case described by Chabot, the distinction between euthanasia and suicide may be blurred, but it is clear that both are distinct from death arising from a terminal disease. On the other hand, these are all forms of death in which dying is a predictable outcome.

Unpredicted death

It will be clear by now that there are many different forms of predicted death, and degrees to which death can be predicted. The truly unpredicted death, with no illness or warning beforehand, is quite rare, but such deaths when they do occur are among the most distressing for those left behind. This is not just because of the suddenness of the event; it is also because such deaths are often of younger people. Such deaths (often by 'accident' as discussed in Chapter 5) in a society where death is largely confined to old age are commonly felt to be unfair. The following account (the author's own, previously unpublished) illustrates the shock of one such death:

My brother died when he was fourteen. He went for a walk, having asked me to go with him. I have felt very guilty about my refusal, as he would still be here if I had said yes. He climbed up an electricity pylon and either jumped or fell off. No one really knew why—no drugs were found in his body, and he was not unhappy. Perhaps he just really fell, but then why did he climb up there? I learned about it when I was woken by the sound of the doorbell that night. It kept on ringing and no one was answering. Two policemen were at the door, and they told me that my mother was wandering around the streets crying out and distressed. Not understanding what was happening, I went up to get my father who was lying on his bed, asleep on his back, fully clothed. He jumped up, and told me what had happened: 'He's had a terrible accident' and then in response to my questions, 'No, he's dead'. I remember nothing else except my father then saying anxiously to me 'Are you alright?' as he went out to the policemen. I think I said yes, I was alright. It was the start of the most intense distress I have ever experienced.

Yet death by injury and poisoning accounted for only 3 per cent of deaths in 1993 (OPCS, 1993). Far more common, accounting for 26.3 per cent of deaths in the same year, is death from ischaemic heart disease, which often involves a heart 'attack'.[5] Such deaths are rarely totally unexpected, in that they are usually preceded by some history of known heart trouble. There may be a general awareness that the disease may result in death, but its timing is less easy to predict than many deaths from cancer. Such uncertainty may allow people to persuade themselves that their illness may not be as serious as it is. Thus, a 68-year-old man who died of myocardial infarction (heart attack) was said by his wife to have had chest pains, but he

> ... wouldn't go to the doctor. He ... had a terrible job to breathe [but] I don't know whether he told [the doctors]. If he didn't, they couldn't prescribe could they? ... He kept a lot of things to himself ... He never said anything

[5]Heart disease is the subject of a case study in *Dilemmas in Health Care*, Chapter 10.

about his health ... he didn't like to worry me. He left me a lovely letter. I think he must have known he was really ill.

Unpredictable deaths can also occur in people who live alone, sometimes because they have become so socially isolated that no one else is affected by the ending of their lives. Such people may be found dead in their homes long after they have died, as was this 58-year-old man whose circumstances are described by his neighbour.

> He was a loner. He had worked [as a sailor] and the Foreign Legion, but had decided to come back to England to live. He had a ... flat next door, and one day he suddenly knocked on my door and introduced himself and said he wanted to be friends. He used to come in here for a coffee and a natter ... He never asked you in; he always came here. I would see him regularly and then all of a sudden you wouldn't see him for five or six weeks. But that was his way; he just seemed to want to be on his own occasionally. [When he] had an operation because he had angina I visited him in the hospital and he thanked me for seeing him. He said I was his family because he didn't have any family ... time went on and I used to go into my back bedroom and there was an awful smell in there. I reported it to housing ... Then I came home one afternoon and my wife said the police had been. [They had broken in] ... They found his body, badly decomposed. It was black. They reckon he'd been dead for five or six weeks.

In such cases, officials from local councils may have to try to discover whether the person had relatives who can be informed of the death and take responsibility for funeral arrangements and the affairs of the deceased. Sometimes no one can be found, and burial takes place with the attendance of officials only, the modern form of a 'pauper's burial', in which the poverty of the dead person's life, measured by lack of human contact, is reflected in the lack of funeral ceremony (see photo *overleaf*).

Dying, then, is experienced in a variety of ways. A major cause of variation is the degree to which death is expected, and knowledge of this can vary between the person who dies and those close to him or her. The medical prediction that death will inevitably occur may be possible some time before serious physical decline has occurred in some diseases—as in certain cancers—but such prediction is the experience of only a minority of people who die. Far more common is the experience of

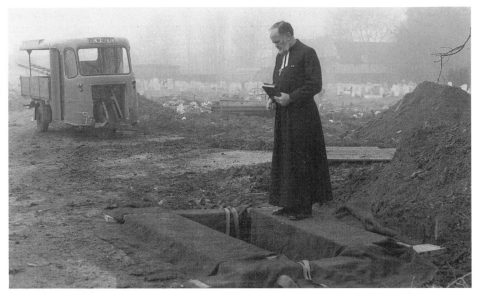

The burial of an unidentified woman, referred to only as DB16 in police records, took place on Christmas Eve 1992 in East London; she was estimated to have been about 45 years old when she died. (Photo: Anne Parisio)

uncertainty about the timing of death, either because physical decline is a gradual process associated with old age, or because the eventual cause of death is a disease, such as heart disease or stroke, whose course is unpredictable. Age is associated with variations in causes of death, of symptoms and restrictions, and in the experience of care. Wholly unpredicted death is rare.

Death and institutional care

Hospitals

Hospitals are busy places, largely geared to curing people of disease, or rehabilitating people with disabling conditions. They are not, on the whole, places where people go expecting to die. Yet the hospital environment is the single most common place of death, with nearly two-thirds of all deaths occurring there. Table 12.2 shows how death in hospital and other institutions compares with death in other places, according to cause of death.

   ☐ How might the predictability of these deaths, and the age at death, influence where they occur?

   ■ Fatal accidents are the most unpredictable form of death, and are likely to occur in public places, such as the road or a place of work. The pattern for circulatory disease, which includes a small propor-

tion of people who collapse and die with heart attacks, may explain why a higher than average proportion occur in 'other places'. Pneumonia is often recorded as the cause of death in very old people, which may explain the high proportion of such deaths in residential homes. Death from cancer is cited on death certificates in a somewhat younger group of people than average, so they are quite likely to have family members who can care for them at home. Thus, cancer is less likely to occur in residential homes where older people live, and less likely in the main site of unpredictable death—'other places'.

Studies of the experience of people who die in hospitals have sometimes found that impersonal routines can get in the way of humane care. Jeanne Quint Benoliel, who has studied a variety of hospital settings where people die, has described the character of intensive care units where, typically, there may be a high proportion of deaths from heart disease and where patients who die often do so within a short period of time.

> Because these settings are organized to prevent death, they are spatially arranged so that the doctors and nurses can easily maintain observation of all the patients assigned there. To accomplish this goal, privacy for the patients gives way to the need for constant vigilance, and contacts with patients are done mainly for

Table 12.2 Place of death by cause, 1991, England and Wales (includes only deaths of people aged 28 days and over)

Cause of death	Hospital	Other institution*	Deceased's own home	Other private home and other places	Number of deaths
	%	%	%	%	100%
neoplasms (cancer)	68.2	3.5	25.9	2.4	145 355
circulatory (e.g. ischaemic heart disease, strokes)	61.4	8.1	25.5	5.0	261 834
respiratory (e.g. broncho-pneumonia)	67.3	13.5	17.4	1.8	63 273
injury/poison (e.g. accidents, suicide)	48.3	1.2	21.6	20.0	17 286
other (e.g. digestive, nervous, genito-urinary systems)	75.0	11.2	12.2	1.6	79 244
all causes	65.3	7.7	22.7	4.3	566 992

*Includes residential homes for older people (Data calculated from Office of Population Censuses and Surveys, 1993e, *Mortality Statistics: General. Review of the Registrar-General on Deaths in England and Wales, 1991*, Series DH1, No. 26, HMSO, London, Table 7, pp. 16–21)

the implementation of technical tasks and the performance of medical procedures ... The unit regulations are commonly designed to minimize disruption of staff activities by controlling the family's presence at the bedside, and disclosure of information to the family by members of the staff is more likely than not to be minimal and controlled ... These ... conditions create a depersonalizing situation for many patients. (Benoliel, 1988, p. 174)

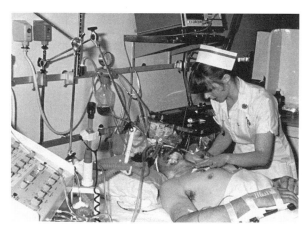

The need for constant vigilance in intensive therapy units makes it difficult to give patients and families any privacy. (© John Watney)

Deaths that take a longer time, but may similarly be expected, are those of patients with certain kinds of cancer. These too, on occasion, may be treated impersonally, with hospital staff on busy wards often finding it hard to spend time understanding dying patients' concerns and, in some cases, actively avoiding contact, or deflecting direct questions. However, not all hospital settings are like this. You should now read David Field's article ' "We didn't want him to die on his own"—nurses' accounts of nursing dying patients'.[b]

☐ What were the nurses' preferences with regard to 'awareness contexts' and what were the consequences of this?

■ Most of the nurses preferred 'open awareness' where all parties, including the patient, knew that the patient was dying. Where this applied, nurses became emotionally involved in patients' care, grieving at their deaths, and sometimes maintaining contact with relatives after a death. Although this created emotional stress for nurses, they saw it as bringing them closer to the ideals of good nursing care, and in caring for the 'whole person'.

[b]In *Health and Disease: A Reader* (second edition, Open University Press, 1995).

□ What characteristics of relations between staff facilitated this form of nursing?

■ Hierarchical distinctions between senior and junior nurses, and between doctors and nurses, were not emphasised (unlike a nearby surgical ward). Relationships between staff involved mutual support, informality, and freedom for nurses to make decisions regarding disclosure.

A variety of forms of death, then, occur in hospital. Although hospitals may be seen by the general public as impersonal settings in which to die, Field's example shows that this need not always be the case.

Hospice care

Hospices arose in reaction to what many saw as the excessive *medicalisation* of dying concerning, in particular, the cancer patient dying in hospital. Thus Cicely Saunders, who in 1967 founded St Christopher's Hospice in London as the first modern hospice, had experiences of the hospital care of dying people which her biographer described in the following terms:

> Medicine was about cure, if they couldn't cure doctors felt they had failed; it was about having answers, they had no answers for the dying. Doctors did not consider it their job to ease the process of dying beyond prescribing pain-killing drugs; as far as possible they avoided dying patients, embarrassed by what they saw as failure. (du Boulay, 1984, pp. 9–10)

Hospices, broadly speaking, have sought to adopt the following approach in reaction to these perceived deficiencies:

1 *Palliative* medical care which emphasises symptom relief, particularly pain control, rather than 'heroic' attempts at cure at the expense of the patient.

2 Since closed awareness and a 'conspiracy of silence' is an abandonment of patients, open awareness of death and counselling is preferred, together with emphasis on informed patient choice regarding treatment.

3 A preference for supported death at home if possible, with hospice beds for respite or crisis care. Domiciliary support from nurses specialising in terminal care is a widespread means of achieving this.

4 Involvement of the patient's family in care, and concern for bereavement. This means that hospices often contain a bereavement counselling service.

5 A weakening of the traditional line of authority from doctor to nurse and other care workers associated with a greater stress on mutual support by staff.

6 Involvement of volunteers and 'the community' in providing care.

This is reminiscent of the characteristics of the hospital ward described by David Field. Field's study reminds us that hospices are not the only setting where this style of care may occur, although it may be more difficult to achieve these conditions in a traditional hospital setting. In the years since 1967, the hospice movement has grown rapidly in the United Kingdom and Ireland, so that by 1993 there were 193 in-patient hospices with 2 993 beds in these countries, along with over 400 'home care' teams (St Christopher's Hospice, 1993). Nevertheless, only a small proportion of people who die receive hospice services. In Seale and Cartwright's (1994) study of a representative sample of deaths in England and Wales in 1987, 2.9 per cent of people died in a hospice, and 6.9 per cent received some form of hospice care in the year before death. Field and James (1993) estimate that about 4 per cent of deaths occur in a hospice.

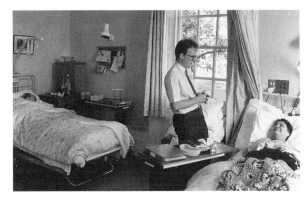

Hospice care seeks to address the physical, emotional and spiritual pains of dying. The Hospice of Our Lady and St John, Willen, Milton Keynes. (Photo: Mike Levers)

Hospices espouse a model of care largely suited to patients with fatal forms of cancer, since an essential condition for the sort of awareness that hospices are premised on is the presence of a disease that is known to be fatal. Some hospices admit people with *motor neurone disease*, a fairly rare terminal illness, and there are facilities for people with AIDS that give hospice-style care, but the mainstream hospice movement remains associated with cancer care. The movement has raised the social status of terminal cancer patients from their previous low status in medical thinking (as revealed in the quote from du Boulay). However, the needs of people dying in other circumstances, such as extreme old age, are not the focus of hospice efforts.

Conclusion

This chapter has sought to convey something of the variation in the experience of people who die in the United Kingdom today. It has emphasised a perspective on dying that recognises that for many people death is an intensification and end-point of the experience of old age— occurring, for the most part, in institutional settings. At the same time, there are significant variations from this dominant pattern, in that some deaths occur to younger people, and at home. The stress that caring for people who die at home can involve, as well as its rewards, have been described.

In the comparison of predicted and unpredicted death, it became clear that this distinction primarily lies in the eye of the beholder. People possess varying degrees of knowledge about their own and others' impending deaths; it is only in very rare circumstances that death occurs in a completely unpredictable way. Indeed, we might say that no death is wholly unpredictable, as we all know that we must die and, at a philosophical or religious level, life itself can be understood as a preparation for death.

The discussion of institutional care revealed some of the strengths as well as the weaknesses of hospital care, with the potential for overcoming the impersonal and routinised care that so many fear from hospitals being illustrated by David Field's account. The example of the hospice movement in relation to the care of terminal cancer patients and their families demonstrates a potential for transforming the experience of dying from cancer, which points to the possibilities for a similar transformation in the experience of death in extreme old age.

OBJECTIVES FOR CHAPTER 12

When you have studied this chapter, you should be able to:

12.1 Describe when and where people die in the United Kingdom in recent years, indicating the relative balance between home and institutional care.

12.2 Describe how variation in the experience of dying involves variation in the sort of care and support people need and receive.

12.3 Assess the advantages and disadvantages of the institutional (particularly hospital) care of people who are dying, relative to other forms of terminal care.

QUESTIONS FOR CHAPTER 12

Question 1 (*Objective 12.1*)

It is estimated (by Seale and Cartwright, 1994) that in 1986 approximately 22 per cent of all occupied NHS-hospital-bed days were devoted to the care of people who would be dead within twelve months.

This compares with an estimate of between 25 and 30 per cent for 1969 (Cartwright, Hockey and Anderson, 1973). Yet more people died in hospital at the later date. What might explain this apparent discrepancy, and what does this mean for the balance between community and institutional care?

Question 2 (*Objective 12.2*)

'Dying' is only experienced by a proportion of people who die. How do these people's needs vary from those of others who die?

Question 3 (*Objective 12.3*)

Field and James (1993) claim that in hospitals:

It is often difficult for doctors to switch from the active management of disease towards a pattern of care in which the concerns and quality of life of the patient become paramount. (p. 12)

How accurate is this statement in relation to the care of people who die, and how does hospice care contrast with this?

13 Society and death

During your study of this chapter you will be asked to read an article by Sally Vincent entitled 'Exits', which appears in the Reader.[1]

The author of this chapter, Clive Seale, is a Lecturer in Medical Sociology at Goldmiths' College, University of London; his principal research interests concern the experience of terminal illness, hospice care, euthanasia and old age.

Introduction

It has become very common, in books and articles about death, dying and bereavement, to read that we live in a society that denies death. Sometimes it is said that death is a taboo subject, in the way that sexuality once was but is presumed to be no longer. Yet writing about death, and discussing dying and grief, has become quite a widespread activity. It may not have quite the same appeal as the contemplation of sex, but there is undoubtedly a steady stream of media representations of these matters. We frequently see violent or sudden death displayed on television screens or in newspaper headlines; there is much media interest—sometimes condemned as

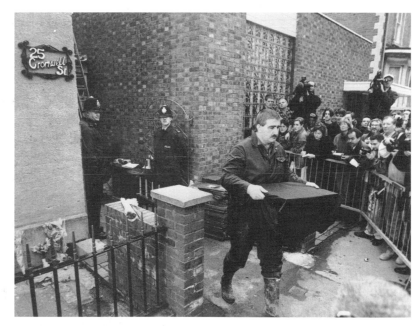

Massed ranks of photographers wait for front-page pictures outside the house of Frederick West in Gloucester in 1994, where police were excavating the bodies of at least nine of the women West was accused of murdering. Here a policeman emerges carrying a box (rumoured to be a tool box) draped in black cloth, obligingly satisfying the media's appetite for images of death. (Photo: Guardian Syndication)

[1]In *Health and Disease: A Reader* (second edition, Open University Press, 1995).

prurient—in the reactions of those who are suddenly bereaved. In the more 'serious' media, there are many accounts of dying and mourning, with a notable interest in accounts of death from AIDS.

In view of this fairly widespread public awareness of death, in what sense can the United Kingdom in the 1990s still be said to be a death-denying society? This chapter begins by outlining the arguments put forward by historians and sociologists to support the **denial of death thesis**. Some more recent social movements (in addition to that of the hospice movement described in the previous chapter) that have emphasised the perception that death is denied are then described, and then some critiques of the denial of death thesis are considered. The chapter then gives an account of bereavement and mourning, focusing particularly on the varying social and emotional value placed on the deaths of people of different ages. The chapter concludes with a discussion of euthanasia.

The approach of this chapter towards death shows that people's experiences of points in the lifespan are influenced by social values that are themselves the product of historical changes. Other people in other societies, or at other times, may not experience dying, bereavement, or indeed childhood, adolescence, middle and old age, in the way that people do in the United Kingdom of the 1990s.

The denial of death thesis

The main components of the denial of death thesis are as follows: that we live in a society where death is hidden away in hospitals and institutions, that we no longer know how to talk about death, or mourn for the dead, and this produces loneliness and abandonment in dying and bereaved people.

A key writer who argues this view is the French historian Philippe Ariès, who contrasts what he calls the 'tamed' death of early medieval times with today's 'forbidden' death (Ariès, 1976, 1981). In earlier times, he claims, individuals were familiar with death, in the sense that they knew and tended for people who died, saw their deaths happen, and experienced less fear and feelings of loss when individuals died (Figure 13.1). Medical science, however, increasingly gave people the hope that nature, and therefore illness, could be controlled. Gradually the doctor rather than the priest came to be seen as interceding on behalf of the dying person to resist the onslaught of death.

In his account of 'forbidden' death, which he sees as characterising modern society, Ariès sees the logical conclusion of this reliance on doctors. Because, ultimately, medicine cannot save us, death is segregated, removed from social life in institutions in an attempt to banish what

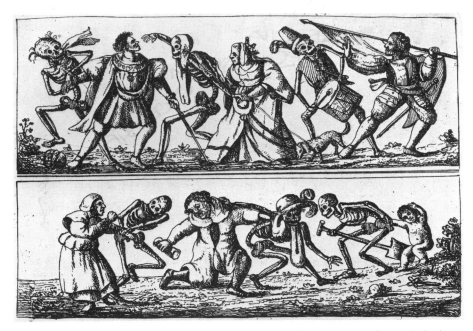

Figure 13.1 *A medieval 'dance of death', in which skeletal images of death are seen mingling with the living. In early medieval times death was seen as a part of life. (Source: Mary Evans Picture Library)*

is beyond control. In avoiding open discussion of death with those who are dying, and often placing dying patients in a side-room off the main ward, hospital staff contribute to this segregation. Funeral rituals are increasingly taken over by professionals and lack personal content. Through these means death is made hygienic, and nature is held at bay.

The sociologist Norbert Elias has expanded on this theme in his book, *The Loneliness of the Dying*, written in his own old age:

> Closely bound up, in our day, with the greatest possible exclusion of death and dying from social life, and with the screening-off of dying people from others ... is a peculiar embarrassment felt by the living in the presence of dying people. They often do not know what to say ... Feelings of embarrassment hold words back. For the dying this can be a bitter experience. (p. 23) ... It is not always easy to show to people on their way to death that they have not lost their meaning for other people ... If this happens, if a person must feel while dying that, though still alive, he or she has scarcely any significance for other people, that person is truly alone. (Elias, 1985, p. 64)

Loneliness and isolation, but in this case of the bereaved, is also the theme of a third writer important in the development of the denial of death thesis. The anthropologist Geoffrey Gorer's influential book, *Death, Grief and Mourning in Contemporary Britain* (Gorer, 1965), is based on a survey of bereaved people. He describes the relative absence of mourning rituals, contrasting this with mourning in Victorian times and the early twentieth century. Locating a primary cause of this in the decline of religious belief, he argues that the occurrence of a death, from being widely noted in the earlier period, was now much more difficult for mourners to display to others. He gives an example of this contrast in the case of his own mother, after his father died in 1915, compared with his own experience after the death of his brother:

> ... [My mother] followed scrupulously the modification of her outdoor costume, the shortening and abandoning of the veil, the addition of a touch of white at proper calendrical moments. It would have been unthinkable at that date for a respectable woman to do otherwise. In early 1917, when she could otherwise have worn some colour, her father died at a ripe old age and she had to return to black for a further six months. (Gorer, 1965, p. 5)

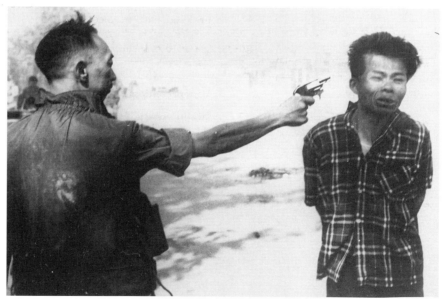

This photograph of Brigadier General Nguyen Ngoc Loan executing a Viet Cong officer in Saigon during the Vietnamese War in 1968 received such widespread publicity that it has become one of the most famous images of the late twentieth century. Is this evidence for a 'pornography of death'? (Associated Press Photo)

[After my brother died] a couple of times I refused invitations to cocktail parties, explaining that I was in mourning; the people who invited me responded to this statement with shocked embarrassment, as if I had voiced some appalling obscenity ... educated and sophisticated as they were, [they] mumbled and hurried away. They clearly no longer had any guidance from ritual as to the way to treat a self-confessed mourner; and, I suspect, they were frightened lest I give way to my grief, and involve them in a dreadful upsurge of emotion. (Gorer, 1965, p. 14)

In addition, he claimed in an earlier article (Gorer, 1955) that because of the widespread denial of death in society there is a 'pornography of death' in which people are fascinated by, for example, media representations of violent death. This, Gorer claims, satisfies repressed urges in a manner similar to sexual pornography.

Criticisms of the denial of death thesis

It can be argued that denial that we will die, or at least the constant repression of this knowledge from our day-to-day thoughts, is a necessary condition for continuing in life. To orientate ourselves mentally towards life means that we must constantly turn away from death. Failure to do this is represented by suicide, which threatens the firmness with which we press down our thoughts of mortality. Writers such as Ariès, Elias and Gorer are arguing that this repression is also evident at a societal level. However, there are a number of criticisms that can be made of the denial of death thesis.

Variation and change

The first problem is that these writers tend to describe a society which is rather static, without much potential for variation or change. Variation in views and practices are evident when ethnic and religious groups in the United Kingdom are considered. Thus, a Gujarati woman describes the importance of being present near the time of death:

Nurses should let the family be present when the soul leaves, because if the person dies without the family there, then that person will not be thinking of God, but of his family who weren't there. Not only would the family be affected, but the dying person, who would have to take rebirth. The family couldn't take part in any social occasions or anything because it would always be hanging over them that they hadn't been present at the death ... the person's whole extended family would be affected, uncles, aunts, distant cousins. (Quoted in Firth, 1993, p. 30)

Far from being uninvolved, then, such a family is closely in touch with the experience of the dying family member. Similar examples could have been chosen from the Sikh, Muslim or Jewish communities. Religious belief, in particular, can provide the believer with a way of talking with others about his or her experience of dying or of bereavement. Emotional support is provided by participation in religious ritual, or in just the physical presence of others when extreme moments in the experience of dying and grief are anticipated, experienced or remembered.

That society is capable of change is shown by the rise of the hospice movement, which was described in Chapter 12, which emphasises the importance of open communication about death and effective palliative care. Although both Ariès and Elias mention the efforts of those involved with hospices and the work of Kübler-Ross, neither pay much attention to these developments, or to the multi cultural nature of the population of the United Kingdom.

Misrepresentation of professional care

Misrepresentation of what actually happens in the care and attention received by dying and bereaved people is the substance of the second main criticism of the denial of death thesis. Apart from the contribution of hospices, which contradicts the view that people are unwilling to become emotionally close to those who are dying, is it really true that hospital care is universally cold, unfeeling and impersonal? You saw in the Reader article associated with Chapter 12 that David Field's account of hospital

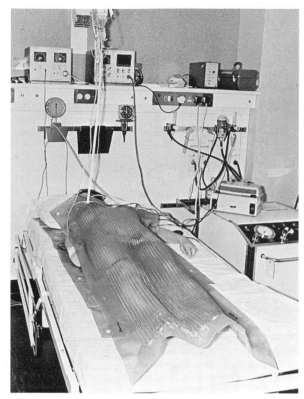

An image of death alone in a modern hospital: but is it really true that hospital care of dying people is unfeeling and impersonal? (Source: Blackwell Biovisual (Videotec Ltd))

care on one ward contrasted strongly with such a negative image. How widespread is this? It is difficult to find conclusive evidence, but Table 13.1 presents some ratings given of the quality of care in hospitals and other settings by relatives, friends and others of people who had died in Seale and Cartwright's (1994) study described in Chapter 12.

☐ What does Table 13.1 show about ratings of the quality of care generally, and of hospital care in particular?

■ The majority of respondents felt that the care of the person who died was excellent, good or kind and

understanding from all sources, with only a minority feeling critical. There are no marked differences between ratings of hospital staff compared with care received from GPs or community nurses; care from nurses is rated more highly than that from doctors.

The table suggests that caution is appropriate before adopting the generalisation that all hospital care towards those who die and who are bereaved is impersonal.

☐ What objection might be raised to the argument that the increasing proportion of deaths in institutions (as shown in the previous chapter, in Table 12.1) gives support to the denial of death thesis?

■ It remains the case that the majority of care for those who die in institutions occurs at home, and is given by the family and sometimes the friends of the person who dies.

Official surveillance of death

A third criticism of the denial of death thesis is that there is a sense in which modern society makes death *more* visible than in the past. The public, official realm of death certification and registration, and the presentation of mortality statistics in official documents and reports, has been described by the sociologist Lindsey Prior as the means by which 'death in the modern world is made visible' (Prior, 1989, p. 1). He contrasts this public face of death with the private realm of care, sentiments and funeral rituals with which the denial of death thesis is concerned. In the early medieval period of Ariès' 'tamed death', such official surveillance of population mortality did not exist; it is very much a product of modern conditions.

Intimately connected with governmental surveillance of the population is the perspective of medical science. Where once the presence of a priest to give last rites was considered essential, now it is a legal requirement that all deaths must be certified by a qualified medical practitioner. In completing a death certificate, the doctor plays both a medical and a legal role.

Sometimes the contrast between the medical view and those of other parties raises political issues. Here are

Table 13.1 Ratings by relatives and friends of quality of care given to a dying person in the year before death, Great Britain, 1987

Relatives/friends responding	Overall ratings of quality of care from:			
	General practitioners %	Hospital doctors %	Hospital nurses %	Community nurses %
excellent	44	43	58	51
good	36	44	30	35
fair	14	10	8	11
poor	8	4	3	2
total[*] (=100%)	(525)	(501)	(516)	(285)

Rating of how staff at hospital treated respondent at time of death[†]	%
very kind and understanding	87
fairly kind and understanding	11
not very kind and understanding	2
total[†] (=100%)	(306)

[*]Totals refer to number of people who died in the care of general practitioners, and number of care episodes for others. A care episode is defined as a series of admissions to a single hospital, or a series of visits to the home by a particular type of community nurse. Thus an individual could have been admitted to more than one hospital, or had more than one type of nurse visiting the home (e.g. district nurse and specialist cancer care nurse). [†]Includes only respondents reporting for people who died in hospitals. (Data from C. Seale, 1995, not previously published)

two accounts of a death which occurred in Northern Ireland, before and then after relatives of the deceased had brought a successful legal action to change the official record of the cause:

> *Cause of death:* Bruising and Oedema of Brain associated with Fractures of the Skull.

> Died as a result of injuries received after having been struck by a plastic bullet, and we believe her to have been an innocent victim. (Prior, 1989, p. 65)

Legally, a purpose of death certification is to identify causes of 'unnatural death', and the activities of pathologists and coroners become important here. If a doctor has not attended a person who dies within 14 days prior to the death (28 days in Northern Ireland), the death is referred to a coroner who may require a post-mortem. These procedures are designed to guard against the possibility of murder remaining undetected, and to monitor deaths by suicide, or occurring as the result of medical or other forms of accident.

The investigation of the health of populations by analysis of data derived from death certificates is made possible as a by-product of this detailed surveillance and recording of individual causes of death.[2] This represents another combination of the concerns of government with those of medical science, in this case under the umbrella of 'public health'.

The revival of death awareness

A fourth point that can be made about the denial of death thesis is that the appearance of books and articles saying

[2]Extensive use is made of epidemiological data based on mortality records in *World Health and Disease*.

ISLE COLLEGE
RESOURCES CENTRE

that we live in a death-denying society is itself a sign of movement in social attitudes towards death. A bibliography of writings in the English language on death listed over 650 books on the subject in 1979; by 1987 a further 1 700 books were added (Simpson, 1987, quoted by Walter, 1993). It is no coincidence that this upsurge of interest on the part of writers has coincided with the growth of the hospice movement both in the United Kingdom and the USA (described in Chapter 12).

At the same time there has been a growth of counselling and communication expertise in relation to dying people and those who are bereaved. Elisabeth Kübler-Ross's work (see Chapter 12) epitomises this in relation to people who are terminally ill; the psychology of grief and the counselling of the bereaved will be described later in this chapter.

These various developments—the upsurge of writing about death, the growth of the hospice movement and counselling expertise in relation to dying and bereaved people—have been described by Tony Walter, a sociologist, as part of a *revivalist* movement (Walter, 1994). Walter has contrasted this with two previous sets of attitudes towards death, which he calls the *traditional* and the *modern*. A scheme for understanding this is given in Table 13.2.

With this scheme, it is possible to understand those who argue that we live in a death-defying society as being critical of the 'modern' treatment of death. The 'revivalists' tend to share certain common themes: not to abandon dying and grieving people, to seek to accompany them on their journey in dying or grief, to relieve and learn from their suffering, to mistrust the modern medical and bureaucratised expertise that has produced the alienating hospital, medicalised death, and professionalised funerals.

□ Why does Walter call the third set of attitudes 'revivalist'?

■ Because to some extent they are (or believe they are) reviving traditions of the past: emphasising the private and personal meaning of death, and the importance of family and community values.

Revivalist ideas, however, are in some respects different from those of the past. Although many in the hospice movement are religious, and spiritual awareness is spoken of in revivalist literature, the person preparing for death in the revivalist paradigm is not so much making peace with God, but with Self. Thus Kübler-Ross entitled one of her books *Death: The Final Stage of Growth* (Kübler-Ross, 1975) in a reference to psychological development at this time of life.

Much revivalism has been associated with changes in the attitudes and practices of professional health-care workers, such as doctors and nurses. Although the hospice movement began with a message that was explicitly opposed to the values and practices of mainstream health care, it has now become firmly established as a new medical and nursing specialty within the National Health Service, albeit with some funding from charitable sources. Psychotherapy and counselling have similarly attained the status of recognition as an integral part of modern health-care practice.

Discussion of death and dying is undoubtedly more open in modern society than is suggested by the denial of death thesis. Perhaps it is accurate to say that discussion is conducted in a context of *expertise*, outside of which there is a fairly widespread lack of involvement with death. Death experts may claim that their skill lies in helping others to discover their own truths, through

Table 13.2 Walter's three forms of death

	Traditional	Modern	Revivalist
death is:	passage of soul	end of body	psychological process
social context:	community	public/private split	public and private invade each other
source of knowledge:	tradition/religion	medicine	self
meaning:	given/communal	abolished	interpersonal, private meaning celebrated
institution:	church	hospital	hospice/counselling
the good death is:	conscious, ready to meet Maker	unconscious, sudden, painless	aware, finish business, painless

(Adapted from Walter, T., 1994, *The Revival of Death*, Routledge, London.)

adopting a listening attitude, but it seems that these truths will often not emerge unaided. In a sense, we do live in a society that denies and hides death away in certain places, but these places are no longer represented solely by an alienating, medicalised hospital. Hospices, humanised hospital wards, bereavement self-help groups, academic courses such as the one you are reading now, are all institutional settings for the modern discussion of death. In less formal settings, as where the nurse visits the home, or where the dying or grieving person who describes his or her experience in the language of popular psychology that is nowadays so readily available to all of us, we may also see traces of revivalist expertise.

More broadly, psychological expertise in a modern society such as that of the United Kingdom also shapes our experience of the other points of the life span discussed in this book. Our understanding of childhood and adolescence is informed by a host of child development and parenting manuals; we are offered continual advice on the management of our sexual lives by professional and media experts; occupational psychology proposes a variety of models of worker motivation for the enlightenment of management teams, and discussion of therapies for the mid-life crisis and the challenges of retirement are the stuff of popular magazines.[3] Dying is just another area for colonisation by expertise; bereavement is, of course, another.

Bereavement and mourning

With the decline of elaborate, formalised mourning rituals in many parts of modern society, a counselling approach to bereavement can be experienced as particularly helpful. Bereavement support groups can provide a setting in which people who have lost someone close to them have that loss recognised by others, and in which their loss can be understood by comparing experiences. Here is one woman's account:

> My close friends and family were absolutely wonderful when Ernest died. But other people I knew well would cross the road if they saw me coming, and if they did have to speak and ask me how I was, I learned to my cost that I mustn't really tell. They wanted me to say just, 'I'm fine' … The most helpful thing people can do is listen, just let you talk and be compassionate.

[3] The growing influence of psychological expertise in all areas of personal life during the twentieth century is discussed in Rose, 1989.

People think it will hurt you to talk, but talking keeps the person alive for you. Or they fear they will be reminding you—as if you had forgotten.

> It is an absolute safety valve to be allowed to talk, which is why I joined CRUSE, the support group for widows and widowers. There people can cry because everyone understands, but you'll hear gales of laughter too. (Jean Baker, quoted in Albery et al., 1993, p. 191)

In an attempt to understand the psychology of grieving, a number of theorists have proposed *models* of the grieving process, suggesting, for example, that in grieving people are likely to pass through certain stages. Such *stage theories* are quite similar to the stage theory proposed by Elisabeth Kübler-Ross (see Chapter 12) to help understand the reaction to learning that one has a terminal illness. One influential model has been proposed by Worden (1983) and is outlined below. Worden saw grieving as a sequence of four stages, described in terms of *tasks* that mourners work through.

> **Stage 1** *To accept the reality of the loss*
> People who have not done this may, for example, forget that the person is not there and lay the table for them, or hear their voice.
>
> **Stage 2** *To experience the pain of grief*
> This involves anguished feelings and sometimes anger at people who had cared for the person who died, or guilt about things done or not done.
>
> **Stage 3** *To adjust to an environment in which the deceased is missing*
> This task can involve anxiety about coping alone, and a struggle against loss of confidence.
>
> **Stage 4** *To withdraw emotional energy from the lost one and reinvest it in other relationships*
> Letting go of the lost person and ceasing to be obsessed with their memory is dominant.
>
> (Adapted from Worden, 1983)

Associated with such models has been the idea that some people experience *pathological grief*, where the mourner fails to work through a stage, becoming psychologically 'stuck'. Consider the following description, written by her psychotherapist, of a woman called Sarah whose 10-year-old son died when he was hit by a lorry coming home from school:

> … her grief was intense and compounded by a terrible resignation—fatalism—about the loss

... she sank into a deeper and deeper depression, slowly losing touch with rational values until it became clear that she was somehow taking upon herself the blame for all the ills in the world; every war, famine and disaster was somehow linked to her, appropriated by her as part of the tragedy that was her life ... therapy eventually reached feelings of intense pain and guilt at the death of her mother some years previously ... [for which] she had always felt to blame ... It was not until some of these feelings were to be unravelled that Sarah managed to reveal the additional burden of guilt she was carrying—that she had caused her son's death also, by her insistence that he should always hurry home from school each day ... In blaming herself she had hidden from herself the immense personal power that she assumed in 'being able' to bring about the death of both her mother and her son; but this power had started to show itself in her assumption of responsibility for all other ills in the world. (Ridley, 1993, p. 265)

☐ Which of Worden's stages is Sarah 'stuck' at (at least in her psychotherapist's view)?

■ She is struggling with the tasks of the second stage, allowing her self-blame to become the dominant feature of her life.

The identification of pathology, in terms of deviation from what is considered normal, is an important part of the modern medical definition of disease.[4] In assessing Sarah in terms of Worden's stages the model is taken to be a description of normality, in a manner similar to that of the pathologist who compares the appearance of diseased organs with what is known of the appearance of healthy ones. The obligation to conform to stages of 'healthy' grieving is not always accepted, however, and a common criticism of such models is heard from those who interpret the exhortation to reinvest in other relationships as a requirement to forget about people they have loved.

Another criticism of psychological stage theories is that they are culture-bound, not recognising that grief may take different forms in people who adhere to beliefs and practices alien to those of the psychologist. Here is an example of a Christian Scientist who was interviewed some six months after her 89-year-old mother had died:

We don't believe in death—it may appear one dies but you go on to find out that life is eternal. What we understand is that materiality is a dream that man has conjured up for himself. [There are] a lot of beliefs to overcome when you get old. We work on the basis of man's perfection. But medical practitioners are working on the idea of things being wrong. We're spiritual—they're physical ... [I] take for granted that we rejoice over what [a dead person has] done in their time. I have no feelings of needing comfort—I've got that in the books we study ... [My feelings] definitely wouldn't have been the same if I hadn't had that [Christian Science] to fall on.[5]

Such powerfully held beliefs about the nature of death are unusual in a society where religion now competes with a variety of other systems of knowledge, but they were once more current in the United Kingdom, and are widely adhered to in some other cultures, many of which are present in various ethnic groups in the United Kingdom. In Worden's terms, this woman might be understood as being stuck in the first stage, unable to accept the reality of the death, but this interpretation can only be applied if the validity of her religious beliefs is denied. One then begins to enter the dangerous territory of defining religious belief itself as a sign of pathology.

The social distribution of grief

Another danger with psychological accounts of grief is that they may lead us to believe that everyone is grieved for, or indeed that grief is usually felt when someone close dies. First, there are reasons to believe that the expression of grief—and perhaps the subjective experience of grief—is determined by social custom as well as purely psychological factors. In 1899, *The Lady* magazine offered advice to its readers on the proper length of time for wearing mourning clothes, suggesting that a woman should mourn the death of her child for three months, but that of a grand-parent for nine months (reported in

[4]The medical view of disease is discussed extensively in *Medical Knowledge: Doubt and Certainty* (second edition, Open University Press, 1994).

[5]Previously unpublished account collected during the fieldwork for the survey reported by Seale and Cartwright (1994).

Morley, 1971). If mourning clothes were worn now, there is no doubt that these timescales would be reversed, as the loss of children is nowadays grieved for more intensely than the loss of many older people.

◻ Why might this be so?

◼ Infant mortality was higher in 1899, so most families could expect to experience the death of a child. Familiarity may have bred fortitude, if not lessened sensitivity, to the loss. Additionally, the veneration of one's forebears and of older people in general was greater then that it has become in the 1990s (as Chapter 10 revealed).

Second, it is the case that not everyone who dies has someone close to them, in the sense that they see them regularly and have an emotional presence in their lives. As was shown in Chapter 2, more elderly people live alone or in institutions than in previous times. Social and emotional isolation is a problem for a proportion of older people while alive, and is reflected in there being no one left to miss them when they are dead.

Third, closeness, where it occurs, can sometimes breed resentment and irritation, leaving only feelings of relief when a person dies, although the expression of such feelings is, on the whole, socially unacceptable.

Euthanasia

Some aspects of the debate about the legalisation of voluntary euthanasia reflect conflicting feelings of relief and loss, and the guilt that this can bring. Sally Vincent, a journalist, wrote an article about euthanasia, entitled 'Exits'; it is in the Reader[6] and you should read it now.

◻ What situations does she describe where voluntary euthanasia might be desirable?

◼ The case of Mrs Boyes, who was experiencing intolerable pain before her doctor administered an injection that may have ended her life, and Anthony Bland, who lay in a persistent vegetative state until his parents gave their permission for doctors to cease life-sustaining treatment.

◻ What arguments against euthanasia does she make?

◼ In a society where there are increasing numbers of dependent older people, there may be a temptation to opt for euthanasia out of a concern to save resources.

[6]*Health and Disease: A Reader* (second edition, Open University Press, 1995).

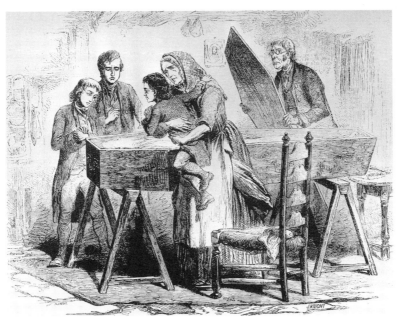

Children viewing their father's corpse in a nineteenth-century illustration: does this suggest a more open acceptance of death and bereavement as a part of life than we have today? (Source: Mary Evans Picture Library)

Evidence exists (Ogg and Bennett, 1992) to suggest that a proportion of elderly people are subjected to physical and financial abuse by their relatives. In addition, older people—particularly older women—are less likely to have spouses close to them who place particular value on the continuation of their lives (Seale and Addington-Hall, 1995). Grief and loss are intimately bound up with the social value placed on people's lives, with each influencing the other. The House of Lords Select Committee on Medical Ethics, referred to by Vincent, concluded in 1994 that if medically-assisted euthanasia were legalised it would prove very difficult to guard against undue pressure on older people to opt for death when they felt they were a burden on those around them.

Conclusion

This chapter has considered evidence for and against the argument that we live in a 'death-denying' society. Clearly, there is a sense in which this is true. Dying people, and dead bodies, are physically more hidden away than they once were; the increasing association of death with old age may also have enabled younger people to avoid thinking about dying. With the decline in organised religion, mourning ritual has atrophied. Yet it has been shown that the generalisations contained in the denial of death thesis hide a more complex reality. Those who propose that death is denied are themselves part of a revivalist social movement, and may have presented a somewhat distorted picture. This movement has involved hospices, counsellors and others who have advocated an opening up of awareness about death and bereavement, albeit one that is often achieved under the enabling gaze of the psychologically-informed, professional health worker.

The final part of the chapter has returned to a theme introduced in Chapter 12, that death can be understood, for the most part, as an end point in the experience of ageing. The extent to which older people are missed when they die was discussed in the context of psychological theories of grief. This, and the decline in the social power of older people, was then related to the issue of euthanasia, which represents one solution—albeit a controversial one—to the suffering and loss of control that many people are so afraid will happen when they die.

OBJECTIVES FOR CHAPTER 13

When you have studied this chapter, you should be able to:

13.1 Give a critical account of the denial of death thesis.

13.2 Identify the themes of those advocating a revival of death awareness.

13.3 Distinguish psychological from social aspects of grief.

QUESTIONS FOR CHAPTER 13

Question 1 (*Objectives 13.1 and 13.2*)

> We live in a society in which dying is not part of the business of living … we find that there are … barriers between Us, the bystanders, and Them, our friends who are facing death. I think it is very important to recognise that many of those barriers were not created by us individually, and they are not our fault. Once you realise that you are struggling to overcome a block that society has put in your way, it gets a little easier to step around it. (Buckman, 1988, pp. xiv, xviii)

This comes from the introduction of a book for people wanting to help and support a dying person. Similar statements might have been taken from any one of a number of books about death that have appeared over the past 20 years. Why have such statements become so common?

Question 2 (*Objective 13.3*)

> For most parents the possibility of the death of a child is the most terrifying loss they can imagine. The pain that parents suffer is almost impossible to describe. When a parent says something like, 'I wish I could change places and die in place of my child', there's no doubt in my mind that he or she means it … Children are not *meant* to die before their parents … (Buckman, 1988, p. 136)

Why is such an expression of grief more typical of the present day than of the past?

14 Health in transition

The life course revisited

Now that you have studied some of the major health issues affecting people of all ages living in the United Kingdom in the 1990s, we can look back on the life course as a whole and emphasise, on the one hand, its integrity and continuity, and on the other, its variability and shifting character. This chapter aims first to illustrate some of the ways in which the traditional 'stages of life' are becoming less sharply defined, and second to stress the value of longitudinal research which seeks to illuminate the shifting patterns of health and disease as the life course unfolds.

In the preceding chapters, with their diverse authorship and focus, we have inevitably tended to present the life course as a series of apparently discrete stages, corresponding to what sociologists call **age grades**: infancy, childhood, adolescence, adulthood, middle age and old age. In reality, as we all know from personal experience, the life course is not as neatly 'packaged' as these widely-recognised divisions imply. The definition of these age grades changes over time, and varies from one place to another; different ethnic groups within the same community may view the progression of the life course in different ways; and individuals who share all the standard demographic variables can nonetheless display sharply differing personal interpretations of what (say) being a teenager or a pensioner means to them.

It could be argued that chronological age is becoming less reliable as a measure of a person's 'position' in the trajectory from birth to old age. Part of the explanation for this trend may be because relatively few **rites of passage** survive in modern Western culture—rituals symbolising a transition from one stage of life to another have all but disappeared in secular society. Those that remain in the United Kingdom are to be found primarily within religious ceremonies such as first Catholic Communion and the Jewish Bar-Mitzvah, and lie outside the experience of most of the non-religious population. The majority are left with small private symbols: the first day at school, the first bra, the first shave, the gold watch at retirement. Even the twenty-first birthday party has been 'upstaged' as the entry to adulthood by the reduction of legal voting age to 18. The only large-scale public rite of passage left to most people is to get married for the first time, which—regardless of whether it is celebrated with a civil or a religious wedding ceremony—is still the most powerful symbolic confirmation of entry into adult status.

However, the symbolic significance of marriage as the key 'life course transition' to adulthood may be in decline. Marriage is legally sanctioned only for heterosexual couples, so a significant minority of the population have never been able to marry even if they wished to do so, but a growing proportion of heterosexual couples prefer to cohabit without marrying (as Chapter 2 described). Young people with jobs are increasingly delaying marriage until their late 20s and early 30s—often several years after they have established themselves as adult wage-earners, financially independent of their family of origin. At the same time, the start of adulthood may be delayed for the less fortunate who cannot afford to leave home, let alone marry, as jobs for school leavers become more scarce and a growing proportion of young people remain dependent on their parents until well into their twenties.

As a consequence of these and other changes in modern culture and social relationships, the traditional stages of the life course are becoming more blurred at the edges. For example, the span of what we call 'childhood' may decrease if pressure to change the law on juvenile crime results in the assumption of innocence—and with it protection from prosecution—being set at a younger age. As the proportion of people over 65 rises in the population, we may redefine what we consider to be 'old' as more and more of us find the label attached to ourselves.

Retirement may perhaps come to symbolise the arrival at a cross-roads, where some are released from routine labour into decades of leisure and independence, while others have dependency and poverty suddenly imposed upon them. A feature of the United Kingdom in the 1980s and 1990s is that divisions in society have grown wider between those with access to the material resources considered adequate by the majority of the population, and those without this basic living standard.[1]

So it must be acknowledged that the threads contributing to the 'life course' as a general concept, as well as an individual experience, are woven into a more complex tapestry than a superficial reading of the previous chapters in this book might imply. But despite the complexity of real lives, played out over 70 or 80 years, there is considerable value in attempting to investigate the progression from birth to old age. A study of the life course as it unfolds enables us to draw tentative conclusions about the *cumulative* impact on health of events and circumstances, and hence to make limited predictions about the future. Longitudinal research is of particular importance in enriching our knowledge of the antecedents of human health and disease and may enable us to devise better strategies for improving health, or preventing disease, in the remaining portion of our lives. The results may even help us to influence the health of future generations.

It is a commonplace observation that health fluctuates over the course of a lifetime, and that circumstances or events at one point in the lifespan can have health consequences years later. But, even in the 1990s, we have accumulated surprisingly little research data illuminating how past experiences influence present and future health. As you will see in the rest of this chapter, there has been a marked variation in the extent to which different disciplines with an interest in human health and disease have come to recognise the importance of studying the life course as an integrated whole.

Studying the life course

Early influences on psychological development

A man who has been the indisputable favourite of his mother keeps for life the feeling of a conqueror, that confidence of his success that often induces real success. (Sigmund Freud, quoted in Jones, 1984, p. 13)

They fuck you up, your mum and dad,
They may not mean to, but they do.
They fill you with the faults they had
And add some extra, just for you.
(Philip Larkin, lines 1–4 of 'This be the verse', in *High Windows*, 1974)

Larkin's poem demonstrates the strength of belief in the psychodynamic power of parent–child relationships, which has pervaded modern Western culture since Freud made his remark at the beginning of the twentieth century. Few would nowadays dispute the assertion that the quality and character of parenting has a lifelong effect on the child as it grows and develops into an adult. This view is so widespread as to be uncontroversial at the level of social discourse, and is a cornerstone of the disciplines of developmental psychology, psychoanalysis and psychotherapy. However, there has been relatively little systematic investigation of precisely which features of parental behaviour or attitudes towards child-rearing might have an affect on a child's physical or mental health, or of what the outcomes of 'good' or 'bad' parenting might be in later life. In earlier chapters of this book, we referred to examples of research studies that have attempted to shed light on these questions.

❑ Can you describe three of them briefly?

■ In Chapter 3, we referred to research by developmental psychologist Lynne Murray (who also appeared in a television programme associated with this book).[2] She found that babies whose mothers suffered from a prolonged period of clinical postnatal depression showed disruptions in intellectual and psychological development when they were toddlers; this adverse effect on the infants could be alleviated if the mothers were given short-term counselling early enough in their illness (Murray, 1992, 1993).

In Chapter 4, you learnt about research by Naomi Richman and her colleagues which showed that adverse factors in a family, such as a marriage with low mutual support, were associated with behaviour problems in the children; these problems did not disappear if stresses within the family were

---

[1]Relative poverty and its relationship with inequalities in health are discussed in *World Health and Disease*, Chapter 10, and *Dilemmas in Health Care*, Chapter 11.

[2]'First steps to autonomy' was made for Open University students studying this book as part of an undergraduate course.

subsequently reduced (Richman, Stevenson and Graham, 1982).

In Chapter 6, the review by Martin and Moira Plant (1992) of risk-taking among adolescents, pointed to convincing evidence from a number of studies that teenagers who become dependent on alcohol tend to come from homes where at least one parent is also a heavy drinker.

All of these studies focus on potentially-damaging aspects of the psychodynamic relationship between parent and child. This focus on pathology is common to authorities on child development from Freud to the present day, and dominates modern research agendas. Far less research has been conducted on the protective or health-promoting features of successful parenting—despite the mountain of self-help books for parents on the subject from theorists such as Dr Spock.

However, although infants' health is profoundly affected by the quality of care provided by their primary caregivers, even during the first months of life the influence of the infants themselves on the care they receive can be glimpsed. For example, recent research by Lynne Murray (1993b) suggests that the temperament of even very young babies affects how their caregivers behave towards them: infants with poor motor coordination who are also 'irritable' (i.e. easy to arouse, but hard to calm) may be found difficult to relate to by their mothers. This may precipitate an episode of post-natal depression in mothers who are already at risk, if there is additional stress on the mother–child relationship as a result of socio-economic factors such as poor housing, low income, etc. This example shows how the determination of infant health is a 'transactional' process (as Chapter 4 concluded), in which both the infant and environmental factors act together to affect its long-term psychological development. Parenting is of prime importance but cannot be seen as the sole determinant of later psychological function.

One aspect of the psychological consequences of different styles of parenting that has attracted more attention than most concerns differences in parental attitudes and behaviours towards male and female children. In Chapter 5, we discussed the idea that parents may be more likely to encourage or condone assertive or aggressive behaviour among boys than they would tolerate from girls, and that this in turn might contribute to the greater confidence that boys show in taking risks during play. For example, parents have been shown to allow their sons to cross roads and to cycle on main roads at an earlier age

than their daughters (Hillman, *et al.,*1990). The effect of attitudes such as this on gender differences in psychological development may partly underlie the higher accident rates suffered by males at all ages from one year into their 30s; it *may* also influence risk-taking behaviours from reckless driving to drug abuse, as Chapter 6 suggests—but we cannot say for sure without systematic research on the matter.

By comparison with the disciplines of psychoanalysis and psychology, which have their roots in the last decades of the nineteenth century, epidemiologists and social scientists with an interest in human health were relative late-comers to the view that the long-term effects of events and circumstances in youth were important antecedents of disease in later life.

Epidemiological analysis of the life course

The massive social and political changes that took place in the United Kingdom in the wake of World War II have been discussed elsewhere in this series.[3] The 1940s saw major reforms in education, housing, wages and the conditions of work, and in the welfare state, including the setting up of the first National Health Service in 1948. It was recognised by policy makers of the time that the effects of these profound shifts in the relationship between the state and its citizens had to be monitored and evaluated, particularly so in terms of health outcomes and the potential use of the new health services. One of the methods chosen was an ambitious study of maternity services, home help during pregnancy and after childbirth, and the costs of childbirth, which involved interviewing 13 687 women who gave birth in England, Scotland or Wales in the week of 3–9 March 1946. This represented 91 per cent of the women who gave birth in this period.

As the years passed, the babies born to these women became one of the most intensively researched **birth cohorts** in the Western world: by the start of the 1990s, almost 200 publications had appeared about them. The survivors are now in their late 40s and have been tracked through more than half their predicted lifespans; they will continue to provide a rich source of data on the cumulative effects of events and circumstances on health and well-being, disease, disability and death across the whole of their life course. Many of them have had children of their own, so the study has entered its second generation

[3]See *Caring for Health: History and Diversity* (second edition, 1993), Chapter 6.

and comparisons are increasingly being made between the health of the original cohort in childhood and that of their offspring. The key findings have been summarised by Mike Wadsworth, a leading member of the team presently investigating the 1946 cohort and their children, in his book *The Imprint of Time: Childhood, History and Adult Life* (1991).

More than a decade after the first national cohort was recruited, a second longitudinal study of a birth cohort began: the Perinatal Mortality Survey obtained information on almost all of the 17 000 babies born between 3 and 9 March 1958. This subsequently became the National Child Development Study, which gathered data on these babies when they reached the ages of 7, 11 and 16 years. In 1991, Chris Power and her colleagues Orly Manor and John Fox, published their analysis of social inequalities and health in this cohort at the age of 23 (in 1981), and a follow-up is under way on data collected when they were 33.

Several other important longitudinal studies of representative samples of the adult population have also been undertaken, two of which were mentioned earlier in this book. In 1984–5, a random sample of 9 003 adults aged over 18 and living in Britain were recruited into the 'Health and Lifestyles' survey, and 5 352 of them were traced for a follow-up study seven years later (see Cox, *et al.,*1987; Blaxter, 1990; and Cox, Huppert and Whichelow, 1993). A rather different method was chosen for the 'West of Scotland Twenty-07 Study: Health in the Community', which began in 1987–8 by contacting three **age cohorts**, each of about 1 000 individuals, who were then aged 15, 35 or 55 years, living in the Central Clydesdale area in and around Glasgow (see the *Annual Reports* from the MRC (Medical Research Council) Medical Sociology Unit at the University of Glasgow for a comprehensive list of publications). The intention is that these age cohorts will be studied throughout their lives.

The value of comparing age cohorts has been eloquently expressed by a leading exponent of the method, Mike Wadsworth.

> Just as a core sample of glacial ice or pond mud can show layers of matter deposited at earlier times, when climate and foliage were not as they are today, so an age slice through the population reveals the differences in impacts of influences from earlier times, in the same way that layers of earlier influences accumulate and interact in the individual. (Wadsworth, 1991, p. 203)

Although there are some differences in the aims of these (and other) longitudinal studies, all of them point to one

over-riding conclusion: social and material disadvantage has a profound *cumulative* effect on individuals from birth to old age, which leads to a widening 'health gap'— particularly after middle age—between people at the top of the social hierarchy and people at the bottom. The gap is apparent at birth and during childhood, but seems to narrow somewhat during adolescence, before widening again. The results confirm the social-class gradients in mortality and morbidity which have been apparent from the far more numerous cross-sectional studies of the population, several of which have been discussed in previous chapters of this book and elsewhere in this series.[4]

❑ What is the main advantage of longitudinal studies such as the ones described above, compared with cross-sectional surveys that also show an association between health status, social class and material circumstances?

■ Longitudinal studies follow the same individuals through time, enabling the researchers to identify how health and social circumstances are related in each person as they age; the *direction* of cause–effect relationships between two factors can be more clearly distinguished. Cross-sectional studies look at a sample of the population at a single point in time, so they cannot tell us what happens to those individuals as their lives progress; they show whether one factor is statistically associated with another at that time point, but cannot show whether they are causally related nor reveal the direction of cause–effect relationships.

❑ Longitudinal studies of birth or age cohorts do have one limitation (apart from their huge cost) which must be born in mind when interpreting the results. What is it? (It was mentioned in Chapter 2.)

■ Each cohort is affected by certain unique features of the surrounding cultural, political, economic and demographic characteristics of the period in which these individuals were born and grew up, grew old and died. For example, as Chapter 2 pointed out, some cohorts are more 'crowded' than others as a

[4]Reviewed in *World Health and Disease*, Chapters 9 and 10, and *Dilemmas in Health Care*, Chapter 11. Open University students are also referred to an optional article in *Health and Disease: A Reader* (second edition, 1995) by J. N. Morris, entitled 'Inequalities in health: ten years and little further on', which appeared originally as an editorial in the *Lancet* in 1990.

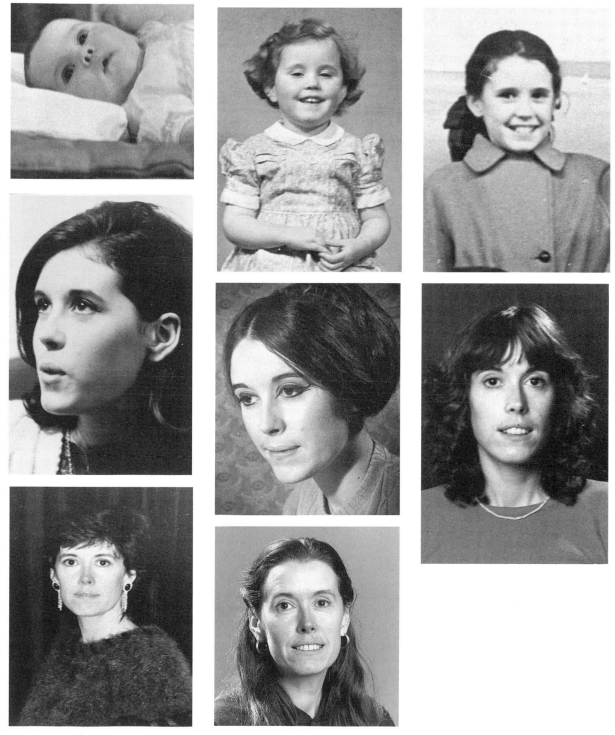

Studying the same individual at sequential points in their life course can yield important insights into the cumulative effects of earlier experiences on health. (Photos: courtesy of Basiro Davey)

result of fluctuations in the birth rate, and this can have a marked effect on the availability of services, education and jobs, with consequent impacts on the relative health of two cohorts which might have been born only a few years apart. Unique features of each cohort must be kept in mind when interpreting the results.

Two examples serve to illustrate this point. In his book about the 1946 cohort, Mike Wadsworth notes that during their childhood 20 per 1 000 of these children were admitted to hospital for surgery to remove their tonsils or adenoids; in the 1958 cohort, the rate had fallen to 7 per 1 000 (Calnan et al., 1978). This fall is believed to be due to changes in medical 'fashion' in the treatment of persistent nose and throat infections in children, rather than to any major improvement in the rate of illness. However, the fall in lower respiratory tract infections in children below the age of 2 years, from 250 per 1 000 in the 1946 cohort to 130 per 1 000 in their first-born children, is believed to be due to a genuine fall in the rate of infection (Mann, Wadsworth and Colley, 1992).

❑ Can you suggest some possible contributors to this marked improvement in respiratory health?

■ You may have considered the possible impact of the Clean Air Act of 1956, which restricted the burning of coal in domestic fires and industrial processes,[5] and the falling popularity of cigarette smoking by the time the second generation was born. Urban children in the 1946 cohort grew up in a far smokier atmosphere than their own offspring experienced.

Improvements such as these between one generation and the next can be seen in a wide range of mortality and morbidity statistics (for example, in perinatal and infant mortality rates, Chapters 3 and 4; childhood accident rates, Chapter 5), and also in more general indicators of health such as adult height. Children born into the 1958 cohort grew taller than those born in 1946, and in their turn the children of the 1958 cohort grew taller than their parents (Kuh and Wadsworth, 1989; Kuh, Power and Rodgers, 1991). These trends are thought to be due to improvements in nutrition and reductions in persistent childhood infections which may 'stunt' growth (Chapter 4).

[5]See Caring for Health: History and Diversity (second edition), Chapter 6.

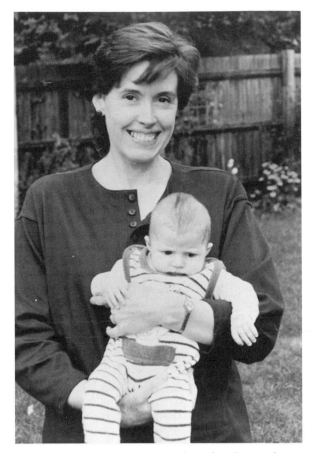

This woman, born in 1947 in a working-class district of London, suffered repeatedly from bronchitis and pneumonia in the winter 'smogs' of her childhood. Her daughter, born on the edge of countryside in Milton Keynes, has had a very different experience of atmospheric pollution and respiratory illness. (Photo: Mike Wibberley)

But despite this background of steady advances in health, social-class differences have not only persisted within each cohort, they have become more marked over time— the gap between people who grew up in auspicious material circumstances and those whose early life experience was relatively deprived has grown wider as the twentieth century has progressed. Longitudinal studies of the life course have shed light on how early disadvantages can exacerbate later ones, leading to cumulative damage to health and wellbeing. We do not have the space to review all of the evidence here, but one important and well-researched example illustrates the more general findings.

It derives from the study of respiratory infection by Mann, Wadsworth and Colley, mentioned earlier.

Exposure to atmospheric pollution during the first 11 years of life were calculated for the children in the 1946 cohort, based on the consumption of domestic coal; 22 per cent of them were found to live in heavily polluted districts. Not surprisingly, these children were predominantly from lower-social-class families; their homes were more likely to be overcrowded and damp and their parents were also more likely to suffer from persistent chest infections and to be smokers. These children not only experienced more numerous and more serious episodes of respiratory illness in childhood than their contemporaries from better domestic circumstances, but they were also significantly more likely to do so in adolescence and in adulthood. It remains to be seen what the longer-term outcome will be on their respiratory vulnerability as they age, but the prediction is obvious.

Early biological influences on later health

Finally, we return to a strand of research which has been mentioned before in this book—the so-called 'programming hypothesis', which suggests that experiences during embryonic and fetal development and in the first year of life may have an irreversible effect on biological growth and development. The evidence collected by David Barker's team at the University of Southampton (1990, 1992) has been reviewed elsewhere in this series.[6] They obtained the birth and infant records of several thousand babies born in the early decades of this century, and traced the survivors who are in their 50s and 60s, or the death certificates of those who had already died. In brief, a strong statistical association was found between the relative weight of the baby and the placenta at birth (a low-weight baby with a heavy placenta is considered to be evidence of poor fetal growth), the infant's weight at one year, and the incidence of certain chronic degenerative diseases of later life, such as coronary heart disease, stroke and late-onset diabetes.

Barker has proposed an underlying biological mechanism for these findings, which requires further investigation: he suggests that poor nutrition during pregnancy leads to poor fetal growth, particularly in the development of the circulatory system, which renders the individual vulnerable to certain chronic degenerative diseases in later life. Poor nutrition is a well-established feature of social deprivation, which may not only damage

the health of the woman during pregnancy, but have an adverse effect on her offspring's development. These early biological effects can be exacerbated by poor material circumstances in infancy and childhood. Obviously, caution is essential in attributing illness in later life to the effects of early life experiences, without taking into account the circumstances of the intervening 50 or more years. But Barker's findings are in line with other studies on inter-generational effects on pregnancy outcomes: girls who were not well-nourished in childhood and who failed to reach their predicted adult height, are at greater risk of complications during pregnancy and are more likely to give birth to low-weight babies, who in their turn suffer more health problems (Illsley and Mitchell, 1984; Emanuel, 1986).

In conclusion

We can summarise the evidence of all the epidemiological studies discussed in this chapter in the words of one leading researcher into the life course:

> ... health, like education, is an investment in childhood which has long-term consequences both for the individual and for future national well-being ... Without better knowledge of the population's health and education, particularly in childhood, many of the important questions of the 1940s remain the important questions of today, and answers are as difficult to find now as they were then. (Wadsworth, 1991, pp. 11 and 206)

But each life course is more than the cumulative influence of individual health status and education. It is also lived out in a social and political context; it is shaped by cultural norms which label certain states (such as adolescence or the menopause) as problematic, and others as desirable (e.g. motherhood); personal freedoms are subject to ethical constraints, as in the debate about euthanasia; the individual is also a member of a collective. In looking back over your own life, you may wish to reflect on whether this book has altered your perceptions of the influences you have experienced from birth to your present age.

[6]See *Studying Health and Disease* (second edition), Chapter 10, and the audiotape for Open University students which is associated with it.

OBJECTIVES FOR CHAPTER 14

When you have studied this chapter, you should be able to:

14.1 Give examples from this book or from general knowledge of forces that seem to be blurring the boundaries of traditional age grades in the life courses of people living in the United Kingdom in the 1990s.

14.2 Comment on the strengths and weaknesses of longitudinal and cross-sectional studies of the life course, drawing on examples from anywhere in this book or from external sources.

14.3 Discuss evidence from research which points to a cumulative effect on health of events and circumstances throughout life, with possible repercussions on the health of future generations.

QUESTIONS FOR CHAPTER 14

Question 1 *(Objective 14.1)*

The period we refer to as 'adolescence' was not identified as a distinct stage of the life course until the late nineteenth century. What forces have contributed to the increasing recognition of adolescence in the twentieth century and how have they affected its duration?

Question 2 *(Objective 14.2)*

The 'Health and Lifestyles' survey began in 1984–5 with a random sample of just over 9 000 adults of all ages. Seven years later, 5 352 of these people were traced and surveyed again. What common weakness of longitudinal studies does the follow-up study illustrate, and why is this of particular importance in a study such as this, which began with a random sample across a wide age-range?

Question 3 *(Objective 14.3)*

Analysis of data from the 1958 birth cohort at the ages of 7, 11, 16 and 23 years showed a strong statistical association between birth weight and later socio-economic circumstances (Bartley *et al.,* 1994). The relationship was 'graded'—a term used by epidemiologists to signify that it held across the whole range of birth weights: the heaviest 20 per cent of babies suffered the least socio-economic disadvantage at all the later age-points surveyed, and the lightest 20 per cent suffered the most, with the three remaining 20 per cent bands falling sequentially in between these extremes. Socio-economic disadvantage was assessed in terms of the child living in overcrowded housing, lacking (or sharing) the basic amenities of an inside toilet, hot water supply and bathroom; having a father in social class IIIN, IV or V; and experiencing financial difficulties indicated by receipt of free school meals before the age of 16, or supplementary or unemployment benefit at the age of 23.

Consider this study in the light of other research discussed in Chapter 14. Taken together, what do they suggest about the possible cumulative effects of events in the life course up to the age of 23 years, which might influence later health—not only in the 1958 cohort but possibly also in their children?

Appendix

Table of abbreviations used in this book

Abbreviation	What it stands for
A&E	Accident and Emergency (hospital casualty department)
ABILITIES	audition intellectual functioning limbs communication muscles physical health structural status
AID	artificial insemination using donated sperm
AIDS	acquired immune deficiency syndrome
AIMS	Association for Improvements in Maternity Services
AZT	3'-azido-3'-deoxythymidine (also known as Zidovudine)
CAPT	Child Accident Prevention Trust
CBI	Confederation of British Industry
CHD	coronary heart disease
DHSS	Department of Health and Social Security
DoH	Department of Health
DoT	Department of Transport
EFM	electronic fetal monitoring
EU	European Union
GHQ	General Health Questionnaire
GHS	General Household Survey
GNP	Gross National Product
GP	general practitioner

Abbreviation	What it stands for
HFEA	Human Fertilisation and Embryology Authority
HIV	human immunodeficiency virus
HRT	hormone replacement therapy
IA	intermittent auscultation
ICD	International Classification of Diseases
IDDM	insulin-dependent diabetes mellitus
IMR	infant mortality rate
IQ	intelligence quotient
IT	information technology
IUCD	intra-uterine contraceptive device
IV	intravenous drip
IVF	*in-vitro* fertilisation
MRC	Medical Research Council
NAHA	National Association of Health Authorities
NHS	National Health Service
OHE	Office of Health Economics
OPCS	Office of Population Censuses and Surveys
PKU	phenylketonuria
PNMR	perinatal mortality rate
RNIB	Royal National Institute for the Blind
RoSPA	Royal Society for the Prevention of Accidents
UPIAS	Union of the Physically Impaired Against Segregation
VDU	visual display unit
WHO	World Health Organisation
YTS	youth training scheme

References and further reading

References

Abdulrahim, D., White, D., Phillips, K., Boyd, G., Nicholson, J. and Elliott, J. (1994) *Ethnicity and Drug Use, Volume I, Executive Summary and Recommendations*, North Thames Regional Health Authority, London.

Abrams, D., Abraham, C., Spears, R. and Marks, D. (1990) AIDS invulnerability: relationships, sexual behaviour and attitudes among 16–19-year-olds, Chapter 3, pp. 35–51, in Aggleton, P., Davies, P. and Hart, G. (eds) *AIDS: Individual, Cultural and Policy Dimensions*, The Falmer Press, Basingstoke.

Age Concern (1994) Transport—older drivers survey, *Age Concern Information Circular*, October, p. 12.

Albery, N., Elliott, G. and Elliott, J. (1993) *The Natural Death Handbook*, Virgin, London.

Alderson, P. (1993) *Children's Consent to Surgery*, Open University Press, Buckingham.

Alwash, R. and McCarthy, M. (1988) Accidents in the home among children under five: ethnic differences or social disadvantage?, *British Medical Journal*, **296**, pp. 1450–3.

Anderson, H. R. and Strachan, D. P. (1991) Asthma mortality in England and Wales, 1979–89, *British Medical Journal*, **337**, p. 1357.

Anderson, M. (1980) *Approaches to the History of the Western Family 1500–1914*, Macmillan, London.

Annual Abstract of Statistics (1994) HMSO, London.

Aquilina Ross, G. (1984) *How to Survive The Male Menopause*, Elm Tree Books, London.

Arber, S. (1991) Class, paid employment and family roles: making sense of structural disadvantage, gender and health status, *Social Science and Medicine*, **32**, pp. 425–36.

Arber, S. and Gilbert, N. (1992) Re-assessing women's working lives: an introductory essay, in Arber, S. and Gilbert, N. (eds) *Women and Working Lives: Divisions and Change*, Macmillan, London.

Arber, S. and Ginn, J. (1991) *Gender and Later Life: A Sociological Analysis of Resources and Constraints*, Sage, London.

Ariès, P. (1976) *Western Attitudes Towards Death*, Marion Boyars, London.

Ariès, P. (1981) *The Hour of our Death*, Penguin, Harmondsworth.

Avis, N. E. and McKinlay, S. M. (1991) A longitudinal analysis of women's attitudes toward the menopause: results from the Massachusetts Women's Health Study, *Maturitas*, **13**, pp. 65–79.

Babb, P. (1993) Teenage conceptions and fertility in England and Wales, 1971–91, *Population Trends*, No. 74, Winter, OPCS, London, pp. 12–17.

Bailey, D. B., Simeonsson, R. J., Buysse, V. and Smith, T. (1993) Reliability of an index of child characteristics, *Developmental Medicine and Child Neurology*, **35**(9), pp. 806–15.

Barker, D. J. P. (ed.) (1992) *Fetal and Infant Origins of Adult Disease*, BMJ Publications, London.

Barker, D. J. P., Bull, A. R., Osmond, C. and Simmonds, S. J. (1990) Fetal and placental size and risk of hypertension in adult life, *British Medical Journal*, **301**, pp. 259–62.

Barnard, M. and McKeganey, N. (1990) Adolescents, sex and injecting drug use: risks for HIV infection, *AIDS Care*, **2**(2), pp. 103–16.

Baron, R. A. (1986) *Behavior in Organisations*, Allyn and Bacon, Newton, Massachusetts.

Bartley, M., Power, C., Blane, D., Davey Smith, G. and Shipley, M. (1994) Birth weight and later socioeconomic disadvantage: evidence from the 1958 British cohort study, *British Medical Journal*, **309**, pp. 1475–9.

Bennett, G. J. and Ebrahim, S. (1992) *The Essentials of Health Care of the Elderly*, Edward Arnold, London.

Benoliel, J. Q. (1988) Institutional dying: a convergence of cultural values, technology, and social organization, in Wass, H., Berardo, F. M. and Neimeyer, R. A. (eds) *Dying: Facing the Facts*, Hemisphere, Washington.

Berer, M. (1994) Meeting consumers' needs: a reproductive health perspective, *Journal of the National Association of Family Planning Nurses*, **26**, pp. 80–5.

Bernard, M. and Meade, K. (1993) *Women Come of Age: Perspectives on the Lives of Older Women*, E. Arnold, Sevenoaks, Kent.

Bijur, P., Golding, J., Haslum, M. and Kurzon, M. (1988) Behavioral predictors of injury in school-age children, *American Journal of Diseases of Children*, **142**, pp. 1307–12.

Blair, E. and Stanley, F. J. (1988) Intrapartum asphyxia: a rare cause of cerebral palsy, *Journal of Pediatrics*, **112**, pp. 515–19.

Blakemore, K. and Boneham, M. (1993) *Age, Race and Ethnicity*, Open University Press, Buckingham.

Blaxter, M. (1990) *Health and Lifestyles*, Tavistock–Routledge, London. An extract entitled 'What is health?' appears in Davey, B., Gray, A. and Seale, C. (eds) (1995) *Health and Disease: A Reader*, 2nd edn., Open University Press, Buckingham.

BMA (1936) The BMA and maternity services, *British Medical Journal*, **i**, p. 656.

BMA, GMSC, HEA, Brook Advisory Centres, FPA, RCGP (1994) *Confidentiality and People under 16*, Health Education Authority, London.

Bogin, B. (1993) Why must I be a teenager at all? *New Scientist*, 6th March, pp. 34–8. An edited extract appears in Davey, B., Gray, A. and Seale, C. (eds) (1995) *Health and Disease: A Reader* (2nd edn), Open University Press, Buckingham.

Bone, M. and Meltzer, H. (1989) *The Prevalence of Disability among Children*, OPCS Surveys of Disability in Great Britain, report 3, HMSO, London.

Botting, B. (1991) Trends in abortion, *Population Trends*, No. 64, Summer, OPCS, London, pp. 19–29.

Bowskill, D. and Linacre, A. (1976) *The 'Male' Menopause*, Frederick Muller, London.

Brazier, M. (1992) *Medicine, Patients and the Law*, Penguin, Harmondsworth.

Brecher, E. M. (1984) *Love, Sex, and Aging: A Consumer's Union Report*, Little, Brown and Company, Boston, USA.

Breslow, L. and Buell, P. (1960) Mortality from coronary heart disease and physical activity of work in California, *Journal of Chronic Diseases*, **11**, pp. 615–26.

Brindle, D. (1994) 'Study charts further fall in family fortunes', *Guardian*, 26 January, p. 4.

British Gas (1991) *The British Gas Report on Attitudes to Ageing 1991*, British Gas, London.

British Medical Journal (1994) (editorial) HIV in childhood, *British Medical Journal*, **308** (12 February), p. 425.

British Society for Population Studies (1983) *The Family*, Occasional Paper 31, OPCS, London.

Brooksbank, D. J. (1985) Suicide and parasuicide in childhood and early adolescence, *British Journal of Psychiatry*, **146**, pp. 159–63.

Brown, G. W. and Davidson, S. (1978) Social class, psychiatric disorder of mother and accidents to children, *Lancet*, **i**, pp. 378–80.

Bruce, I., McKennell, A. and Walker, E. (1991) *Blind and Partially Sighted Adults in Britain: The RNIB Survey*, HMSO, London.

Bucher, H. C. and Schmidt, J. G. (1993) Does routine ultrasound scanning improve outcome in pregnancy? Meta-analysis of various outcome measures, *British Medical Journal*, **307**, pp. 13–17.

Buckman, R. (1988) *'I Don't Know What to Say': How to Help and Support Someone who is Dying*, MacMillan, London.

Burghes, L. (1994) *Lone Parenthood and Family Disruption: The Outcomes for Children*, Family Policy Studies Centre, London.

Burke, R. J. and McKeen, C. A. (1995) Work and career experiences and emotional well-being of managerial and professional women, *Stress Medicine*, **11**, pp. 51–60.

Burnie, J. (1994) Why men don't act their age!, *Daily Record*, 4 May, p. 21.

Bury, M. (1988), Meanings at risk with arthritis, in Bury, M. and Anderson, R. (eds) *Living with Chronic Illness: The Experience of Patients and their Families*, Unwin Hyman, London.

Bury, M. and Holme, A. (1991) *Life After Ninety*, Routledge, London.

Butler, C. (ed.) (1994) *If not a Mother*, published by Claire Butler, 72 Lynton Rd, Chesham, Bucks.

Calnan, M., Douglas, J. W. B. and Goldstein, H. (1978) Tonsillectomy and circumcision: comparison of two cohorts, *International Journal of Epidemiology*, **7**, pp. 79–85.

Campbell, R. and Macfarlane, A. (1994) *Where to be Born? The Debate and the Evidence*, 2nd edn, National Perinatal Epidemiology Unit, Oxford (1st edn 1987).

Campbell, R., Davies, I. M., Macfarlane, A. and Beral, V. (1984) Home births in England and Wales, 1979: perinatal mortality according to intended place of delivery, *British Medical Journal*, **289**, pp. 721–4.

CAPT (Child Accident Prevention Trust) (1989) *Basic Principles of Child Accident Prevention: A Guide to Action*, Child Accident Prevention Trust, London.

Carter, Y. H. and Jones, P. W. (1993) Accidents among children under five years old: a general practice based study in north Staffordshire, *British Journal of General Practice*, **43**, pp. 159–63.

Cartwright, A., Hockey, L. and Anderson, J. L. (1973) *Life Before Death*, Routledge and Kegan Paul, London.

Cavalli-Sforza, L. and Bodmer, W. (1971) *Human Genetics*, Oxford University Press, Oxford.

Central Statistical Office (1987) *Social Trends* 17, HMSO, London.

Central Statistical Office (1994a) *Annual Abstract of Statistics 1994*, HMSO, London.

Central Statistical Office (1994b) *Social Trends* 24, HMSO, London.

Centre for Disease Control (1990) Comorbidity of chronic conditions and disability among older persons—United States, 1984, *Journal of the American Medical Association*, **263**(2), pp. 209–10.

Challis, J. and Elliman, O. (1979) *Child Workers Today*, Quatermaine House, Sunbury, Middlesex.

Chalmers, I., Enkin, M. and Keirse, M. J. N. C. (eds) (1989) *Effective Care in Pregnancy and Childbirth*, 2 vols, Oxford University Press, Oxford.

Chen, I. (1994) Hormone replacement for men?, *Hippocrates*, September, pp. 22 and 25.

Choquet, M. and Menke, H. (1987) Development of self-perceived risk behaviour and psychosomatic symptoms in adolescents: a longitudinal approach, *Journal of Adolescence*, **10**(3), pp. 291–308.

Cliff, K. S. (1984) *Accidents: Causes, Prevention and Services*, Croom Helm, London.

Cochrane, A. L. (1972) *Effectiveness and Efficiency: Random Reflections on the Health Service*, Nuffield Provincial Hospitals Trust, London. (Reprinted in 1989 as a joint publication of the British Medical Journal and the Nuffield Provincial Hospitals Trust.)

Cohen, R.Y., Brownell, K. D. and Felox, M. R. (1990) Age and sex differences in health habits and beliefs of school children, *Health Psychology*, **9**(2), pp. 208–24.

Cole, T. R. (1992) *The Journey of Life: A Cultural History of Ageing in America*, Cambridge University Press, Cambridge.

Coleman, A. and Chiva, A. (1991) *Coping With Change: Focus on Retirement*, Health Education Authority, London.

Coleman, D. and Salt, J. (1992) *The British Population: Patterns, Trends and Processes*, Oxford University Press, Oxford.

Coleman, J. (1979) Who leads who astray? Causes of anti-social behaviour in adolescence, *Journal of Adolescence*, **2**(3), pp. 179–85.

Combes, G. (1991) *'You can't watch them twenty four hours a day': Parents' and Children's Perceptions, Understanding and Experience of Accidents and Accident Prevention*, Child Accident Prevention Trust, London.

Confederation of British Industry (CBI) (1994) *Managing Absence in Sickness and in Health*, CBI, London.

Confederation of British Industry (CBI) and Department of Health (1992) *Prevention of Mental Ill Health at Work: A CBI and Department of Health Conference Report*, HMSO, London.

Cooper, C. L. (1986) Job distress: recent research and the emerging role of the clinical occupational psychologist, *Bulletin of the British Psychological Society,* **39**, pp. 325–31.

Cooper, C. L. and Faragher, E. B. (1993) Psychosocial stress and breast cancer: the inter-relationship between stress events, coping strategies and personality, *Psychological Medicine*, **23**, pp. 653–62.

Cooper, C. L., Faragher, E. B., Bray, C. L. and Ramsdale, D. R. (1985) The significance of psychosocial factors in predicting coronary disease in patients with valvular heart disease, *Social Science and Medicine*, **20**(4), pp. 315–8.

Cooper, P. J., Campbell, E. A., Day, A., Kennerly, H. and Bond, A. (1988) Non-psychotic psychiatric disorder after childbirth: a prospective study of prevalence, incidence, course and nature, *British Journal of Psychiatry*, **152**, pp. 799–806.

Cowling, A. G., Stanworth, M. J. K., Bennett, R. D., Curran, J. and Lyons, P. (1988) *Behavioural Sciences for Managers*, Edward Arnold, London.

Cox. B. D. *et al.* (1987) *The Health and Lifestyle Survey*, The Health Promotion Research Trust, London.

Cox, B. D., Huppert, F. A. and Whichelow, M. J. (1993) *The Health and Lifestyle Survey: Seven Years On*, Dartmouth Publishing Co. Ltd, Aldershot.

Cox, J. L., Holden, J. M. and Sagovsky, R. (1987) Detection of post-natal depression: development of the Edinburgh Postnatal Depression Scale, *British Journal of Psychiatry*, **150**, pp. 782–6.

Cox, T. (1985) *Stress*, Macmillan, London.

Cox, T. (1993) *Stress Research and Stress Management: Putting Theory to Work*, Health and Safety Executive (HSE) Contract Research Report No. 61, HMSO, London.

Croft, A. and Sibert, J. (1992) Accident prevention: environmental change and education, in Sibert, J. (ed.) *Accidents and Emergencies in Childhood*, Royal College of Physicians, London.

Crown, S. and Crisp, A. H. (1979) *Manual of the Crown–Crisp Experiential Index*, Hodder and Stoughton, Sevenoaks, Kent.

Daly, E., Roche, M., Barlow, D., Gray, A., McPherson, K. and Vessey, M. (1992) HRT: an analysis of benefits, risks and costs, *British Medical Bulletin*, **48**(2), pp. 368–400.

Department of Health (1990) *Health and Personal Social Services Statistics for England 1990*, HMSO, London.

Department of Health (1991) *The Health of the Nation: A Consultative Document for Health in England,* Cmd. 1523, HMSO, London.

Department of Health (1992a) *The Health of the Nation: A Strategy for Health in England*, Cmd. 1986, HMSO, London.

Department of Health (1992b) *The Health of the Nation: A Summary of the Strategy for Health in England*, HMSO, London.

Department of Health (1993) *Changing Childbirth, Part 1. Report of the Expert Maternity Group*, HMSO, London (the 'Cumberlege Report').

Department of Health (1994) *Report on Confidential Enquiries into Maternal Deaths in the UK 1988–90*, HMSO, London.

Department of Health and Social Security (1974) *Family Planning Memorandum of Guidance 1974*, DHSS, London.

Department of Health and Social Security (1980) *Inequalities in Health*, Report of a Working Group, DHSS, London (the 'Black Report').

Department of Health and Social Security (1982) *Health and Personal Social Services Statistics for England 1982*, HMSO, London.

Department of Transport (1985) *Compulsory Seat Belt Wearing*, HMSO, London.

Department of Transport (1992) *Accident Fact Sheet No. 5*, Department of Transport, London.

Department of Transport (1993) *Road Accidents Great Britain 1992: The Casualty Report*, HMSO, London.

Diamond, J. (1992) How menopausal men go mad, *She*, March, p. 89.

Dixon, S. (1991) *Autonomy and Dependence in Residential Care*, Age Concern England, London.

Donovan, J. E., Lessor, R. and Costa, F. M. (1991) Adolescent health behavior and conventionality-unconventionality: an extension of problem-behavior theory, *Health Psychology*, **10**(1), pp. 52–61.

Doress, P. B., Siegal, D. L. and Shapiro, J. (eds) and the Midlife and Older Women Book Project in co-operation with the Boston Women's Health Book Collective (1989) *Ourselves, Growing Older: Women Ageing with Knowledge and Power*, British edition, Fontana, London.

du Boulay, S. (1984) *Cicely Saunders: Founder of the Modern Hospice Movement*, Hodder and Stoughton, London.

Duval Smith, A. (1994) Shamrock pink, *Guardian,* 8 February, p. 16.

Easterlin, R. (1980) *Birth and Fortune: The Impact of Numbers on Personal Welfare*, Grant McIntyre, London.

Easterlin, R., Schaeffer, C. and Macunovich, D. (1993) Will the baby boomers be less well off than their parents? Income, wealth, and family circumstances over the life cycle in the United States, *Population and Development Review*, **19**(3), pp. 497–522.

Edwards, R. and Steptoe, P. (1981) *A Matter of Life: The Story of a Medical Breakthrough*, Sphere Books Ltd, London.

Elborn, J. S., Shale, D. J. and Britton, J. R. (1992) Cystic fibrosis: current survival and population estimates to the year 2000, *Thorax*, **46**, pp. 881–5.

Elias, N. (1985) *The Loneliness of the Dying*, Blackwell, Oxford.

Elkind, D. (1967) Egocentrism in adolescence, *Child Development*, **30**, pp. 1025–34.

Emanuel, I. (1986) Maternal health during childhood and later reproductive performance, *Annals of the New York Academy of Sciences*, **477**, pp. 27–39.

Enkin, M., Keirse, M. J. N. C., Renfrew, M. and Neilson, J. (1995) *A Guide to Effective Care in Pregnancy and Childbirth*, 2nd edn, Oxford University Press, Oxford (1st edn edited by Chalmers, Enkin and Keirse, 1989; see above).

Evans, J. G. (1991) Challenge of aging, *British Medical Journal*, **303** (6799), pp. 408–9.

Ewigman, B. G., Crane, J. P., Frigoletto, F. D., LeFevre, M. L., Bain, R. P., McNellis, D. and the RADIUS Study Group (1993) Effect of prenatal ultrasound screening on perinatal outcome, *New England Journal of Medicine*, **329**, pp. 821–7.

Fabricius, J. (1993) Psychodynamic perspectives, in Wright, H. and Giddey, M. (eds) *Mental Health Nursing*, Chapman & Hall, London.

Feldman, H. A., Goldstein, I., Hatzichristou, D. G., Krane, R. J. and McKinlay, J. B. (1994) Impotence and its medical and psychosocial correlates: results from the Massachusetts Male Aging Study, *The Journal of Urology*, **151**, pp. 54–61.

Fennell, G., Phillipson, C. and Evers, H. (1988) *The Sociology of Old Age*, Open University Press, Milton Keynes.

Field, D. and James, N. (1993) Where and how people die, in Clarke, D. (ed.) *The Future for Palliative Care*, Open University Press, Buckingham.

Firth, S. (1993) Approaches to death in Hindu and Sikh communities in Britain, pp. 26–32, in Dickenson, D. and Johnson, M. (eds) *Death, Dying and Bereavement*, Sage, London.

Foreman, J. (1993) Male menopause: much ado about nothing? *The Boston Globe*, October, pp. 31 and 55.

Foster, K., Wilmot, A. and Dobbs, J. (1990) *General Household Survey*, HMSO, London.

Garcia, J., Corry, M., MacDonald, D., Elbourne, D. and Grant, A. (1985) Mothers' views of continuous electronic fetal monitoring and intermittent auscultation in a randomised controlled trial, *Birth*, **12**, pp. 79–85.

Glazener, C., Templeton, A. and Russell, I. (1992) *Postnatal Care: Empirical Evidence from Grampian*, Health Services Research Unit, University of Aberdeen, Aberdeen.

Glendenning, C. (1992) *The Costs of Informal Care: Looking Inside the Household*, HMSO, London.

Goddard, E. (1991) *Drinking in England and Wales in the Late 1980s*, HMSO, London.

Gordon, T. (1991) Childless parents, *Issue*, No. 23, Autumn, p.4.

Gorer, G. (1955) The pornography of death, *Encounter*, October, pp. 49–53.

Gorer, G. (1965) *Death, Grief and Mourning in Contemporary Britain*, Cresset, London.

Grant, A., Elbourne, D., Valentin, L. and Alexander S. (1989) Routine formal fetal movement counting and risk of antepartum late death, *Lancet*, **ii**, pp. 345–9.

Grant, A., O'Brien, N., Joy, M-T., Hennessy, E. and MacDonald, D. (1989) Cerebral palsy among children born during the Dublin randomised trial of intrapartum monitoring, *Lancet*, **ii**, pp. 1233–5.

Green, H. (1988) *Informal Carers*, Office of Population Censuses and Surveys (OPCS), Social Survey Division, Series GH5, No. 15, Supplement A, HMSO, London.

Green, J. (1992) The medico-legal production of fatal accidents, *Sociology of Health and Illness*, **14**, pp. 373–90.

Green, J. M. (1990) 'Who is unhappy after childbirth?' Antenatal and intrapartum correlates from a prospective study, *Journal of Reproductive and Infant Psychology*, **8**, pp. 175–83.

Greengross, W. and Greengross, S. (1989) *Living, Loving and Ageing*, Age Concern England, London.

Greer, G. (1991) *The Change: Women, Ageing and The Menopause*, Hamish Hamilton, London.

Groves, D. (1993) Work, poverty and older women, pp. 43–62, in Bernard, M. and Meade, K. (eds) *Women Come of Age*, Edward Arnold, London.

Gunning, J. (1990) *Human IVF, Embryo Research, Fetal Tissue for Research, and Abortion: International Information*, HMSO, London.

Hall, E. M. (1989) Gender, work control, and stress: A theoretical discussion and an empirical test, *International Journal of Health Services*, **19**(4), pp. 725–45.

Hall, M., Macintyre, S. and Porter M. (1985) *Antenatal Care Assessed*, Aberdeen University Press, Aberdeen.

Handy, C. (1990) *The Age of Unreason*, Arrow Books, London.

Hansard (House of Commons Parliamentary Debates) (1993) 1 December, Col. 580, HMSO, London.

Haskey, J. (1993) Trends in the numbers of one-parent families in Great Britain, *Population Trends*, **71**, pp. 26–33.

Hellriegel, D., Slocum, J. W. Jr. and Woodman, R. W. (1992) *Organizational Behavior*, West, St. Paul, Minnesota.

Henwood, M. (1992) *Accident Prevention and Public Health: A Study of the Annual Reports of Directors of Public Health*, RoSPA, Birmingham.

Hepworth, M. (1987) The mid-life phase, in Cohen, G. (ed.) *Social Change and the Life Course*, Tavistock, London.

Hepworth, M. and Featherstone, M. (1982) *Surviving Middle Age*, Basil Blackwell, Oxford.

Hill, A. M. (1993) *Viropause/Andropause: The Male Menopause*, New Horizon Press, Far Hills, New Jersey, USA.

Hillman, M., Adams, J. and Whitelegg, J. (1990) *One False Move … A Study of Children's Independent Mobility*, Policy Studies Institute, London.

Hills, J. (1993) *The Future of the Welfare State: A Guide to the Debate*, Joseph Rowntree Foundation, York.

Hockey, J. and James, A. (1993) *Growing Up and Growing Old: Ageing and Dependence in the Life Course*, Sage, London.

Holland, J., Ramazanoglu, C., Scott, S., Sharpe, S. and Thomson, R. (1990) Sex, gender and power: young women's sexuality in the shadow of AIDS, *Sociology of Health and Illness*, **12**(3), pp. 336–50.

Holland, P. and Rabbitt, P. M. A. (1992) People's awareness of their age-related sensory and cognitive deficits and the implications for road safety, *Applied Cognitive Psychology*, **6**(3), pp. 217–31.

House of Commons Health Committee (1991–2) *Second Report on Maternity Services*, HMSO, London (the 'Winterton Report').

Human Fertilisation and Embryology Authority (1993a) *Code of Practice*, HFEA, London.

Human Fertilisation and Embryology Authority (1993b) *Second Annual Report*, HFEA, London.

Hunt, A. and Davies, P. (1991) What is a sexual encounter?, in Aggleton, P., Hart, G. and Davies, P. (eds) *AIDS: Responses, Interventions and Care*, The Falmer Press, London.

Hunt, K. and Annandale, E. (1993) Just the Job? Is the relationship between health and domestic and paid work gender-specific? *Sociology of Health and Illness*, **15**(5), pp. 632–64.

Hunter, P. and Houghton, D. M. (1993) Nurse teacher stress in Northern Ireland, *Journal of Advanced Nursing*, **18**(8), pp. 1315–23.

Illsley, R. and Mitchell, R. G. (1984) *Low Birth Weight*, Wiley, Chichester.

Irwin, C. E. (1989) Risk-taking behaviours in the adolescent patient. Are they impulsive? *Paediatric Annals*, **18**, pp. 122–33.

Jaques, E. (1965) Death and The Mid-Life Crisis, *International Journal of Psychoanalysis*, October, **46**, pp. 502–14.

Johnson, J. (1993), Does group living work?, in Johnson, J. and Slater, R. (eds), *Ageing and Later Life*, Sage, London.

Johnson, P. and Falkingham, J. (1992) *Ageing and Economic Welfare*, Sage, London.

Johnson, S. B., Fruend, A., Silverstein, J., Hansen, C. A. and Malone, J. (1990) Adherence-health status relationships in childhood diabetes, *Health Psychology*, **9**(5), pp. 606–31.

Jolley, D. (1994) No place for the old and sick, *Guardian* letters page, 19 April.

Jones, E. (1984) *The Life and Work of Sigmund Freud*, Basic Books, New York.

Joshi, H. (ed.) (1989) *The Changing Population of Britain*, Blackwell, Oxford.

Journal of the National Association of Family Planning Nurses (1994) (editorial) Women demand wider range of contraceptives, *Journal National Association of Family Planning Nurses*, **26**.

Kahn, H. and Cooper, C. L. (1986) Computing stress, *Current Psychological Research and Reviews*, **5**(2), pp. 148–62.

Kalache, A. (1993) Ageing in developing countries: has it got anything to do with us?, pp. 339–43, in Johnson, J. and Slater, R. (eds) *Ageing and Later Life*, Sage, London.

Kandel, D. B., Kessler, R. C. and Margulis, R. Z. (1978) Antecedents of adolescent initiation into stages of drug use, *Journal of Youth and Adolescence*, **7**, pp. 13–40.

Karasek, R. and Theorell, T. (1990) *Healthy Work: Stress, Productivity and the Reconstruction of Working Life*, Basic Books, New York.

Kaunitz, A. M., Spence, C., Danielson, T. S., Rochat, R. W. and Grimes, D. A. (1984) Perinatal and maternal mortality in a religious group avoiding obstetric care, *American Journal of Obstetrics and Gynecology*, **150**, pp. 826–31.

Kemp, A. and Sibert, J. R. (1992) Drowning and near drowning in children in the United Kingdom: lessons for prevention, *British Medical Journal*, **304**, pp. 1143–6.

Kiernan, K. (1989) The family: formation and fission, in Joshi, H. (ed.), *The Changing Population of Britain*, Blackwell, Oxford.

Kiernan, K. and Wicks, M. (1990) *Family Change and Future Policy*, Family Policy Studies Centre, London.

Kübler-Ross, E. (1970) *On Death and Dying*, Tavistock, London.

Kübler-Ross, E. (ed.) (1975) *Death: The Final Stage of Growth*, Prentice-Hall, Englewood Cliffs, USA.

Kuh, D. and Wadsworth, M. E. J. (1989) Parental height: childhood environment and subsequent adult height in a national birth cohort, *International Journal of Epidemiology*, **18**, pp. 663–8.

Kuh, D., Power, C. and Rodgers, B. (1991) Secular trends in social class and sex differences in height, *International Journal of Epidemiology*, **20**(4), pp. 1001–9.

Kurtz, Z. (ed.) (1992) *With Health in Mind*, Action for Sick Children, London.

Kutash, I. L., Schlesinger, L. B. and Associates (1980) *Handbook on Stress and Anxiety*, Jossey-Bass, San Francisco.

LaBuda, M. C., Gottesman, I. I. and Pauls, D. L. (1993) Usefulness of twin studies for exploring the etiology of childhood and adolescent psychiatric disorders, *American Journal of Medical Genetics*, **48**(1), pp. 47–59.

Lancet (1989) (editorial) Cerebral palsy, intrapartum care and a shot in the foot, *Lancet*, **ii**, pp. 1251–2.

Lancet (1991) (editorial) Placental localisation in early pregnancy, *Lancet*, **337**, p. 274.

Landale, T. (1989) Addressing stress, *Personnel Today*, 13 June, pp. 34–5.

Larkin, P. (1974) *High Windows*, Faber & Faber, London.

Laslett, P. (1989) A Fresh Map of Life: *The Emergence of the Third Age*, Weidenfeld and Nicolson, London.

Levinson, D. J., Darrow, C., Klein, R., Levinson, M. H. and McKee, B. (1978) *The Seasons of a Man's Life*, Knopf, New York.

Lilford, R. (1987) Clinical experimentation in obstetrics, *British Medical Journal*, **295**, pp. 1298–300.

Lipman, A. and Slater, R. (1977) Homes for old people: toward a positive environment, *The Gerontologist*, **17**(2), pp. 146–56.

Macdonald, B. and Rich, C. (1984) *Look Me in the Eye: Old Women, Aging and Ageism*, The Women's Press, London.

MacDonald, D., Grant, A., Sheridan-Pereira, M., Boylan, P. and Chalmers I. (1985) The Dublin randomised trial of intrapartum fetal monitoring, *American Journal of Obstetrics and Gynecology*, **152**, pp. 524–39.

Mann, S. L., Wadsworth, M. E. J. and Colley, J. R. T. (1992) Accumulation of factors influencing respiratory illness in members of a national birth cohort and their offspring, *Journal of Epidemiology and Community Health*, **46**(3), pp. 286–92.

Margolis, B. L., Kroes, W. H. and Quinn, R. P. (1974) Job stress: an unlisted occupational hazard, *Journal of Occupational Medicine*, **16**, pp. 654–61.

Marmot, M. G. (1986) Social inequalities in mortality: the social environment, in Wilkinson, R. G. (ed.) *Class and Health: Research and Longitudinal Data*, Tavistock, London.

Marmot, M. G., Smith, G. D., Stansfield, S. *et al.* (1991) Health inequalities among British civil servants: The Whitehall II Study, *Lancet*, **i**, pp. 1387–93.

Marshall, W. A. and Tanner, J. M. (1986) The trend in age at menarche in six Western industrialised countries, 1860–1980, in Falkner, F. and Tanner, J. M. (eds) *Human Growth*, volume 2, 2nd edn, Plenum Press, London.

Martin, E. (1987) *The Woman in The Body: A Cultural Analysis of Reproduction*, Open University Press, Milton Keynes.

Martin, J., Meltzer, H. and Elliot, D. (1988) *The Prevalence of Disability among Adults*, OPCS, HMSO, London.

Maternity Services Advisory Committee (1984) *Maternity Care in Action, Part II, Care during childbirth (intrapartum care): a guide to good practice and a plan for action*, HMSO, London.

Matthews, K. A. and Glass, D. C. (1984) Type A behaviour, stressful life events and coronary heart disease, pp. 167–85 in Dohrenwend, B. S. and Dohrenwend, B. P. (eds), *Stressful Life Events and their Contexts*, Rutgers University Press, New Brunswick, USA.

Mayall, B. (1993) Keeping healthy at home and school, *Sociology of Health and Illness*, **15**, pp. 447–63.

Melia, R. J. W., Morrell, D. C., Swan, A. V. and Bartholomew, J. (1989) A health visitor investigation of home accidents in pre-school children, *Health Visitor*, June, **62**, pp. 181–3.

Midwinter, E. (1992) *Report on Leisure for the Carnegie Inquiry into the Third Age*, Centre for Policy on Ageing, London.

Miller, A. M. (1994) *Young People: Sex Education and Sexual Activity*, Centre for Consumer Education and Research, Liverpool John Moores University, Liverpool.

Ministry of Health (1959) *Report of the Maternity Services Committee (Chairman Lord Cranbrook)*, HMSO, London.

Morgan, B. M., Bulpitt, C. J., Clifton, P. and Lewis, P. J. (1982) Analgesia and satisfaction in childbirth (The Queen Charlotte's 1000 Mother Survey), *Lancet*, **ii**, p. 808.

Morley, J. (1971) *Death, Heaven and the Victorian*, Studio Vista, London.

Morris, J. (1993) *Community Care or Independent Living?*, Joseph Rowntree Foundation (in association with Community Care), York.

Morris, J. N. (1990) Inequalities is health: ten years and little further on, *Lancet*, **336**, pp. 491–3. (Also appears in full in Davey, B., Gray, A. and Seale, C. (eds) (1995) *Health and Disease: A Reader*, 2nd edn, Open University Press, Buckingham.)

MRC Medical Sociology Unit at the University of Glasgow (various years) *Annual Reports*, MRC Medical Sociology Unit, Glasgow.

Murphy, E. (1993) *Dementia and Mental Illness in Older People*, Papermac, London.

Murphy, J. F., Dauncey, M., Gray, O. P. and Chalmers, I. (1984) Planned and unplanned deliveries at home: implications of a changing ratio, *British Medical Journal*, **288**, pp. 1429–32.

Murray, L. (1992) The impact of postnatal depression on infant development, *Journal of Child Psychology and Psychiatry*, **33**, pp. 543–61.

Murray, L. (1993a) Prevention of adverse effects of parental depression on the infant with brief psychotherapy: a treatment trial, paper presented at the 3rd International Psychoanalytic Association Conference on Psychoanalytic Research, UCL London, March 1993.

Murray, L. (1993b) The role of infant irritability in postnatal depression in a Cambridge (UK) community population, in Nugent, J. K., Brazelton, T. B. and Lester, B. M. (eds) *The Cultural Context of Infancy, Volume 3*, Ablex, New Jersey.

Musgrove, F. (1964) *Youth and the Social Order*, Routledge and Kegan Paul, London.

Musgrove, F. and Middleton, R. (1981) Rites of passage and the meaning of age in three contrasted social groups, *British Journal of Sociology*, **32**, pp. 39–55.

NAHA/RoSPA Strategy Group (1990) *Action on Accidents*, NAHA/RoSPA, Birmingham.

Nelson, D. L. and Quick, J. C. (1994) *Organizational Behavior: Foundations, Realities and Challenges*, West, St. Paul, Minnesota.

Nelson, K. (1988) What proportion of cerebral palsy is related to birth asphyxia? *Journal of Pediatrics*, **112**, pp. 572–3.

Nicholson, A. and Alberman, E. (1992) Cerebral palsy—an increasing contributor to severe mental retardation? *Archives of Disease in Childhood*, **67**, pp. 1050–5.

North, F., Syme, S. L., Feeney, A., Head, J., Shipley, M. J. and Marmot, M. G. (1993) Explaining socioeconomic differences in sickness absence: the Whitehall II study, *British Medical Journal*, **306**, pp. 361–6.

Northern Regional Health Authority (1994) *Regional Maternity Survey Office Report*, Northern Regional Health Authority, Newcastle.

Oakley, A. (1980) *Women Confined: Towards a Sociology of Childbirth*, Martin Robinson, Oxford.

Office of Health Economics (1994) *Eating Disorders: Anorexia nervosa and Bulimia nervosa*, OHE, London.

Ogg, J. and Bennett, G. (1992) Elder abuse in Britain, *British Medical Journal*, **305**, pp. 998–9.

Oliver, M. (1990) *The Politics of Disablement*, Macmillan, Basingstoke.

O'Malley, J. E. and Koocher, G. P. (1977) Psychological consultation in a pediatric oncology unit: obstacles to effective intervention, *Journal of Pediatric Psychology*, **2**(2), pp. 54–7.

OPCS (1982) Studies of Sudden Infant Death, in *Studies on Medical and Population Subjects*, No. 45, HMSO, London.

OPCS (1984) *Mortality Statistics 1981, England and Wales, Childhood*, series DH3 No. 10, HMSO, London.

OPCS (1988) *Occupational Mortality: Childhood Supplement*, series DS No. 8, HMSO, London.

OPCS (1992a) *Mortality Statistics, England and Wales, Serial Tables*, series DH1 No. 25, HMSO, London.

OPCS (1992b) *Mortality Statistics 1990, England and Wales, Perinatal and Infant: Social and Biological Factors,* series DH3 No. 24, HMSO, London.

OPCS (1993a) *Birth Statistics 1991, England and Wales,* series FM1 No. 20, HMSO, London.

OPCS (1993b) *Mortality Statistics 1991, England and Wales, Childhood,* series DH6 No. 5, HMSO, London.

OPCS (1993c) *Mortality Statistics 1991, England and Wales, Perinatal and Infant: Social and Biological Factors,* series DH3 No. 25, HMSO, London.

OPCS (1993d) *1991 Morbidity Statistics: Childhood,* series DH6 No. 5, HMSO, London.

OPCS (1993e) *Mortality Statistics: General. Review of the Registrar General on Deaths in England and Wales, 1991,* Series DH1, No. 26, HMSO, London.

Open University (1992) *Life and Death,* 'Death and Dying' Workbook 1, School of Health and Social Welfare, Open University, Milton Keynes.

Paykel, E. S., Emms, E. M., Fletcher, J. and Rossaby, E. S. (1980) Life events and social support in puerperal depression, *British Journal of Psychiatry,* **136,** pp. 339–46.

Pfeffer, N. (1985) The hidden pathology of the male reproductive system, pp. 30–44, in Homans, H. (ed.) *The Sexual Politics of Reproduction,* Gower, Aldershot.

Pharaoh, P. O. D., Cooke, T., Cooke, R. W. I. and Rosenbloom, L. (1990) Birthweight specific trends in cerebral palsy, *Archives of Disease in Childhood,* **65,** pp. 602–6.

Phillipson, C. (1993) The sociology of retirement, pp. 180–99, in Bond, J., Coleman, P. and Peace, S. (eds) *Ageing in Society: An Introduction to Social Gerontology,* 2nd edn, Sage, London.

Piaget, J. (1930) *The Child's Conception of Physical Causality* (translated by M. Gabain), Kegan Paul, Trench, Trubner and Co., London.

Pinder, R. (1988) Striking balances: living with Parkinson's disease, in Bury, M. and Anderson, R. (eds) *Living with Chronic Illness: The Experience of Patients and their Families,* Unwin Hyman, London.

Plant, M. A., Bagnall, G., Foster, J. and Sales, J. (1990) Young people and drinking: results of an English national survey, *Alcohol and Alcoholism,* **25,** pp. 685–90.

Plant, M. and Plant, M. (1992) *Risktakers, Alcohol, Drugs, Sex and Youth,* Routledge, London.

Plomin, R. and Bergeman, C. S. (1991). The nature of nurture: genetic influence on 'environmental' measures, *Behavioral and Brain Sciences,* **14,** pp. 373–427.

Popay, J. and Young, A. (eds) (1993) *Reducing Accidental Death and Injury in Children: A Report produced for NWRHA Public Health Working Group on Child Accidents,* Public Health Research and Resources Centre, Salford.

Porter, M., Penney, G., Russell, D., Russell, E., and Templeton, A. (1994) *A Population-based Study of Women's Perceptions of the Menopause,* Final report submitted to the Scottish Home and Health Dept., Edinburgh. Copies obtainable from the Department of Obstetrics and Gynaecology, Aberdeen University.

Power, C., Manor, O. and Fox, J. (1991) *Health and Class: The Early Years,* Chapman & Hall, London.

Prior, L. (1989) *The Social Organization of Death: Medical Discourse and Social Practices in Belfast,* MacMillan, London.

Qureshi, H. and Walker, A. (1989) *The Caring Relationship: Elderly People and their Families,* London, Macmillan.

R v R (rape: marital exemption) [1991] All England Reports.

Registrar General (1929) *Registrar General's Statistical Review for the Year 1927,* HMSO, London.

Richman, N., Stevenson, J. and Graham, P. (1982) *Preschool to School: A Behavioural Study,* Academic Press, London.

Ridley, S. (1993) Psychological defence mechanisms and coping strategies, pp. 262–7 in Dickenson, D. and Johnson, M. (eds) *Death, Dying and Bereavement,* Sage, London.

Roberts, A. (1989) Sexuality in later life, *Nursing Times,* **85** (24), Systems of Life series No. 172, Senior Systems No. 37.

Roberts, H., Smith, S. and Bryce, C. (1993) Prevention is better …, *Sociology of Health and Illness,* **15,** pp. 447–63; extract reprinted in Davey, B., Gray, A. and Seale, C. (1995) *Health and Disease: A Reader,* 2nd edn, Open University Press, Buckingham.

Roberts, H., Smith, S. and Lloyd, M. (1992) Safety as social value: a community approach, in Scott, S., Williams, G., Platt, S. and Thomas, H. (eds) *Private Risks and Public Dangers,* Avebury, Aldershot.

Roberts, I. (1993) Why have pedestrian death rates fallen? *British Medical Journal,* **306,** pp. 1737–9.

Robinson, D. (1994) Derek Jarman: obituary, *Guardian,* 21 February, pp. 4–5.

Rose, N. (1989) *Governing the Soul,* Routledge, London.

Rosenman, R. H. and Friedman, M. (1983) Relationship of Type A behavior pattern to coronary heart disease, in Selye, H. (ed.) *Selye's Guide to Stress Research,* Volume 2, Van Nostrand, New York.

Ross, E. and Rapp, R. (1984) Sex and society: a research note from social history and anthropology, in Snitow, A., Stansell, C. and Thompson, S. (eds) *Desire: The Politics of Sexuality,* Virago, London.

Ross, R. R. and Altmaier, E. M. (1994) *Intervention in Occupational Stress,* Sage, London.

Rosser, C. and Harris, C. C. (1965) *The Family and Social Change: A Study of Family and Kinship in a South Wales Town,* Routledge and Kegan Paul, London.

Royal College of Physicians (1992) *Smoking and the Young,* RCP, London.

Rutter, M., Graham, P., Chadwick, O. F. D. and Yule, W. (1976) Adolescent turmoil: fact or fiction, *Journal of Child Psychology and Psychiatry,* **17,** pp. 35–56.

Saari-Kemppainen, A., Karjalainen, O., Ylostals, P. and Heinonen, O.P. (1990) Ultrasound screening and perinatal mortality: the Helsinki Ultrasound Trial, *Lancet,* **336,** pp. 387–91.

Salvesen, K. A., Vatten, L. J., Eik-Nes, S. H., Hugdahl, K., and Bakketeig L. S. (1993) Routine ultrasonography in utero and subsequent handedness and neurological development, *British Medical Journal,* **307,** pp. 159–64.

Sangala, V., Dunster, G., Bohin, S. and Osborne J. P. (1990) Perinatal mortality rates in isolated GP units, *British Medical Journal*, **301**, pp. 418–20.

Sarton, M. (1992) *Endgame: A Journal of the Seventy-ninth Year*, The Women's Press, London.

Schröder, F. H. (1993) Prostate cancer: to screen or not to screen?, *British Medical Journal*, **306**, 13 February, pp. 407–8.

Seabrook, J. (1980) *The Way We Are: Old People Talk about Themselves*, Age Concern, Mitcham, Surrey.

Seale, C. F. and Addington-Hall, J. (1995) Dying at the best time, *Social Science and Medicine*, **40** (5), pp. 589–95.

Seale, C. F. and Cartwright, A. (1994) *The Year Before Death*, Avebury, Aldershot.

Sears, E. (1986) *The Ages of Man: Medieval Interpretations of The Life Cycle*, Princeton University Press, Princeton, New Jersey.

Shapiro, J. (ed.) (1989) *Ourselves Growing Older: Women Ageing with Knowledge and Power*, Fontana/Collins, London.

Sheehy, G. (1993) The unspeakable passage: is there a male menopause?, *Vanity Fair*, April, pp. 72–5 and 118–26.

Sibert, J. R., Maddocks, G. B. and Brown, B. M. (1981) Childhood accidents—an endemic of epidemic proportion, *Archives of Diseases in Childhood*, **56**, pp. 225–34.

Sidell, M. (1995) *Health in Old Age: Myth, Mystery and Management*, Open University Press, Buckingham.

Simpson, M. (1987) *Dying, Death and Grief: A Critical Bibliography*, University of Philadelphia Press, Philadelphia.

Sixsmith, A. (1990) The meaning and experience of 'home' in later life, in Bytheway, B. and Johnson, J. (eds) *Welfare and the Ageing Experience*, Avebury, Aldershot.

Sloan, S. J. and Cooper, C. L. (1987) Sources of stress in the modern office, in Gale, A. and Christie, B. (eds) *Psychophysiology and the Electronic Workplace*, Wiley, Chichester.

Smith, C. (1992) Do combined oral contraceptive users know how to take their pill correctly? *British Journal of Family Planning*, **17**, pp. 18–20.

Spiegel, C. N. and Lindaman, F. C. (1977) Children can't fly: a program to prevent childhood morbidity and mortality from window falls, *American Journal of Public Health*, **67**, pp. 1143–7.

Spencer, J. A. D. and Ward, R. H. T. (eds) (1993) *Intrapartum Fetal Surveillance*, RCOG Press, London.

St. Christopher's Hospice (1993) *1993 Directory of Hospice Services*, Hospice Information Service, London.

Steer, P. (1993) Rituals in antenatal care—do we need them? *British Medical Journal*, **307**, pp. 697–8.

Steffey, B. D. and Jones, J. W. (1988) Workplace stress and indicators of coronary-disease risk, *Academy of Management Journal*, **31**(3), pp. 686–98.

Sullivan, P. J. (1993) Occupational stress in psychiatric nursing, *Journal of Advanced Nursing*, **18**, pp. 591–601.

Sutherland, R. (1992) Preventing child traffic injuries, in Sibert, J. (ed.) *Accidents and Emergencies in Childhood*, Royal College of Physicians, London.

Sutherland, V. J. and Cooper, C. L. (1990) *Understanding Stress: A Psychological Perspective for Health Professionals*, Chapman & Hall, London.

Tabor, A., Philip, J., Madsen, M., Bang, J., Obel, E. B. and Nørgaard-Pedersen, B. (1986) Randomised controlled trial of genetic amniocentesis in 4606 low-risk women, *Lancet*, **i**, pp. 1289–93.

Tackling Drugs Together: A Consultation Document on a Strategy for England, 1995–1998 (1994) presented to Parliament by the Lord President of the Council and Leader of the House of Commons, the Secretary of State for the Home Department, the Secretary of State for Health, the Secretary of State for Education and the Paymaster General, Cmd. 267, October, HMSO, London.

Tanner, J. M. (1992) Human growth and development, Chapter 2.13, pp. 98–105 in Jones, S., Martin, R., Pilbeam, D. and Bunney, S. (eds) *The Cambridge Encyclopedia of Human Evolution*, Cambridge University Press, Cambridge.

Taylor Made Films (1992) *Time Management: MORI Poll*, Taylor Made Films, London.

Tew, M. (1985) Place of birth and perinatal mortality, *Journal of the Royal College of General Practitioners*, **35**, pp. 390–4.

Thompson, P., Itzin, C. and Abendstern, M. (1990) *I Don't Feel Old: Understanding the Experience of Later Life*, Oxford University Press, Oxford.

Thomson, M. and Westreich, R. (1989) Restriction of mother–infant contact in the immediate postnatal period, pp. 1322–30 in Chalmers, I. Enkin, M. and Keirse, M. J. N. C. (eds) *Effective Care in Pregnancy and Childbirth*, Oxford University Press, Oxford.

Tonks, A. (1994) Pregnancy's toll in the developing world, *British Medical Journal*, **308**, pp. 353–4.

Torrey, T. W. (1971) *Morphogenesis of the Vertebrates*, 3rd edn, John Wiley & Sons, New York.

Tovey, S. J. and Bonell, C. P. (1993) Condoms: a wider range needed, *British Medical Journal*, **307**, p. 987.

Townsend, P. (1962) *The Last Refuge*, Routledge and Kegan Paul, London.

Townsend, P. (1979) *Poverty in the United Kingdom*, Penguin Books, Harmondsworth.

Townsend, P. (1981) The structured dependency of the elderly, *Ageing and Society*, **1** (1), pp. 5–28.

Tromp, J. (1993) The right to die, *Guardian 2*, 3 December, p. 16.

Tudor Hart, J. (1971) The Inverse Care Law, *Lancet*, **i**, pp. 405–12.

United Nations (1991) *United Nations Demographic Yearbook 1989*, UN, New York.

Union of the Physically Impaired Against Segregation (1976) *Fundamental Principles of Disability*, UPIAS, London.

van Alten, D., Eskes, M. and Treffers, P. (1989) Midwifery in the Netherlands: The Wormerveer Study, *British Journal of Obstetrics and Gynaecology*, **96**, pp. 656–62.

van Keep, P. A., Serr, D. M., and Greenblatt, R. B. (1979) *Female and Male Climacteric: Current Opinion*, MTP Press, Lancaster.

Victor, C. (1991) Continuity or change: inequalities in health in later life, *Ageing and Society*, **11**(1), pp. 23–40.

215

Vincent, S. (1994) Exits, *The Guardian Weekend*, February 19th, pp. 6–10 and 52; an edited extract appears as pp. 406–11 in Davey, B., Gray, A. and Seale, C. (eds) (1995) *Health and Disease: A Reader*, Open University Press, Buckingham.

Wadsworth, M. (1991) *The Imprint of Time: Childhood, History and Adult Life*, Clarendon Press, Oxford.

Walker, A. (1993) Poverty and inequality in old age, in Bond, J., Coleman, P. and Peace, S. (eds) *Ageing in Society*, 2nd edn, Sage, London.

Walter, T. (1993) Modern death: taboo or not taboo?, pp. 33–44, in Dickenson, D. and Johnson, M. (eds) (1993) *Death, Dying and Bereavement*, Sage, London.

Walter, T. (1994) *The Revival of Death*, Routledge, London.

Wellings, K. and Wadsworth, J. (1990) AIDS and the moral climate, in Jowell, R., Witherspoon, S. and Brook, L. with Taylor, B. (eds) *British Social Attitudes: the 7th Report*, Gower, Aldershot.

Wellings, K., Field, J., Johnson, A. M. and Wadsworth, J. (1994) *Sexual Behaviour in Britain: The National Survey of Sexual Attitudes and Lifestyles*, Penguin, Harmondsworth.

West, P. (1994) Future imperfect: teenagers and health, *MRC News*, No. 63, Summer, pp. 36–40.

White, E. (1993) Life, love and death, *Guardian 2*, 30 November, p. 3.

Williams, R. (1990) *A Protestant Legacy: Attitudes to Death and Illness among Older Aberdonians*, Clarendon Press, Oxford.

Wilson, R. (1983) The Louisville Twin Study: developmental synchronies in behavior, *Child Development*, **54**(2), pp. 298–316.

Wiltshire Health Care Trust (1991) *Data on Maternity Units*, Wiltshire Health Care Trust, St John's Hospital, Trowbridge, BA14 0QU.

Winston, R. (1982) The quads: nothing to apologise for, *Observer*, May 13th.

Woodroffe, C., Glickman, M., Barker, M. and Power, C. (1993) *Children, Teenagers and Health: The Key Data*, Open University Press, Buckingham.

Worden, J. W. (1983) *Grief Counselling and Grief Therapy*, Tavistock, London.

World Health Organisation (1958) *Constitution of the World Health Organisation*, WHO, Geneva.

World Health Organisation (1980) *International Classification of Impairments, Disabilities and Handicaps*, WHO, Geneva.

World Health Organisation (1981) *Psychosocial Factors Related to Accidents in Childhood and Adolescence*, WHO, Geneva.

World Health Organisation (1994) *International Classification of Diseases—10th Edition*, WHO, Geneva.

Young, M. and Schuller, T. (1991) *Life After Work: The Arrival of the Ageless Society*, HarperCollins, London.

Zarb, G. (1993) Forgotten but not gone, in Arber, S. and Evandrou, M. (eds), *Ageing, Independence and the Life Course*, Jessica Kingsley, London.

Further reading

Chapters 1 and 14

Barker, D. J. P. (ed.) (1992) *Fetal and Infant Origins of Adult Disease*, BMJ Publications, London. In this collection of 31 articles by David Barker and his colleagues, the evidence for the 'programming hypothesis' is convincingly presented. Data from a number of different sources are brought together, including birth records from the first quarter of this century and physiological measurements on the same individuals traced after retirement age.

Blaxter, M. (1990) *Health and Lifestyles,* Tavistock–Routledge, London. In this book, a leading sociologist analyses lay health beliefs and behaviours from the results of a large-scale survey of over 9 000 adults conducted in Britain in 1984–5. An extract is 'set reading' for Chapter 1, but the whole book is accessible and informative, and has become a classic for the author's thoroughness in data analysis and her perceptive commentary on the results.

Cox, B. D., Huppert, F. A. and Whichelow, M. J. (1993) *The Health and Lifestyle Survey: Seven Years On,* Dartmouth Publishing Co. Ltd., Aldershot. Brian Cox heads the multidisciplinary team which conducted the original 'Health and Lifestyles' survey in 1984–5; in this book, the authors report the results of a follow-up study of over 5 000 of the adults who were first surveyed seven years earlier. The longitudinal design of this study and the collection of data on health behaviours, smoking and alcohol, family circumstances, income, employment and education, together with measurements of height, weight, blood pressure, respiratory function and other physiological parameters, have given the authors a unique insight into the nation's health and the relationship with 'lifestyle'.

Power, C., Manor, O. and Fox, J. (1991) *Health and Class: The Early Years*, Chapman & Hall, London. Chris Power and her colleagues have analysed data on the health and social circumstances of 12 537 young adults, all aged 23 years in 1981, who were entered into the National Child Development Study at their birth in the same week of March 1958. The authors interpret these data in the light of earlier studies of the same cohort conducted when the children were 7, 11 and 16 years old. Their purpose is to shed light on the factors contributing to the significant inequalities in health which can be detected even in this relatively young cohort.

Wadsworth, M. (1991) *The Imprint of Time: Childhood, History and Adult Life*, Clarendon Press, Oxford. In this clearly presented review of over 40 years' research on a cohort of 5 362 people born in Britain in one week in 1946, Mike Wadsworth reveals the strength of longitudinal studies of the life course, and the unique characteristics of the first post-war, post-NHS generation. This is a most readable and wide-ranging social history, as well as a clear exposition of the data collected from this cohort; the author pays great attention to the social and political environment in which these individuals were growing up.

Chapter 2

Burghes, L. (1994) *Lone Parenthood and Family Disruption: The Outcomes for Children*, Family Policy Studies Centre, London. Louie Burghes provides a lucid review of one of the issues in Chapter 2—lone parenthood—summarising a large amount of previous research.

Joshi, H. (ed.) (1989) *The Changing Population of Britain*, Blackwell Publishers, Oxford. This collection of readings, edited by Heather Joshi, gives a broad introduction to a range of topics associated with the life course and demographic change.

Wadsworth, M. (1991) *The Imprint of Time: Childhood, History and Adult Life*, Clarendon Press, Oxford (see entry under Chapter 1).

Chapter 3

Campbell, R. and Macfarlane, A. (1994) *Where to be Born? The Debate and the Evidence*, 2nd edn, National Perinatal Epidemiology Unit, Oxford (paperback). This book outlines the available evidence on safety, costs, parents' preference, and other aspects of the debate that lies behind policy changes on place of birth. It is aimed at users of health care as well as professional carers, and it provides a clear overview of this controversial area.

Chalmers, I., Enkin, M. and Keirse, M. J. N. C. (eds.) (1989) *Effective Care in Pregnancy and Childbirth*, 2 vols, Oxford University Press, Oxford. An influential and important book consisting of authoritative summaries of the available evidence on effective care in all aspects of pregnancy and childbirth. However, it is becoming out of date as new evidence becomes available, and the information is now available and being regularly updated in electronic form (CD-ROM and via the Internet).

Department of Health (1993) *Changing Childbirth, Part 1. Report of the Expert Maternity Group*, HMSO, London (paperback). This report, known as the Cumberlege Report after its chairperson, was produced by a group of experts from a range of professions and groups connected with pregnancy and childbirth. It provides a thorough yet readable review of policy and practice in NHS maternity care, based firmly round the principle that 'the woman must be the focus of maternity care'.

Enkin, M., Keirse, M. J. N. C., Renfrew, M. and Neilson, J. (1995) *A Guide to Effective Care in Pregnancy and Childbirth*, 2nd edn, Oxford University Press, Oxford (paperback). This is a considerably smaller (and cheaper) single volume than the definitive two-volume version by Chalmers *et al.* (above), which is much more accessible for the non-medical reader and provides interpretation of the evidence without listing the sources. It has also been updated more recently. Both books have had an influence wider than the area of care in pregnancy and childbirth, by strongly promoting the view that choice of care should be based on firm evidence about effectiveness.

Johnson, M. H. and Everitt, B. J. (1988) *Essential Reproduction*, 3rd edn (paperback), Blackwell Scientific Publications, Oxford. This is the standard biological textbook of reproduction and is clearly written, comprehensive and interesting. It covers the topic in an integrated way, including biochemical, physiological and behavioural aspects, and is not limited to a discussion of human reproduction, but also deals with other mammals.

Oakley, A. (1986) *The Captive Womb: A History of the Medical Care of Pregnant Women*, Blackwell Publishers, Oxford (paperback). This book supplements the discussion of maternity care in Chapter 3 by providing a history of how the existing system of care developed historically. Sadly, it is out of print so you cannot buy it, but it is well worth borrowing through your local library.

Chapter 4

Brazelton, T. B. (1992) *Touchpoints: Your Child's Emotional and Behavioural Development*, Viking, Harmondsworth. Written by one of the world's foremost paediatricians, this book describes developmental pathways during the first six years of a child's life. 'Touchpoints' are the major milestones in development during this period: predictable spurts of development which are often associated with difficult periods of regression. Dr Brazelton shows how an understanding of these points can help parents and others foster children's healthy development.

Oates, J. (ed.) (1994) *The Foundations of Child Development*, Blackwell Publishers/The Open University, Oxford. This fully-illustrated paperback is the first book in an Open University course on child development, and is edited and part-authored by John Oates, one of the authors of Chapter 4. It provides a broad, accessible and up-to-date introduction to theory and research; key areas of early childhood development are discussed, including perceptual abilities, social relationships, individuality and object knowledge. Particular attention is paid to images of children and childhood from historical and cross-cultural perspectives.

Rutter, M. and Rutter, M. (1992) *Developing Minds: Challenge and Continuity across the Life-span*, Penguin, Harmondsworth. This book draws on the authors' comprehensive experience in research and practice associated with children's social and emotional development and gives a detailed account of how various factors in children's lives affect their health and development.

Woodroffe, C., Glickman, M., Barker, M. and Power, C. (1993) *Children, Teenagers and Health: The Key Data*, Open University Press, Buckingham. This book provides a wealth of detail on the state of children's health at the beginning of the 1990s.

Chapter 5

Child Accident Prevention Trust (CAPT) (1989) *Basic Principles of Child Accident Prevention: Guide to Action*, CAPT, London. Written for health visitors and other professionals concerned with accident prevention, this paperback provides a good overview of the 'problem' and how to address it.

Hillman, M., Adams, J. and Whitelegg, J. (1990) *One False Move … A Study of Children's Independent Mobility*, Policy Studies Institute, London. This is the report of a comparative study of children's independent mobility in Britain and Germany. The researchers looked at different road accident rates in the two countries and asked parents about the ages at which their children were allowed to cross roads alone, go out to play and cycle on the main roads. The study raises many issues about transport policy, the prevention of accidents to children, and the impact of cultural differences on children's independence.

James, A. and Prout, A. (1990) *Constructing and Reconstructing Childhood: Contemporary Issues in Sociology of Childhood*, Falmer Press, London. This book signalled the inclusion of 'childhood' on the sociological agenda as a topic of theoretical study. A collection of chapters by various sociologists who have worked in the area, it is a good introduction to some of the issues raised by seeing childhood as a socially constructed period, and by treating children's culture as worthy of study in its own right.

Roberts, H., Smith, S. J. and Bryce, C. (in press, scheduled for publication December 1995) *Children at Risk?—Safety as a Social Value,* Open University Press, Buckingham. The authors examine a range of survey data to explore the causes, consequences and policy implications of child accidents in Britain, and make a range of practical suggestions on how parents and professionals might best keep children safe.

Woodroff, C., Glickman, M., Barker, M. and Power, C. (1993) *Children, Teenagers and Health: The Key Data,* Open University Press, Buckingham. A good overview of current statistics on the health of children and young people, with a chapter on the distribution of fatal and non fatal accidents. Excellent source of data for reference (also cited as Further Reading for Chapter 4).

Wyke, S. and Hewison, J. (1991) *Child Health Matters,* Open University Press, Buckingham. A collection of research-based chapters on various aspects of children's health and health care, including use of services, health beliefs and the impact of material factors on health. The intention of the book is to provide information for those planning and delivering health services, but it also provides an overview of some aspects of children's health that could not be addressed in Chapter 5, which focused on accidents.

Chapter 6

Blos, P. (1962) *On Adolescence,* Free Press of Glencoe. A classic psychodynamic account of the internal worlds of adolescents. It covers the different stages of adolescent development. Best consulted in a public library.

Freud, A. (1966) *Normality and Pathology in Childhood,* The International Psycho-Analytical Library, Hogarth Press and The Institute of Psychoanalysis, London. A Freudian perspective on the course of childhood development. The book goes into great detail on the different psychological forces that make up the whole personality. Best consulted in a public library.

Laufer, M. (1975) *Adolescent Disturbance and Breakdown,* MIND Special, Pelican Books, London. A clearly written and useful book that may be of special interest to parents or to those professionally involved with adolescents. It gives a clear account of the signs indicating normal and more severe difficulties. Best consulted in a public library.

Rutter, M. and Rutter, M. (1992) *Developing Minds: Challenge and Continuity across the Life-span,* Penguin, Harmondsworth. A wide ranging look at human development across the life course covering the relevant psychological, biological and social factors. Extensive use is made of research findings (also cited as Further Reading for Chapter 4).

Chapter 7

Holden, W. (1994) *Unlawful Carnal Knowledge: The True Story of the Irish 'X' Case,* HarperCollins, London. An account of an Irish 14-year-old, pregnant after being raped, who was initially prevented by the Irish courts from travelling to England for an abortion, and who fought the case through the European Court of Justice.

Petchevsky, R. (1986) *Abortion and Woman's Choice: The State, Sexuality and Reproductive Freedom,* Verso, London. A comparative study of the ideology, law and politics behind the struggles around birth control in Britain and the USA in the twentieth century. The author is a leading campaigner for women's reproductive rights in developing and developed countries.

Pfeffer, N. (1992) *The Stork and the Syringe: A Political History of Reproductive Medicine,* Polity Press, Cambridge. A thoroughly-researched and accessible social history by the author of Chapter 7, demonstrating that national politics and the economy have always influenced attitudes towards fertility and infertility as much as the social and moral climate of the day.

Weeks, J. (1981) *Sex, Politics and Society: The Regulation of Sexuality since 1800,* Longman, London. Weeks' comprehensive study of sexuality in Britain explores the social, religious, medical and political concerns which have influenced its control and regulation since the eighteenth century.

Chapter 8

Cox, T. (1993) *Stress Research and Stress Management: Putting Theory to Work,* Health and Safety Executive (HSE) Contract Research Report N. 61/1993, HSE, London. This review of occupational stress research considers early and contemporary studies on the nature of stress at work, its effects on health and the way in which such knowledge is being applied in attempts to manage the problem. It discusses the conceptual frameworks implied in the practice of stress management at work and in health and safety legislation. In particular, it focuses on the utility of the 'control cycle' and problem-solving approaches to the management of stress at work.

Karasek, R. and Theorell, T. (1990) *Healthy Work: Stress Productivity and the Reconstruction of Working Life,* Basic Books, New York. This book is based on a ten-year study of nearly 5 000 workers, and claims to identify a clear connection between work-related illness and workers' lack of participation in the design and outcome of their work. The first half of the book presents a model of psychosocial job structure and stress-related illness. The second part of the book translates these findings into a set of guidelines for the redesign of work. Group processes, the impacts of technology, political conflict at work and the impact of the market and the economy as a whole on stress are addressed.

Petersen, C. L. (1994) Work factors and stress: a critical review, *International Journal of Health Services,* **24**(3), pp. 495–519. This substantial review focuses on the need for a comprehensive framework for occupational stress research, which encompasses both psychological and sociological approaches. The author reviews the literature from both these orientations and argues that each has serious limitations when work factors and stress are addressed from within the constraints of a single discipline.

Ross, R. R. and Altmaier, E. M. (1994) *Intervention in Occupational Stress,* Sage, London. This practical guide focuses on the intervention strategies that can be employed by counsellors to help individuals suffering from the emotional and physiological stresses engendered in the workplace. The authors define the nature of stress at work and discuss the factors that can influence the problem: the individual, the work setting, and the wider social context. Coping strategies at the individual and workplace levels are reviewed, together with methods for the evaluation of possible interventions.

Sutherland, V. J. and Cooper, C. L. (1990) *Understanding Stress: A Psychological Perspective for Health Professionals*, Chapman & Hall, London. Health professionals are constantly faced with stressful situations during their working lives. This book is intended to enable this group of employees to understand the sources of stress, their impact on illness and the stress-related problems associated with their own particular occupations. It also discusses how professionals can manage their stress by adapting their approaches to work and the workplace.

Chapter 9

Greer G. (1991) *The Change: Women, Ageing and The Menopause*, Hamish Hamilton London (also available as a Penguin paperback). The definitive feminist analysis of the social construction of the menopause. The book is based on comprehensive research into the symptomatology of the menopause and the influence of gender on interpretations of the data. There is a close analysis of hormone replacement therapy (HRT) and a spirited defence of alternative approaches to the ageing process as experienced by women.

Hepworth, M. and Featherstone, M. (1982) *Surviving Middle Age*, Basil Blackwell, Oxford. The title of this book is rather misleading because it focuses on the ways in which images of middle age in popular culture influence our perceptions and expectations of both men and women in mid-life. As a study of images and mid-life, it provides further material on the social construction of the menopause, the male menopause, and mid-life crises.

Kitzinger, S. (1985) *Women's Experience of Sex*, Penguin, Harmondsworth. A highly accessible, jargon-free exploration and explanation of women's experience of sex through the life course. Contains a valuable discussion of the pros and cons of HRT, and the influence of social attitudes on growing older. Well referenced and profusely illustrated.

Pfeffer, N. (1985) The hidden pathology of the male reproductive system, pp. 30–44 in Homans, H. (ed.) *The Sexual Politics of Reproduction*, Gower, Aldershot. This article (by the author of Chapter 7) compares variations in the medical treatment of age-associated changes in the reproductive systems of men and women, and relates these variations to the belief that the reproductive systems of women are more complex than those of men. The author argues that this belief leads to the expectation that women's reproductive systems are likely to develop problems in later life, and the tendency to ignore the pathology suffered by men (e.g. prostate problems).

Chapter 10

Blakemore, K. and Boneham, M. (1993) *Age, Race and Ethnicity*, Open University Press, Buckingham. This is a comprehensive overview of the research on ageing among black and Asian people in Britain and it includes the authors' own research on the subject. It offers valuable insights into health and illness in Asian and Afro-Caribbean communities and their use of health services.

Bytheway, B. (1995) *Ageism*, Open University Press, Buckingham. The literature on ageism and age prejudice is reviewed and a wide range of settings in which ageism is clearly apparent are considered, for example, the use of chronological age to ration health services. The author discusses many aspects

of power, language, relationships and the organisation of services, and concludes with the argument that the terms 'elderly' and 'old age' be abandoned.

Sidell, M. (1995) *Health in Old Age: Myths, Mystery and Management*, Open University Press, Buckingham. This book addresses a variety of issues relating to health in later life: why do many older people rate their health as good when 'objective' evidence suggests the opposite? How do different perspectives on health inform our understanding of health in later life? What are the policy implications for ensuring a healthy life for older people?

Chapter 11

Arber, S. and Evandrou, M. (eds) (1993) *Ageing, Independence and the Life Course*, Jessica Kingsley, London. This collection of articles explores ways in which disadvantages such as low income, poor housing, poor health and disability affect older people. The book adopts a life-course perspective, demonstrating how these disadvantages accumulate over the course of a lifetime. A chapter by Gerry Zarb is included on people who have aged with a life-long disability.

Bury, M. and Holme, A. (1991) *Life After Ninety*, Routledge, London. The authors of this book conducted a unique survey of a representative sample of people aged 90 and over living in Britain. It tells us not only about the objective conditions of their lives but also about the subjective experience of living to such a great age.

Doress, P. B., Siegal, D. L. and Shapiro, J. (eds) and the Midlife and Older Women Book Project in co-operation with the Boston Women's Health Book Collective (1989) *Ourselves, Growing Older: Women Ageing with Knowledge and Power*, British edition, Fontana, London. This practical handbook originated in the USA, but this edition was revised for a British readership. It contains chapters on a wide range of subjects, including work, relationships and health, and is extensively illustrated by personal accounts, photographs and drawings.

Sarton, M. (1983) *As We Are Now*, Women's Press, London. This novel recounts the author's experience of living in a residential care home. It uncovers the sometimes brutal and humiliating aspects of care and dependency.

Williams, R. (1990) *A Protestant Legacy: Attitudes to Death and Illness among Older Aberdonians*, Clarendon Press, Oxford. Rory Williams interviewed a sample of older Aberdonians about how they deal with illness and death. His interview material is eloquently used to illustrate how this is strongly related to their own biography and religious traditions.

Chapters 12 and 13

Albery, N., Elliott, G. and Elliott, J. (1993) *The Natural Death Handbook*, Virgin Press, London. A radical statement of 'revivalism' written by members of a pressure group with similar aims in relation to dying as the Natural Childbirth movement had for birth.

British Medical Association (1988) *Euthanasia*, BMA, London. A pamphlet outlining the BMA's view on this controversial subject.

Dickenson, D. and Johnson M. (eds) (1993) *Death, Dying and Bereavement*, Sage, London. This collection is associated with the Open University course (K260) described below and offers a

ISLE COLLEGE
RESOURCES CENTRE

broad range of literature on the subject, from academic research articles to biographical accounts and poetry.

Gomez, C. F. (1991) *Regulating Death: Euthanasia and the case of the Netherlands,* Free Press, New York. Outlines the situation in that country, together with in-depth investigation into particular cases of euthanasia.

Hastings Centre Report (1989) special supplement on 'Euthanasia', No 22. Contains a collection of articles on the topic from various points of view.

House of Lords Select Committee on Medical Ethics (1994) Chairman, The Lord Walton of Detchant, House of Lords Papers, Session 1993–94, 21-I/III, HMSO, London. This report focuses on the implications of medical involvement in voluntary euthanasia, if it were ever legalised in the United Kingdom, and concluded that the potential dangers outweigh the potential benefits to those patients who ask for euthanasia to end intolerable suffering.

Kübler-Ross, E. (1975) *Death: The Final Stage of Growth,* Prentice-Hall, Englewood Cliffs, USA. A discussion of the issues involved in awareness of dying, with the author's famous account of stages of grief.

Law Commission (1995) *Mental Incapacity,* Report No. 231, HMSO, London. The Law Commission's report to the government includes advice on the legality of medical decisions to comply with or ignore an advance directive ('living will'), made by a person in sound mind and body, directing their medical attendants to withdraw life-maintaining treatments and procedures in the event of terminal illness and the patient's mental incapacity to refuse consent to these procedures.

Maas, P. J., Delden, J. J. M., Pijneborg, L. and Looman, C. W. N. (1991) Euthanasia and other medical decisions concerning the end of life, *Lancet,* **338**, pp. 669–74. Reports a national survey of practice in the Netherlands.

The Open University, School of Health and Social Welfare (1993) *Death, Dying and Bereavement* (K260). This course is available for study by Associate Students of the Open University (outside the Undergraduate programme), and as a stand-alone study pack. It is designed for both academic and professional study, as well as for the needs of people who simply have a general interest in the topic. Workbooks, audiotapes and videos are all included.

Seale, C. and Cartwright, A. (1994) *The Year Before Death,* Avebury, Aldershot. This book reports the complete findings of the survey (discussed briefly by Clive Seale in Chapter 12) of the last year of life of a nationally representative sample of people who had died in 1987, using interviews with their relatives, friends and others who knew them.

Worden, J. W. (1983) *Grief Counselling and Grief Therapy,* Tavistock, London. Outlines the author's analysis of bereavement and a series of tasks facing bereaved people, written from a counselling point of view.

Answers to self-assessment questions

Chapter 2

1   It is true that patterns of marriage in Britain have changed significantly in recent decades, with more cohabitation, older age of marriage, higher divorce rates, fewer children and more lone parents. However, as Table 2.1 shows, the quote is slightly inaccurate, as the 'one in four households' should refer to couples *with dependent children*. In fact, at any point in time around one in three households and more than half the population can be described as couples with children, and a higher proportion of the population pass through this stage at some point in their life course. Moreover, as the chapter suggests, the concept of the 'conventional family pattern' may not be a very helpful guide to the past patterns which the author claims have been eroded: in the nineteenth century, for example, many marriages were broken and lone parents created by the death of a spouse.

2   The main difference is that, at all points in the life course, the participation rate among women is lower than among men, peaking at 77 per cent for women but at 95 per cent for men. In addition, there is a slight decline in the female participation rate between the ages of 25 and 30, attributable mainly to child-bearing and child-rearing.

3   Such profiles of participation rates or of earnings over the life course are normally compiled from cross-sectional data based on the experience of different people of different ages, rather than the same people over time. But it is possible, indeed likely, that the life course of successive birth cohorts will be different. For example, the fact that 55–9 year-old women in 1992 had a participation rate of around 50 per cent does not necessarily mean that women aged 25–9 in 1992 will also have a participation rate of 50 per cent in 30 years' time, when they also are aged 55–9.

4   Figure 2.7 shows that the need for social security, education and health services varies tremendously over the life course and, in particular, that spending on education is mainly directed towards young people and spending on health services is mainly directed to people from the age of 65 onwards. In general, these welfare services are most needed at times when individuals have not begun employment or have retired; consequently they cannot pay for them out of current income. By levying taxes during the working life and providing services primarily before and after the working life, the welfare state acts like a 'savings bank', redistributing people's own money over their life course. This 'savings bank' function accounts for about three-quarters of all welfare spending.

Chapter 3

1   As blood pressure rises in the aorta it offers high resistance to blood entering it from the ductus arteriosus, so less blood bypasses the lungs. At the same time, blood pressure falls in the lungs, allowing much more blood to flow through them, so again less blood reaches the ductus. Thus blood flow in the ductus is very much reduced (which is what leads to its gradual collapse until it finally seals up). *Note* You may be interested to know that if the ductus arteriosus remains open, blood flow along it gradually reverses as the increasing blood pressure in the aorta forces blood back down the ductus into the heart. This can lead to heart failure as the child grows.

2   Around seven days after conception, about 50 per cent of early embryos fail to implant in the womb and are lost in the next menstrual period.

3   The chapter makes it clear that evidence from fairly recent clinical trials does not support the hypothesis that routine ultrasound scanning improves perinatal outcomes. This is not to say that ultrasound has no place in medical practice. There is evidence that in selected circumstances it has important uses. However, it is clear from evidence discussed in the chapter that, even at the time of writing, the circumstances in which ultrasound is useful have not been clearly defined. There are many disadvantages of introducing an intervention before full evaluation has taken place. The intervention may turn out to be harmful on balance. Even if it is not specifically harmful, resources spent on the intervention are resources that are unavailable elsewhere—the benefits from the intervention must be worth its costs, and without proper evaluation it is not possible to tell whether this is

true. However, evaluation takes time and money, and proper evaluation may delay the introduction of an intervention that eventually turns out to be of benefit.

4 (i) In many areas of the country, the only maternity care easily available is in large maternity hospitals, because pressure from some health professions and previous governments (and in the past some consumers' groups) has led to the concentration of care there.

(ii) The Winterton Report of 1992 led to the Cumberlege Expert Group report of 1993, which advocated a cessation of the policy to concentrate maternity care in large units, and its replacement by a policy of providing a wider range of types and locations for maternity care.

(iii) There are several reasons why a trial would be difficult. First, women participating in the trial would need to accept randomisation to different places of birth. Many parents have strong feelings about their choice of place of birth and would be unlikely to accept randomisation. Second, because such a trial would probably concentrate on women who appeared to be at low risk, and because unfavourable outcomes at birth are uncommon in the United Kingdom for women at low risk, the number of women in the trial would have to be huge. (Lilford estimated that half a million women would need to be involved.) Third, partly because of the strong feelings held by health professionals and others on this topic, it might well prove impossible to design a trial that would be ethically acceptable.

5 There are advantages going on into childhood in terms of reductions in allergies and in diseases of the digestive system. There are disadvantages in that the mother is more likely to suffer from tiredness or late post-natal depression, and research such as that of Murray has indicated that post-natal depression may have consequences for the child in later life.

Chapter 4

1 This would make a good starting point for a definition. Children whose biological makeup or early experience results in a failure to maintain the normal patterns of growth and development are more likely to experience ill-health. It is important to recognise that this developmental perspective on health needs to encompass both mental as well as physical health. There are limitations to this definition in that a normally-developing child may have periods of infectious illness which cause a temporary lag in growth, followed by a period of 'catching up' (see Figure 4.1); states of ill-health such as these are

not usefully described as disorders of growth or development. This developmental approach to the definition of health is difficult to apply to later stages in the lifespan; in adults, growth and development has largely been completed and illness occurs as a consequence of the dysfunction of developed physiological systems.

2 The infectious diseases have become less prevalent, through the effects of immunisation and improvements in nutrition and public health measures; their threat to children's health has been diminished by the advent of antibiotics. The exception is HIV infection, which has appeared (albeit in very low numbers) among babies and young children since the 1980s. There has been a shift in the major threats to children's quality of life, which are now primarily chronic physical diseases and disabilities, many of which are disorders of growth and development with a genetic basis (or a genetic component). A few chronic disorders, such as asthma and other respiratory illnesses, seem to be influenced by changes in the modern industrial environment. The high level of psychological morbidity has been increasingly recognised in recent years; mental health problems include disability stemming from limitations in intellectual abilities and from psychiatric disturbance.

3 Not exactly. There is a progression through increasing self-regulation and autonomy in decision making in areas that have an influence on health (e.g. choice of diet, risk taking, compliance with medical treatment, etc.). However, as children are given greater freedom to make choices on matters of lifestyle that relate to health, so in adolescence they become more prone to reject convention, including medical advice. This has been shown to be true both for chronically ill children and the general population. Another factor that has to be considered is the possibility that genetic inheritance has an increasing influence on children's behaviour as they grow up and, in acquiring more autonomy, any genetic tendency to behave in certain ways or to seek out certain experiences or environments will become more marked. Evidence from twin studies suggests that aggressive and antisocial behaviour may have a genetic component, which could adversely affect the ability of an affected child to become more competent at looking after his or her health as genetic influences strengthen with age.

Chapter 5

1 Pedestrian accidents to children are unequally distributed by age, gender and social class (based on

occupation of the child's father). Although adolescents have the highest rate of road traffic accident deaths (all types combined), younger children are most at risk as pedestrians: for example, the child was a pedestrian in two-thirds of the road accident deaths in 1990 among children aged under 15 years (Woodroffe *et al.,* 1993). The likely explanation for this is that as children become more independent they spend more time playing outdoors, but in the younger age-groups they may not have developed the necessary abilities to judge traffic speed and distance adequately when crossing roads.

Boys are more likely to experience a traffic accident than girls at all ages, and this may be partly because parents are more likely to allow them to go out without adult supervision. There is also speculation about whether personality traits such as aggression and hyperactivity might be commoner among boys and, if so, whether these might contribute to greater levels of risk-taking behaviour. Children, particularly boys with a father from social class V, are most at risk of pedestrian accidents and this is likely to be in part the result of inadequate play spaces in working-class areas, and because their families are the least likely to have access to a car, so children have to walk to school and elsewhere.

You could speculate that Britain has been slower to adopt 'traffic-calming' measures in residential areas than other European countries, and has fewer schemes to separate children from traffic.

2   The main reason for caution concerns doubts about the representativeness (a) of this small sample of children, (b) of this general practice in north Staffordshire, and (c) of accidents that lead to GP consultation.

(a)   The size of the sample is of concern (just 100 children) and the fact that they are not a *random* sample of children under five, even within this practice's catchment area. The small sample size produces very low numbers of accidents in most categories other than falls; this means that even a few more or a few less incidents could markedly change the apparent profile of hazards to the under fives.

(b)   A single general practice could never be representative of the United Kingdom as a whole; for example, it could not cover both an inner city area and a rural district. To take account of biases in the representativeness of this general practice we would at least need to know about the demographic characteristics of people in the catchment area, and the general nature of the environment (e.g. rural/urban, traffic flow, play areas, etc.).

(c)   Several factors affect the decision to take an injured child to a GP and hence affect the representativeness of the cases seen in the surgery. Many minor accidents are treated at home and would go unrecorded in this study; conversely, some accidents will bypass the GP and end up in a hospital A&E department, either because they were thought to be serious (even if they subsequently proved to be minor) or they occurred 'out of surgery hours'; the distance to the nearest A&E department might influence the results. It seems unlikely that the true incidence of scalds and bicycle accidents is represented in this study.

The main conclusion we can draw from this study is that falls are overwhelmingly the main cause of accidents to young children of those that *were* taken to these GPs. Falls are not a major cause of fatal accidents in this age-group and might therefore be overlooked as a serious hazard without studies such as this one.

3   Although education has a role to play, particularly in sensitising people to the hazards children face in an environment designed for adults, much of the research suggests that education strategies *alone* have little impact on accident rates. The interventions that have had most success in the past are either engineering strategies, i.e. those that improved the safety of the environment (e.g. child-proof drug containers), or enforcement strategies that made safer behaviours compulsory (e.g. seat-belt legislation). Engineering and enforcement strategies inevitably impose greater regulation on businesses and individuals.

Chapter 6

1   The psychodynamic perspective identifies three major psychological tasks facing adolescents in making the transition to adulthood. These tasks are highly interacting and involve:

(a)   *sexual development*, the incorporation of a sexual reproductive body into the individual's sense of self, reflected in an increased interest in personal appearance, growth of sexual fantasies, wishes, hopes and fears;

(b)   *separation* from the family of origin: balancing progressive and regressive impulses such as the increased wish for independence alongside a need for continued dependency and support; taking increasing responsibility for decision-making, e.g. in relation to personal health and education;

(c)   *individuation*, the formation of a unique and stable sense of 'self', with the ability to resolve inner conflicts and manage the anxiety that the transition to adulthood generates.

2   The extent of mortality among older adolescents from injury, poisoning, drug abuse and suicide (Table 6.1 and Figure 6.1) suggests that this phase of the life course is a time of psychological turmoil, serious enough to precipitate acts of recklessness or self-harm. This view of adolescence as a time of unmanageable internal conflict is reinforced by the prevalence of self-inflicted injury and depression, aggression and other psychosomatic symptoms and, particularly among teenage girls, anorexia nervosa, revealed by studies such as the one by West (1994) in Scotland. However, critics of this view point out that a minority—sometimes a very small percentage—of adolescents show such extreme signs of difficulty; the impact of their problems is inflated by the strength of concern that adults feel when a young person suffers severe harm.

3   The trend in Figure 6.5 is of steadily falling age at menarche across the entire period in all the countries shown, from about 16 years in 1860 to about 12.5 years in 1980. The most likely reason for this downward trend is the steady improvement in standards of nutrition and general health. Menarche is a significant event in the process of physical changes during puberty, and the falling age at which girls are faced with coming to terms with those changes may have an impact on their ability to manage the anxieties they generate. In the nineteenth century, puberty occurred at an age when girls would be considered as already entering adulthood (adolescence was not recognised as a distinct phase of the life course until the late nineteenth century), whereas in the late twentieth century puberty marks the 'beginning of the end' of childhood. It may be more difficult for young people to resolve their feelings of growing interest in sexuality in a society which considers them to be children.

4   (a) The prevalence of drug use among Haringay teenagers is comparable to that quoted nationally in the government report *Tackling Drugs Together* (1994). It confirms the view that drug use is widespread among young people and is a common part of the social environment even of those adolescents who have never used illegal drugs. However, in contrast to adult perceptions of drug use as a major risk, it is not perceived as problematic by the majority of young people themselves, who tend to think of it as an enjoyable and exciting activity rather than as 'taking a risk' with their health or 'acting out' unmanagable feelings of anxiety, depression or boredom.

(b)   The reasons given by the high proportion of sexually-active 14–15 year olds who did not use contraception during their first experience of intercourse reveal that they have a very inaccurate understanding of the risks involved. The influence of embarrassment, lack of knowledge and availability are also clearly seen. Adults have a greater understanding of the risks of unprotected sex and may see teenagers as behaving recklessly and wilfully taking sexual risks.

5   The most important influences on self-esteem are the family context and the social environment. Adolescents from families which express a high level of conflict are more likely to suffer from difficulties in managing the anxieties that the transition to adulthood brings (a point also made in relation to younger children in Chapter 4); parents who cannot face 'letting go' of their teenage children make their task of healthy separation more problematic. Social conditions which offer little hope of secure employment for school-leavers also contribute to a sense of hopelessness. Teenagers with low self-esteem are more likely to engage in persistent or serious acts of risk taking, or to suffer from poor mental health.

Chapter 7

1   Table 7.3 shows a wide variation in what kinds of sexual behaviour these men 'counted' as defining their contact with a sexual partner. For example, genital contact was mentioned by less than half the respondents; about a quarter considered that orgasm was an essential aspect of a sexual encounter and/or that they had to go to bed with or sleep naked with a person before thinking of them as a sexual partner; a few men felt they had to see a person more than once before they would 'count'. The authors of the study comment:

> The notion of the sexual encounter is central to the study of sexual behaviour in general … The question 'How many sexual partners have you had?' is asked explicitly or implicitly in all studies of sexual behaviour. A moment's thought should, however, suffice to convince that the question, 'who is a partner?' begs the question, 'what counts as sex?' However, the meaning of 'sexual partner' is usually taken for granted and very few of these studies define what is meant. (Hunt and Davies, 1991, p. 43)

2   The variation in the legal age of consent to sexual intercourse between European countries suggests that they are largely determined by social forces which differ between countries: for example, the youngest age at which a person can consent to heterosexual sex is 12

years (in Spain) and the oldest is 18 (in Malta). The range is equally large in the age at which men and women can consent to homosexual sex (except in Cyprus where sex between men is illegal). Although most countries set the same age of consent for heterosexual and homosexual sex, a few countries (including the United Kingdom) set a higher age for homosexual sex between men, despite the lower age at which males reach biological maturity. It could be argued, however, that some notice is being taken of biological development in that most countries set the age of consent within the relatively few years during which puberty is completed for the majority of young people; thus the ability to consent to sexual intercourse is (loosely) related to reproductive maturity.

3   The language chosen by the authors of this account suggests that Edwards (a doctor) and Steptoe (a medical scientist) have taken the place of the prospective parents; one supplies the eggs, the other tries to fertilise them and feels deflated when conception fails. This is an example of the unprecedented increase in recent years in the authority of doctors and medical scientists in the management of fertility, both in controlling infertility treatments (as in this example) and as the 'gatekeepers' of legal abortion and forms of contraception which require medical prescription (e.g. the 'pill') or medical supervision (e.g. the 'coil').

4   Greater autonomy in control of one's own fertility would be enhanced by policies that increase the *availability* and the *accessibility* of *appropriate* education and health services dealing with contraception, abortion and infertility. In the 1990s, these services are highly variable in their distribution across the country and some techniques are unavailable in some places, unless paid for privately; available services and techniques are not always acceptable to the people who want them, for reasons of personal ethics, religion or 'taste'; nor are they always accessible, either because of the expense involved or because the person is considered 'unfit' to receive them, e.g. some doctors might not give advice on contraception to girls under age 16; infertility treatment can be withheld from parents who fail the vetting procedure or who are considered to be 'too old'.

Chapter 8

1   Jeff, the porter, says he needs the money he earns to survive, but he shows a *solidaristic* orientation to his job when he says: 'I mean, we're here to serve the public. We are public service workers. We're not here to feather our own nests, do you know what I mean?'. Later in the interview he makes this statement of 'solidarity' with his immediate workmates: 'I chose the two colleagues that I have with me on a permanent basis. I chose them carefully in respect that, 1, they could do their job and, 2, that we could all get on together. And we are all very supportive of one another and it works, it does work.'

2   In the published report of his study (1993), Sullivan drew attention to several weaknesses of his research method, which he considered were cause for caution but did not invalidate his conclusions. First, he noted that the 78 nurses were not a random sample of all psychiatric nurses, although they were *all* of the nurses in two health authorities. Second, the use of self-completed questionnaires and interviews has certain drawbacks, most notably the assumption that all respondents have interpreted the questions in the same way and have answered honestly. Questionnaires are generally not good at revealing complex emotions, where the respondent is 'torn' between feelings going in opposite directions. More specifically, questions about performance at work can elicit defensive answers which bias the outcome. Third, two of the questionnaires were devised by the researcher for this study, so they had not been validated previously on larger samples or by other researchers. Fourth, the generally accepted practice of *measuring* stress by simply asking subjects to comment on the level of stress they have experienced, does not resolve differences in their definitions of stress or in their actual ability to cope with it.

3   There are several interacting explanations for the higher rates of sickness absence among blue-collar workers. First, there are the greater *direct physical hazards* of manual work compared with non-manual work, so absence as a result of accidental injuries and illness from, e.g. exposure to fumes, noise, pollution, extremes of temperature, etc. will be greater. Second, manual work has generally lower pay scales than many non-manual occupations (though there are obvious exceptions), and *lower material circumstances* are associated with higher rates of illness through such mediating factors as relatively poor diet and housing. Third, blue-collar workers are more likely than their white-collar counterparts to have *unhealthier 'lifestyles'*, e.g. they tend to smoke more, which contributes to their higher rates of illness. Together, these three explanations seem to account for about 40 per cent of the differences in health experience in the Whitehall Studies by Michael Marmot's team (Marmot, 1986; Marmot *et al.*, 1991; North *et al.*, 1993). Fourth, workers in blue-collar jobs tend to have *lower control over the organisation of their work*, they have

fewer opportunities to participate in decision-making, their work is more likely to be routine and repetitive with little variety, and they are more likely to work unsocial hours or do shiftwork; the decline of heavy industry in the United Kingdom has increased job insecurity among manual workers who have held onto their jobs. These organisational factors are associated with high levels of perceived stressfulness in an occupation and may lead to sickness absence as a consequence of stress-related illness. This is the largest single cause of sickness absence in the national study by Cox, 1993.

Although it falls outside the scope of this chapter, you may have thought of a fifth possibility: there may be differences in the *sickness behaviour* of people in different occupations which result in blue-collar workers being more likely to take time off for a minor illness than their white-collar counterparts. Finally, you might have considered the possibility that sickness absence is more accurately recorded for blue-collar workers and that a proportion of 'days off sick' among white-collar workers (particularly in the higher grades) never appears in the records.

Chapter 9

1   There is a tendency in modern Western culture for ageing to be regarded negatively and for mid-life to be seen as the 'beginning of the end'. Evidence for this popular belief can be found regularly in magazines and newspapers, for example the extract we quoted from an interview with hormone therapist Michael Carruthers, in which he describes the 'tigers of industry' suddenly turning into 'sheep' when they reach middle age. Certain mid-life changes, notably the menopause, are frequently construed as serious 'problems' which afflict all or most middle-aged women in a negative way. This view is increasingly being applied to men as well as to women, with accounts of the 'male menopause' growing in the media. Such beliefs persist in popular culture despite the lack of epidemiological and sociological evidence that 'all or most' people do experience their middle age as a time of crisis. For example, most women do not appear to experience the menopause as a significant problem in their lives, even though most experience some of the 'classic' symptoms, as the study by Maureen Porter and her colleagues reveals. The pervasive nature of these negative images in popular beliefs tend to dominate personal experience of middle age and the interpretation of mid-life change.

2   Increasing irregularity in the menstrual cycle and complete cessation of menstruation and ovulation in mid-life are associated with the marked decline in levels of the hormones oestrogen and progesterone in middle-aged women. These hormonal changes correlate well with experience of the 'classic' symptoms of the menopause (hot flushes, night sweats, sleep problems and dry/sore vagina), but not with other physical and psychological symptoms, which seem to be associated with pre-existing health status and factors in the woman's personal life and social circumstances. None of the 'symptoms' of the male menopause (the existence of which is itself controversial) are associated with hormonal changes in the great majority of men, nor is there any evidence that experiencing mid-life as a 'crisis' has a biological basis.

3   The psychological model of mid-life change proposed by Elliot Jaques revolves around the growing awareness, in the late 30s, that time is running out and that death is becoming an increasingly inescapable reality. He argued that the mid-life crisis is a turning point in the life course because the awareness of one's biological limitations leads to either a positive or a negative outcome in term's of one's commitment to continued personal growth and creativity in later life.

Daniel Levinson's model presents mid-life as the testing time of a person's 'dream', a period of re-examination of the hopes one had had for one's life and the state of one's plans for realising these hopes. A successful mid-life transition depends on resolving personal disillusionment with those aspects of the dream that have to remain unfulfilled.

Allin Coleman and Tony Chiva's model recognises the diverse range of situations people in the twentieth century experience during mid-life, and the impossibility of generalisation. They view mid-life as a dynamic on-going process of interaction between one's view of changes in one's body and one's position in society. Mid-life change is a creative social process which involves taking stock of one's past life and considering options for the future. In psychological terms, it is a reflective process of self-assessment and adjustment through which individuals actively create their future lives.

Chapter 10

1   People over the age of 60 comprise more than one generation, each with different biographical histories and expectations for later life. Within any generation, there is

a diversity of experience influenced by gender, work, health history, access to resources such as income, adequate housing and support services, education, etc. Consequently age prejudice which characterises 'the elderly' as being (inherently) inactive, sexless, conforming, morose, slow on the uptake, immobile, deaf and daft, etc., is very misleading at best and may foster such characteristics at worst.

2   First and foremost, the future experience of old age could be improved by the widespread recognition that inequality in socio-economic circumstances has a marked differentiating effect on the health and quality of life of older people (as it does in other age-groups). Future generations of more-affluent older people may have a higher expectation of a healthy and active later life and a willingness and ability to exercise influence to achieve it. The outlook for those in poverty, however, may remain grim. Nevertheless, there will be more technology available to reduce (for those with access to it) the limits imposed previously by physical frailty, and new biological knowledge may lead to new treatments for age-associated illnesses, or their prevention. An awareness of being part of an 'ageing society' (i.e. one in which the proportion of older people is increasing) may stimulate a more conscious self-awareness of, and interest in, the processes associated with ageing and the rights and well-being of older people.

3   The short answer is 'not if they don't modify their behaviour to compensate for age-associated physical and mental changes'. Reduced acuity of vision and hearing, slowing of response time when complex decisions have to be made quickly, forgetfulness and reduced ability to attend to a variety of sources of informational input, all require suitable compensatory behaviour if the hazards of driving in later life are not to increase. However, many older drivers seem prepared to make the necessary adjustments, and some surveys of accident rates in the United Kingdom show that older drivers on average have fewer accidents and commit fewer traffic offences (*Age Concern*, 1994), although the picture from American research is not so clear-cut.

Chapter 11

1   The most common physical impairments experienced by older people are arthritis and rheumatism, ear complaints and eye complaints (mainly glaucoma and cataract). The commonest disabilities are problems with mobility (particularly among older women) and with hearing.

2   If the physical limitations that frequently accompany later life, or are carried into later life, were readily acknowledged by society (that is all of us), then, for example, public transport and public buildings would be designed or adapted so that all of us, including older disabled people, could use them; jars would be designed so that all of us, including people with arthritis, could open them. Because society marginalises people with physical impairments by denying them opportunities which are open to others, we can construe society as the disabler rather than the individual impairment.

3   The provision of assistance which ensures (e.g.) access to an adequate income, sound and warm housing, good health care and aids to mobility and other daily living activities, can enable many older people—despite severe physical limitations—to retain a sense of independence and control over their lives. If, however, the help that is provided is overprotective, or denies the opportunity to make choices and decisions, or to reciprocate in some way, then a kind of dependency can be produced which always has the potential to lead to abuse or neglect.

Chapter 12

1   NHS hospital care has increasingly become geared to shorter but more frequent admissions. Thus people with life-threatening illnesses are likely to experience more episodes of hospital care than they used to, but to stay in for a shorter time at each admission. Because admissions are increasingly associated with episodes of crisis, they are also more likely to end in death. Care in private households remains, in quantitative terms, very important, although the role of nursing and residential homes in caring for people who die has also become more important over the years.

2   Describing a person as 'dying' generally involves confirmation of a terminal disease, and helping people to cope with the knowledge of this can then become a major concern, as the priorities of the hospice movement demonstrate. This contrasts with many people who die in extreme old age, having experienced a general bodily decline. In such people, symptoms and restrictions are often of a longer-term nature than for those who die from terminal disease, so they may need long-term personal assistance. However, given their age and the increasing likelihood that they will be living alone, they are most likely to require help from statutory services. Help from family sources may be more readily available for those

dying from a terminal disease such as cancer or AIDs, as such people are generally somewhat younger.

3   Although it is often said that the hospital environment can be impersonal, prioritising technical procedures aimed at saving life (as in Benoliel's description of an intensive care unit), Field's research on a medical ward demonstrates that care that attends to patients' concerns can occur in hospitals. Hospices are sometimes contrasted with hospitals, in that hospice medical care is primarily aimed at the palliation of symptoms rather than extending life. Other aspects of hospice care aim to treat the patient and their family as a whole, attending to their feelings as well the patients' physical needs. Achieving this may also involve a weakening of the authority of the doctor, and strengthening that of the nurse and other health workers in communicating and reaching decisions about care.

Chapter 13

1   In recent times there has been a revival of interest in death and grief, with the production of books advocating an opening up of awareness about death representing a part of this social movement. This revival has involved an interest in exploring the psychology of death and grief, as well as the hospice movement. It is associated with a widespread perception that we live in a death-denying society, and this is claimed routinely, and with some disregard for the evidence, by revivalists.

2   In the past, in the United Kingdom, children were not formally mourned for as long as adults, whereas now it is socially acceptable to grieve for the loss of a child more than that of an older person. This is because of reductions in infant mortality, so that people increasingly feel that the death of a child is unusually unfair and 'unnatural'. Feelings of loss are more intense under these circumstances. We also have far fewer children than formerly, so we invest more in those that we have. Delaying the birth of the first child (Chapter 2) also means that the years of fertility available to 'replace' a dead child are much less than in the past.

Chapter 14

1   Compulsory state education is perhaps the most important force driving the creation of a stage of life between childhood and adulthood. People who are now aged over 70 will almost all have left school at 14 and immediately entered full-time work, but the raising of the school-leaving age (currently set at 16) has prolonged the period of dependency on the family of origin and extended the duration of adolescence. The shortage of jobs for school-leavers in the 1980s and 1990s may extend it still further. Another often-neglected factor is the steady reduction in the age of puberty (Chapter 6), a biological trend driven by improved nutrition in each successive generation. Puberty now begins at around 12–13 years, long before a young person leaves school, whereas in the early generations of the twentieth century puberty and school-leaving age would have roughly coincided. This trend has reinforced the existence of adolescence and extended its duration.

2   Longitudinal studies face the common difficulty of tracing the original subjects between one survey point and the next, usually separated by several years. People move house and change jobs, some leave the United Kingdom, women marry or divorce and change their surnames, a few die and, even if a subject can be traced, he or she may refuse to participate in a follow-up study. (Note that the 'drop-out' between the two phases of the 'Health and Lifestyles' survey was larger than in most longitudinal research because it was originally designed as a single cross-sectional study, so tracing mechanisms were not built in at the outset to enable easier contacting of the subjects at a later date; but all cohort studies experience some 'drop-out' every time the subjects are re-contacted.) Taking account of drop-out is vital because the people who cannot be traced or included in subsequent surveys are unlikely to be randomly distributed across the original sample, so their absence has to be allowed for in interpreting the results of the follow-up study and in making comparisons with earlier data. This is particularly important in an 'all-ages' sample such as the 'Health and Lifestyles' survey, where the drop-out may distort the ages represented in follow-up studies.

3   The graded relationship between birth weight in 1958 and later socio-economic disadvantage found by Bartley *et al.* suggests that these two factors are highly interacting: babies born into poor social circumstances are more likely to have a lower birth weight than their contemporaries born in better material conditions, and are also more likely to remain at a socio-economic disadvantage at least until the age of 23. The 'programming' hypothesis proposed by Barker and co-workers (1992) suggests that babies who did not reach their predicted birth weight will experience the highest risk from certain chronic degenerative diseases in later life, possibly because their vascular system was adversely affected by poor nutrition during

their development in the womb. Numerous studies of social disadvantage reviewed throughout the *Health and Disease* series have concluded that it is consistently associated with greater risks to health at all ages, but most strongly from middle age onwards. (For a review, see the article in *Health and Disease: A Reader*, second edition, by J. N. Morris, 'Inequalities in health: ten years and little further on', which was published originally in the *Lancet* in 1991.)

Thus, the combination of poor fetal growth and material deprivation throughout infancy, childhood, adolescence and early adult life is likely to have an adverse effect on health at later stages of the life course, and may even affect the next generation. Girls who were not well-nourished in childhood, and who failed to reach their predicted adult height, are at greater risk of complications during pregnancy and are more likely to give birth to low-weight babies, who in their turn suffer more health problems as they grow up (Illsley and Mitchell, 1984; Emanuel, 1986). The cycle of deprivation and low birth weight leading to poor growth and inadequate fetal development in the next generation is perpetuated.

ISLE COLLEGE
RESOURCES CENTRE

Acknowledgements

Grateful acknowledgement is made to the following sources for permission to reproduce material in this book:

Text

p. 150 Burnie, J. (1994) 'Why men don't act their age', *Daily Record*, 4 May; *p. 200* Larkin, P. (1974) 'This be the verse', *High Windows*, Faber and Faber Ltd, © 1974 by Philip Larkin. Excerpt from "This be the verse" from *Collected Poems* by Philip Larkin. Copyright © 1988, 1989 by the Estate of Philip Larkin. Reprinted by permission of Farrar, Straus & Giroux, Inc.

Figures

Figure 2.1 Anderson, M. (1980) British Society for Population Studies, *Occasional Paper 31*, OPCS. © Crown Copyright. Reproduced with the permission of the Controller of Her Majesty's Stationery Office; *Figure 2.2* Kiernan, K. and Wicks, M. (1990) *Family Change and Future Policy*, Family Policy Studies Centre; *Figures 2.3 and 2.5* derived from Central Statistical Office (1994) *Social Trends 24* © Crown Copyright. Reproduced with the permission of the Controller of Her Majesty's Stationery Office; *Figure 2.4* Joshi, H. (ed.) (1989) *The Changing Population of Britain*, Basil Blackwell Ltd; *Figure 2.6* derived from Central Statistical Office (1994) Annual Abstract of Statistics, © Crown Copyright. Reproduced with the permission of the Controller of Her Majesty's Stationery Office; *Figures 2.7 and 2.8* Hills, J. (1993) *The Future of the Welfare State: A Guide to the Debate*, Joseph Rowntree Foundation; *Figure 3.3* Professor R. G. Edwards; *Figures 3.4 and 3.6* Carnegie Institution of Washington and the Human Developmental Anatomy Center of the National Museum of Health and Medicine of the Armed Forces Institute of Pathology; *Figure 3.9* Campbell, R. and Macfarlane, A. (1994) *Where to be Born? The Debate and the Evidence*, 2nd edn, National Perinatal Epidemiology Unit, Oxford. Graph based on OPCS mortality statistics, © Crown Copyright. Reproduced with the permission of the Controller of Her Majesty's Stationery Office; *Figure 3.10* Milton Keynes General Hospital; *Figure 3.13(a)* Sally and Richard Greenhill; *Figure 3.13(b)* Science Photo Library; *Figure 3.14* Pharoah, P. O. D., Cooke, T., Cooke, R. W. I. and Rosenbloom, L. (1990) *Archives of Disease in Childhood*, **65**, pp. 602–606, BMJ Publishing Group; *Figures 4.2, 4.3, 4.4, 4.5, 5.1, 6.1* Woodroffe, C. *et al.* (1993), *Children, Teenagers and Health: The Key Data*, Open University Press; *Figures 6.2 and 6.3* Tanner, J. M. (1992) in Jones, S., Martin, R., Pilbeam, D. and Bunney, S. (eds), *The Cambridge Encylopaedia of Human Evolution*, Cambridge University Press, © Professor James M. Tanner; *Figure 6.5* Marshall, W. A. and Tanner, J. M. (1986) in Falkner, F. and Tanner, J. M. (eds), *Human Growth Volume 2*, Plenum Publishing Corporation; *Figure 7.2* Duval Smith, A. (1994) Ages of consent, *Guardian*, 8 February 1994; *Figure 7.3* Babb, P. (1993) Teenage conceptions and fertility in England and Wales, 1971–91, in *Population Trends*, **74**, Winter, OPCS, © Crown Copyright. Reproduced with the permission of the Controller of Her Majesty's Stationery Office; *Figure 8.1* Cooper, C. L. (1986) Job distress: recent research and the emerging role of the clinical occupational psychologist, in the *Bulletin of the British Psychological Society*, **39**, pp. 325–331, The British Psychological Society; *Figure 9.1* The British Library; *Figure 9.2* Bill Bytheway; *Figure 9.3* Coleman, A. and Chiva, A. (1991), *Coping with Change: Focus on Retirement*, reproduced by permission of the Health Education Authority; *Figure 10.1* Roberts, A. (1989), in *Nursing Times*, **85**(24), 14 June, Macmillan Magazines Ltd; *Figure 10.2* Cox, B. D. *et al.* (1987), *The Health and Lifestyle Survey*, University of Cambridge Clinical School; *Figure 11.1* Martin, J., Meltzer, H. and Elliot, D. (1988), *The Prevalence of Disability Among Adults*, OPCS, © Crown Copyright. Reproduced with the permission of the Controller of Her Majesty's Stationery Office; *Figure 13.1* Mary Evans Picture Library.

Tables

Tables 2.1, 2.2 Central Statistical Office (1994) *Social Trends 24*, © Crown Copyright. Reproduced with the permission of the Controller of Her Majesty's Stationery Office; *Table 2.3* Central Statistical Office (1994) *Social Trends 17*, © Crown Copyright. Reproduced with the permission of the Controller of Her Majesty's Stationery

Office; *Table 3.1* Campbell, R., Davies, I. M., Macfarlane, A. and Beral, V. (1984) *British Medical Journal*, **289**, p. 722, BMJ Publishing Group. These data are © Crown Copyright. Reproduced with the permission of the Controller of Her Majesty's Stationery Office; *Table 3.2* Northern Regional Health Authority: Newcastle (1994) *Regional Maternity Survey Office Report*; *Table 4.1* LaBuda, M. C. *et al.* (1993) Usefulness of twin studies for exploring the etiology of childhood and adolescent psychiatric disorders, in the *American Journal of Medical Genetics*, John Wiley and Sons Ltd. Reprinted by permission of John Wiley and Sons Ltd; *Tables 5.1 and 5.2 Action on Accidents*, May 1990, NAHA/ROSPA; *Table 5.3* Carter, Y. H. and Jones, P. W. (1993), *British Journal of General Practitioners*, **43**, p. 161, Royal College of General Practitioners; *Table 5.4* OPCS *Occupational Mortality 1970–72*, quoted in DHSS (1980) *Inequalities in Health* (the 'Black Report'), © Crown Copyright. Reproduced with the permission of the Controller of Her Majesty's Stationery Office; *Table 5.5* OPCS (1988), *Occupational Mortality: childhood supplement: the Registrar General's decennial supplement for England and Wales, 1979–80, 1982–3, Series DS no. 8*, © Crown Copyright. Reproduced with the permission of the Controller of Her Majesty's Stationery Office; *Table 5.6* McCarthy, M. and Alwash, R. (1988) Accidents in the home among children under five years, in the *British Medical Journal*, **296**, BMJ Publishing Group; *Table 6.1* Woodroffe, C. *et al.* (1993), *Children, Teenagers and Health: The Key Data*, Open University Press; *Table 7.1* Botting, B. (1991) Trends in abortion, in *Population Trends*, **64**, Summer, OPCS, © Crown Copyright. Reproduced with the permission of the Controller of Her Majesty's Stationery Office; *Table 7.2* Coleman, D. and Salt, J. (1992), *The British Population: Patterns, Trends and Processes*, by permission of Oxford University Press; *Table 7.3* Aggleton, P., Davies, P., Hart, G. and Hunt, A. (eds) (1991), *Aids: responses, interventions and care*, Falmer Press; *Table 8.1* Handy, C. (1990), *The Age of Unreason*, Arrow Books; *Table 9.1* Porter, M., Penney, G. C., Russell, D., Russell, E. and Templeton, A. (1994), *A Population-based Study of Women's Perceptions of the Menopause*, The Scottish Office; *Tables 11.1 and 11.3* Martin, J., Meltzer, H. and Elliot, D. (1988), *The Prevalence of Disability Amongst Adults*, OPCS, © Crown Copyright. Reproduced with the permission of the Controller of Her Majesty's Stationery Office; *Table 11.2* Victor, C. (1991) Continuity or change: inequalities in health in later life, in *Ageing and Society*, **11**(1), Cambridge University Press; *Table 12.1* OPCS (1962),

The Registrar General's Statistical Review of England and Wales for the Year 1960: Part III Commentary, © Crown Copyright. Reproduced with the permission of the Controller of Her Majesty's Stationery Office; *Table 12.2* OPCS (1993), *Mortality Statistics: General: Review of the Registrar General on Deaths in England and Wales 1991 Series DH1*, **26**, © Crown Copyright. Reproduced with the permission of the Controller of Her Majesty's Stationery Office; *Table 13.2* Walter, T. (1994) *The Revival of Death*, Routledge.

Un-numbered photographs/illustrations

p. 4 courtesy of Tony Boucher; *p. 9* Mike Attwood, print supplied courtesy of Rose Hill; *p. 14* Edward Ede, print supplied courtesy of Christine Randall; *pp. 15, 19, 21(b), 24, 40, 62, 63, 65, 67, 68, 73, 74, 76, 78, 82, 93, 100, 101, 102, 104, 117, 123, 129, 135, 140, 141, 186* Mike Levers, Open University; *p. 21(a)* Rochdale Local Studies Library; *pp. 53(a), 173* Sally and Richard Greenhill; *p. 53(b), 169 (above)* Pam Isherwood/Format; *pp. 86, 106, 127, 134, 136* James McCarthy; *p. 88* courtesy of RoSPA; *p. 89* The Hulton–Deutsch Collection; *p. 96* James Dickson; *p. 107* Centrepiece of a triptych, 'The news comes to town', by Milton Keynes artists Boyd and Evans, gouache, 1985, in the collection of the Open University, courtesy Flowers East; *p. 111* First Response to Pregnancy Planning Experts; *p. 115* Health Education Authority, copy of poster supplied courtesy of Milton Keynes General Hospital; *p. 116* Gerry Free; *p. 118* Daily Express Syndication; *p. 120* Central Office of Information; *p. 130* Nick Baker, *Financial Times*, 23 May 1994. *p. 145* © 1992 Newsweek Inc. All rights reserved. Reprinted by permission; *p. 148* Mirror Syndication International; *pp. 152, 189, 197* Mary Evans Picture Library; *p. 158* Courtesy of Age Concern; *p. 164* E. Hamilton West; *pp. 169 (below), 174* Mo Wilson; *p. 176* Sam Tanner. *p. 184* courtesy of Anne Parisio; *p. 185* © John Watney; *p. 188* Guardian Syndication; *p. 190* Associated Press Photo; *p. 192* Blackwell Biovisual (Videotec Ltd); *pp. 203, 204* courtesy of Basiro Davey; *p. 204* Mike Wibberley.

Cover photographs

Background: Genetic material extracted from coronavirus particles, one of the causative agents of the common cold. (Photo: Heather Davies). *Middleground*: The urban landscape of modern Britain. *Foreground*: From birth to old age. (Photo: Mike Levers)

Index

Entries and page numbers in **bold type** refer to key words which are printed in **bold** in the text. Indexed information on pages indicated by *italics* is carried mainly or wholly in a figure or table.